M. Glantz

Design Concepts in
Nutritional Epidemiology

Design Concepts in Nutritional Epidemiology

Edited by

Barrie M. Margetts
Department of Human Nutrition,
University of Southampton

and

Michael Nelson
Department of Nutrition and Dietetics,
King's College, London

OXFORD   NEW YORK   TOKYO
OXFORD UNIVERSITY PRESS
1991

Oxford University Press, Walton Street, Oxford OX2 6DP

Oxford New York Toronto
Delhi Bombay Calcutta Madras Karachi
Petaling Jaya Singapore Hong Kong Tokyo
Nairobi Dar es Salaam Cape Town
Melbourne Auckland
and associated companies in
Berlin Ibadan

Oxford is a trade mark of Oxford University Press

Published in the United States
by Oxford University Press, New York

A catalogue record for this book is available from the British Library

Library of Congress Cataloging in Publication Data
Design concepts in nutritional epidemiology / edited by Barrie M.
Margetts and Michael Nelson.
p. cm.
1. Nutritionally induced diseases—Epidemiology. 2. Epidemiology-
-Research—Methodology. I. Margetts, Barrie M. II. Nelson,
Michael.
[DNLM: 1. Epidemiologic Methods. 2. Nutrition Surveys.
3. Research Design. QU 145 D457]
RA645.N87D46 616.3'9—dc20 91–3547

ISBN 0–19–261873–3

Set by Footnote Graphics, Warminster, Wiltshire
Printed by in Great Britain by
Dotesios Ltd., Trowbridge, Wiltshire

To Tom, Andrea, and Vanessa

Preface

This book was developed out of individual interests that merged in 1986 when we formed a Nutritional Epidemiology Group in the United Kingdom. Prior to that time, we had worked separately on a number of studies to do with the dietary aetiology of disease, and it resulted in us independently developing a concern about the methodological problems of measuring nutritional variables in epidemiological studies. This led one of us (Barrie Margetts) to organize a workshop in Sydney, Australia in 1981 on dietary methods to be used in epidemiological studies, the aim being to try and reach some agreement on what methods we should use and to acknowledge the limitations in the use of these methods. At the same time, Michael Nelson, working at the MRC Environmental Epidemiology Unit, developed a keen interest in a variety of methods for assessing diet in nutritional epidemiological studies, especially the use and validity of dietary questionnaires.

The formation of the Nutritional Epidemiology Group made us realize two things: one, that there were many people conducting nutritional epidemiological studies in the UK, virtually all of whom were working in relative isolation or as the only nutritionist in a bigger, multidisciplinary group; and two, that there was a general consensus about many issues in nutritional epidemiology and in particular what the main problems were. These factors made us believe that it would be worthwhile setting down some of the key issues that we considered important, as a source book for ourselves and for others.

In 1989 we developed a postgraduate summer course in nutritional epidemiology for which we felt that a course text would be useful. Many of the lecturers on the course have subsequently contributed chapters to this book, and we are grateful to them and to the participants in the courses for their helpful critical feedback on many issues raised in this book. Clearly, an edited book does not exist without the patience and support of all the authors, and we are grateful for their contributions.

We would like to thank a number of people who have helped us in the preparation of this book. Barrie Margetts would like to thank Professor David Barker and other colleagues (David Coggon, Carol Wickham, and Clive Osmond) at the MRC Environmental Epidemiology Unit for support and encouragement while he was working at the MRC Unit; Dr Bruce Armstrong and Dallas English and Professor Alan Jackson for many hours of provocative and helpful discussions. Michael Nelson is grateful to Professor Donald Naismith and colleagues in the Department of Nutrition and Dietetics at King's College, London for their helpful comments and

vii

support; and to the members of the Nutritional Epidemiology Group for their encouragement. We would like to thank Sheila Auger and Lorna Todd for invaluable secretarial support.

September 1990   B.M.M.
                                                           M.N.

Contents

Contributors

Bates, Chris J. *MRC Dunn Nutritional Laboratories, Cambridge*

Bingham, Sheila A. *MRC Dunn Nutritional Laboratories, Cambridge*

Burr, Michael L. *MRC Epidemiology Unit, Cardiff*

Clayton, David *MRC Biostatistics Unit, Cambridge*

Coggon, David *MRC Environmental Epidemiology Unit, University of Southampton, Southampton*

Cole, T. J. *MRC Dunn Nutritional Laboratories, Cambridge*

Gill, Caroline *MRC Biostatistics Unit, Cambridge*

Hiller, Janet E. *Department of Community Medicine, University of Adelaide, South Australia*

Margetts, Barrie M. *Department of Human Nutrition, University of Southampton, Southampton*

McMichael, A. J. *Department of Community Medicine, University of Adelaide, Adelaide, South Australia*

Nelson, Michael *Department of Nutrition and Dietetics, Kings College, London*

Rouse, Ian L. *Department of Health, Perth, Western Australia*

Thurnam, David I. *MRC Dunn Nutritional Laboratories, Cambridge*

van Staveren, W. A. *Department of Human Nutrition, Wageningen Agricultural University, Wageningen, The Netherlands*

Wenlock, R. W. *Nutrition Division, Department of Health, London*

West, C. E. *Department of Human Nutrition, Wageningen Agricultural University, Wageningen, The Netherlands*

Wickham, Carol A. C. *Department of Public Health Medicine and Epidemiology, University Hospital, Queen's Medical Centre, Nottingham*

Introduction

Barrie M. Margetts and Michael Nelson

After the supply of air and water, the supply of food is fundamental to human survival. It has been recognized for centuries that what people eat (or do not eat) affects their health. The relationship between what we eat and our health is very much the concern of nutritional epidemiology.

Much of the history of human civilisation has been concerned with obtaining enough food to avoid deficiencies, and a large part of the world's population is still living under such conditions. In other parts of the world, the emphasis has shifted from a concern about getting enough food to having too much food. Within many countries there is also now a complex mix of excess and deficiency affecting different parts of the community. So the concerns of those responsible for public health differ in different countries and change over time. The decisions about priorities for action should be based upon sound scientific evidence, but in most cases this evidence is at best limited, and at worst it is totally lacking. In many instances, therefore, scarce human and financial resources are being allocated without good evidence of either the need for, or beneficial effect of, the allocation of these resources to a particular programme.

It is our contention that, whenever data that have anything to do with human nutrition and community health are being collected, then nutritional epidemiological principles need to be considered. Further, if a nutrition intervention programme is to be put in place, the effectiveness of that programme must be evaluated following the principles of nutritional epidemiology. While it is beyond the scope of this book to address the major public health issues, it is our intention to set out some guidelines about how evidence that can be used for public health decision-making is gathered.

Our main purpose in this introduction is to define what we mean by nutritional epidemiology, and to consider in broad terms how carefully constructed nutritional epidemiological studies, when properly interpreted, can support the public health debate. We need to be clear about what is unique and important about a nutritional epidemiological approach. The final part of the introduction sets out the organization of the book.

WHAT IS NUTRITIONAL EPIDEMIOLOGY?

Epidemiology has classically been defined as the study of the determinants and distribution of disease frequency in human populations.[1] Nutritional epidemiology may then be defined as the study of the nutritional determinants of disease. This definition implies three aspects: the quantification of the occurrence of disease; a description of who is getting the disease (and where and when); and, leading on from these, a questioning of the dietary determinants of disease, and the development of testable questions. The procedures for formulating, testing, and analysing such questions are the major focus of this book.

Expressed another way, epidemiology seeks to describe the distribution of disease in the human population and then to undertake studies that address specific hypotheses arising from these descriptive studies. Ultimately, it is concerned with understanding how an event causes a disease. We may express this by asking how a particular exposure affects a particular outcome. The exposure may be any variable, and in this book we are focusing on nutritional exposures. The outcome can be a disease state or it can be a classification of a group in relation to the level of a factor such as blood pressure, body mass index, serum cholesterol, or a recommended intake for protein.

In this book we are concerned with relating nutritional exposures to appropriate outcomes. To relate an exposure to an outcome it is essential to be able to take accurate measurements of both the exposure and the outcome. One of the major preoccupations of nutritional epidemiologists is to do this with as little error as possible, and then to spend a lot of time worrying about how well they have been able to achieve this aim! The interpretation of epidemiological research needs to progress carefully with due consideration of the potential effects that chance, bias, and confounding play in affecting the observed relationships.

So far we have talked about the epidemiological side of 'nutritional epidemiology'. It may seem that nutritional epidemiology is simply a special branch of epidemiology, and that nutrition is just another exposure measure of interest. Is this true? What is nutrition? Once we have a concept of what we see as nutrition, we can then begin to discuss the uniquely important role that an appropriate understanding of nutrition has to play in the discipline that we call nutritional epidemiology.

Nutrition has been defined as 'the sum of the processes by which the body utilizes food for energy, maintenance, and growth'.[2] Others have a wider definition:

Nutrition ... is food and its relationship to well being of the human body. It includes (1) the metabolism of foods (2) the nutritive value of foods (3) the qualitative and quantitative requirements of food at different age and development levels to meet physiological changes and activity needs and (4) the economic, psychological, social and cultural factors that affect the selection and eating of foods.[3]

The Council on Foods and Nutrition of the American Medical Association defines nutrition as

the science of food, nutrients and other substances therein, their action, interaction and balance in relation to health and disease and the process by which the organism ingests, digests, absorbs, transports, utilises and excretes food substances.[4]

It is clear that when we talk about nutrition we are talking about a very complex series of processes that operate at many different levels. When we are talking about nutrition, we therefore need to consider not only the effect of the food once it has been eaten, but also the socio-economic, cultural, psychological, and agricultural factors that affect the food getting to the person's mouth. For example, when we talk about vitamin A intake, we need to consider many factors other than the amount of vitamin A said to be in a particular food, or measured in a plasma sample. Equating food intake to a tissue level may be quite misleading. It is also important to be aware that as the study of nutrition deepens, the factors that we are measuring become increasingly complex. For example, fibre, once measured as a crude residue of acid–base digestion of food, is now recognized to be a complex mixture of carbohydrates, each of which may have a different role to play in disease aetiology. And while biological markers of nutritional status may afford more objective ways of assessing dietary exposure, we must not lose sight of the relationship between what people eat and the disease process.

It is therefore a key concern of nutritional epidemiology to consider the complex nature of the exposure measure that is nutritional status. Nutritional status is commonly assessed using dietary; biochemical; anthropometric and clinical measures; and, in broad terms, using vital statistics (such as infant mortality). Most commonly, dietary, biochemical, and anthropometric variables are measured in epidemiological studies, and the general principles of defining the correct exposure apply for whichever of these measures is used. The majority of clinical measures of nutritional status relate to deficiency disease, and therefore have limited application in most epidemiological studies, in which measures that reflect the full spectrum of nutritional status are required.

Vital statistics are more commonly used as outcome variables and, although they have value as measures of exposure, in this role they provide a composite picture of the influence of a number of environmental factors on nutritional status; the same can be said of anthropometric measures. In this sense, vital statistics and anthropometry provide less precise measures of exposure to specific nutritional influences.

Anthropometric measures to assess nutritional status are very commonly used in epidemiological studies because they are considered to be relatively simple to collect with reasonable precision. Where resources are limited they may be the only measures of exposure that can be obtained. For example, they are often used to assess the relationship between the determinants of growth in young children and morbidity and mortality. However, because, for example, there are many factors besides food intake that may affect body weight (or change in weight), it may be misleading to equate anthropometric measures with measures of food and nutrient intake. At the simplest level, weight change can only be considered to indicate an imbalance between energy intake and expenditure. It may indicate little about other specific aspects of nutritional (or dietary) status. However, it may be very useful to measure body weight, for example, in experimental studies where change in weight may indicate poor compliance to the dietary regimen and where adjustment for the potential confounding effects of weight change may give a more accurate estimate of the effect of dietary intervention. As in all epidemiological studies, it is important to consider whether the anthropometric measure proposed is a relevant measure of exposure.

When we describe dietary intake, we are describing food and non-food components of diet and the subsequently derived or measured nutrient (and other) composition of that food. Although throughout the book we will most commonly describe exposure as 'diet' or 'dietary intake', the general principles apply also to anthropometric exposures that we have not referred to in detail. We have chosen not to include a detailed description of anthropometric measures because these have been discussed recently by Willett.[5]

Unlike many other exposures used by epidemiologists, diet is so complicated that special knowledge is required to enable the correct exposure measure to be used. The perspective of nutritional epidemiology thus encompasses factors that influence the availability and consumption of food, on the one hand, to the whole-body expression of disease, on the other. The point(s) along this continuum at which to measure the relevant aspect(s) of diet is a key concern of nutritional epidemiology.

CAUSALITY

The classic studies of the early twentieth century, which led to the discovery of the major dietary determinants of rickets, pellagra, scurvy, beriberi, xerophthalmia, and goitre, set an approach to the study of diet–disease relationships that has, in some respects, hindered our approach to the complex situations that confront us today. This approach has led to a view that a single dietary factor causes a disease and, therefore, the way to determine the aetiology of that disease is to find out what that single factor is. However, even for the nutrient deficiencies described above, a single factor model may not be accurate. For example, Kok and van't Veer[6] have shown that for rickets to occur a child has not only to have a low vitamin D intake, but needs to be growing and to have a low exposure to sunlight. If all three of these factors are not acting together, the outcome—rickets—does not occur. For more complex outcomes, like heart disease or kwashiorkor, the single factor approach is clearly not appropriate.

It is interesting to observe that, in communities where there is either a problem of inadequacy or excess, there are some individuals who seem to be spared from the problems resulting from these inadequacies or excesses. Why is this so? It is the objective of epidemiological research to address this question. An answer to the question usually develops from a description of differences in rates of disease in different places or groups of people and at different times. To be able to undertake epidemiological research it must be assumed that human disease is not randomly distributed in the community and that there are causal and preventive factors that can be identified through carefully conducted research. It is the objective of epidemiological research to try to uncover patterns of disease that are present in the population and then to link these patterns to patterns of exposure, in an attempt to understand the relationship between the two. Thus, the prime concern of epidemiological research is to assess exposure–outcome relationships with minimum error. The patterns that emerge from these studies usually lead to asking more detailed questions about what particular individuals are exposed to.

One of the criticisms often levelled against epidemiological research is that it does not allow you to say with certainty that, for example, all smokers will get lung cancer. Clearly not all smokers do get lung cancer, nor do all women eating a high fat diet get breast cancer. The consistent finding that, on average, if you smoke more, the more likely you are to get lung cancer highlights one of the breaks between an epidemiological approach and that taken by those responsible for the care of an individual patient. It is the shifting from a single patient orientated perspective of health and disease to a population view that characterizes an epidemiological approach.

Epidemiology is thus primarily an activity concerned with human populations, although the principles of epidemiology can be applied to any study of groups of subjects, be they human or monkeys. Many of the principles that have become codified in epidemiology stem from the basic principles of research design developed over many years by scientific disciplines.

There is also an important relationship between animal and human research. Epidemiological studies can never investigate mechanisms in the same way as a scientist working in a laboratory on an animal model. It is difficult to get human volunteers who are prepared to offer up their liver and other organs at the end of an experiment! In many diet–disease states it is only possible to investigate mechanisms and pathways using animal models. The findings of animal experiments often lead to a refinement of the sorts of questions that are addressed by epidemiological studies in humans, and questions of mechanism in causality can often be ethically resolved only through animal experiments.

Epidemiology offers one approach to the study of exposure–outcome relationships. It should be a further objective of epidemiological research to pull together the many disciplines that are involved in studying health/disease and to use these disciplines to gain a better understanding of the way, for example, that diet affects disease. It is essential that research hypotheses are developed in cooperation and consultation with experts in the fields appropriate to the study. Thus, for example, if an investigator aims to assess whether diet affects blood pressure, it is essential that the research is conducted in collaboration with nutritionists, physicians, and biostatisticians, to ensure that both exposure and outcome are measured appropriately.

MEASUREMENTS OF EXPOSURE AND OUTCOME

In the elucidation of causality it is essential to have a specific question that the research will address, and with a good idea about the probable mechanism of action. This means that, in nutritional epidemiological studies, there is a need for a clear definition of the food or nutrient of interest and how this may affect the disease or outcome of interest. From the definitions cited above, it is apparent that to define the food or nutrient of interest requires a wide knowledge of where the food comes from; how it has been grown and processed before being eaten; the constituents of the food and their likely interaction; an understanding of how the food is broken down by the digestive system into its component parts; how these components are subsequently handled by the body; and the effects these components will have on the normal/abnormal functioning of the cells of the body.

A major concern of epidemiology is therefore the validity of the information about exposure and outcome. How precisely can the nutrient of interest and other potential confounders be measured? A particular interest in epidemiology is to look at the differences in exposure levels between persons with and persons without the disease. To determine exposure and outcome requires that these factors can be measured in some way. Neither exposure nor outcome can be measured without error and it is a major concern of nutritional epidemiology that the sources of the measurement error are identified and that the error is minimized. It is also important to have some idea of the likely magnitude of this error, so that some adjustment or account can be taken of this in interpreting the results. If subjects are incorrectly classified as exposed when they are not, then it is likely that a biased estimate of effect will be obtained. This may be a particular problem if the misclassification is different in diseased and non-diseased subjects.

In all research (data collection), the elucidation of the nature of the relationship between an exposure and an outcome measure also requires that other potential confounding factors are considered. It is important to be able to establish whether the association that has been measured is likely to be real or a product of an association with another factor. For example, in a study investigating whether an increase in potassium reduces blood pressure, it is essential to consider the effects that changes in other factors may have on blood pressure. If the potassium is increased by getting subjects to eat potassium-rich foods, such as fruit, vegetables, and cereals, it is also likely that intakes of other nutrients might change. If blood pressure falls on this high potassium diet, it may be that changes in these other nutrients have affected blood pressure. If intakes of these other nutrients have been measured, it may be at least possible to adjust the potassium–blood pressure effect for these other factors (although the adjustment may not be effective because of multicolinearity).

Nutritional epidemiology is thus concerned with the way we approach the aim of the investigation. There are well used and effective epidemiological approaches to designing studies. Each is appropriate in different circumstances and each has strengths and weaknesses. The principles of study design apply whether it is a study of malnourished children in rural Africa or cancer patients in London. The practical issues will be quite different in the different settings, but the theoretical issues are identical. It may be that it is not practical to do a particular study because human and financial resources are limited. It is probably better not to do a study that cannot produce a result that can be interpreted. And it is essential not to allow study design to be compromised by political issues.

A dilemma arises when epidemiology moves into the arena of public health. Some would argue that scientists, and hence epidemiologists, should not be concerned with public health issues but only with mechanisms, cause, and effect. The generalizability of the research should not be a concern. However, this implies that as long as the experiment is carried out properly, and the results are internally valid, it does not matter whether the sample used is representative of the general population, i.e. whether the data have any external validity. But for those concerned with public health issues, the issue of external validity is very important. Public health workers must make general statements and therefore need to base these statements on research that is generalizable to the target population. Nutritional epidemiology must therefore be concerned with both external and internal validity, and the importance of these concepts is discussed in

Chapter 1. Through the rigorous application of scientific principles, and the appropriate testing of hypotheses, we can continue to revise our ideas on the role of nutrition in the causation of disease, and inform and progress the public health debate.

ORGANIZATION OF THE BOOK

The book follows a progression from detailed definitions and clarification of concepts, through identification of the most appropriate methods for measuring exposures and outcomes, to a consideration of the study designs that are best suited to an exploration of hypotheses in nutritional epidemiology.

Part A focuses on the scientific concepts that underlie study design. Chapter 1 provides an overview of the main guiding principles in the design of nutritional epidemiological studies and sets out the definitions of terms that the reader will encounter throughout the book. Chapter 2 looks at sampling and provides important guidelines on the size of a study needed to achieve a given statistical outcome, with appropriate equations to determine power, the likelihood of being able to detect a diet–disease relationship, should one exist, in a study of a given size. Finally, Chapter 3 addresses, in a pragmatic way, the difficult task of how to cope with measurement error in the analysis of experimental results.

Part B concerns measurement of exposure and outcome, looking in detail at the practical aspects of collecting nutritional data in epidemiological studies. Chapter 4 deals with the question of the validity of food composition tables and how their limitations can be addressed and in part overcome. Chapter 5 considers the use of existing nutritional data collected in surveys, the results of which are published for public use. Such information can provide useful databases for the exploration of hypotheses while minimizing the costs usually associated with conducting epidemiological studies. Chapter 6 deals with the difficulties of assessing diet in individuals, paying particular attention to the external validity of such measurements. This applies equally to the so-called 'objective' measures of current intake, such as weighed records, which are now thought to be less objective than was at one time believed, and to the retrospective methods that require proper validation to be of value in epidemiological studies. Chapter 7 sets out the major techniques of assessing and evaluating biochemical markers of nutrient intake and nutritional status for use in nutritional epidemiology. Chapter 8 addresses in detail the task of validation of food frequency questionnaires for use in epidemiological studies, paying particular attention to the design and statistical interpretation of validation studies. Finally, Chapter 9 describes the various measures of disease frequency and effect used in epidemiological studies and considers the pitfalls associated with their use.

Part C covers the design of nutritional epidemiological studies. Chapter 10 explores the use of group data to generate and test nutritional hypotheses, including those situations in which group data may be preferable to individual data. Chapter 11 addresses the particular problems of assessing nutritional causality in case-control and cross-sectional studies, including a thoughtful discussion of factors that influence the equal ascertainment of exposure in both cases and controls. Chapter 12 describes the benefits and limitations of cohort studies in nutritional epidemiology, balancing the advantages and disadvantages against those of ecological and case-control studies. In the last chapter, the authors consider the needs for and the practical execution of experimental studies, and highlight what can and cannot be learned from intervention trials in individuals and communities.

REFERENCES

1. MacMahon, B. and Pugh, T. F. (1970). *An introduction to epidemiology.* Little, Brown and Co., Boston.
2. Poleman, C. M. (1984). *Shackleton's nutrition essentials and diet therapy*, Fifth edition. Saunders, Philadelphia.
3. Krause, M. V. and Mahan, L. K. (1979). *Food, nutrition and diet therapy*, Sixth edition. Saunders, Philadelphia.
4. Guthrie, H. A. (1975). *Introductory nutrition*, Third edition. Mosby Co., St Louis.
5. Willett, W. (1990). *Nutritional epidemiology.* Oxford University Press, Oxford.
6. Kok, F. T. and van't Veer, P. (1989). The strength of relationships which can be detected between diet and disease. In Kohlmeier, L. and Helsing, E. (eds). *Epidemiology, nutrition and health*, pp. 19–29. Smith-Gordon & Co., London.

PART A

The scientific concepts underlying study design

1. Basic issues in designing and interpreting epidemiological research

Barrie M. Margetts

The introduction defined nutrition and epidemiology and showed how the two come together in the study of the nutritional determinants of health or disease. This chapter sets out the basic principles of epidemiology as they apply to the study of relationships between diet and health outcomes.

1.1 OBJECTIVES OF EPIDEMIOLOGICAL RESEARCH

Epidemiological research has three general aims:

1. To describe the distribution and size of disease problems in human populations.
2. To elucidate the aetiology of diseases.
3. To provide the information necessary to manage and plan services for the prevention, control, and treatment of disease. [1]

The primary focus of this book is the design of epidemiological studies that address the first two of these three general aims. The way in which information produced by epidemiological studies is used in the management and planning of services is not discussed. Epidemiological research however, should be designed, conducted, and reported in such a way that it can be critically assessed by those engaged in policy and planning.

The aim in designing epidemiological research is to develop a specific study question and to answer that question as critically as possible. The development of research designs to answer study questions requires that the exposure and outcome measures of interest are clearly articulated and measured with required accuracy.

A major consideration in the design of epidemiological research is the need to reduce bias. Associations between exposure and effect must be interpreted in the context of any biases that may have resulted from inaccurate measurement, and must take into account the uncertainties that arise from random sampling variation. In addition, the influence of other factors on the association between exposure and outcome must be considered. The issues related to measuring exposure and outcome, and interpreting epidemiological research will be covered in more detail in later sections of this chapter.

The design and conduct of epidemiological research are helped by a systematic approach. There are six key steps in this process:

1. Decide what is to be studied. This may derive, for example, from clinical experience, from laboratory experience or from looking at the distribution of disease rates in a community.

2. Refine the broad question of interest into a specific study question.

3. Develop a research protocol that enables the research to be funded and ethically approved.

4. Complete the research in accordance with the protocol.

5. Analyse the study, paying particular attention to any violations of the protocol and to potential effects of other factors.

6. Interpret the results critically and integrate them with the findings of other studies.

The aim of research relating diet/nutrition to disease is to elucidate the nature of the causal relationship between the exposure of interest (such as diet, anthropometric measure or biochemical marker, etc.) and the disease or outcome of interest. The outcome is not always a disease endpoint like gallstones or stomach cancer; it may be body weight, blood pressure or some other physiological process or biochemical marker (Table 1.1). These markers may be intermediate factors in the development of the disease.

However, the principle of the development of the research is the same whatever the outcome variable, and whatever the exposure variable. The

Isn't this a philo/c.a. if they are basically the same. .

Table 1.1 Relationship between measures of exposure and outcome

Exposure measures	Outcome measures
Individual diet	Individual diet
Group diet	RDAs
Biochemical status	Physiological measures, e.g.
Anthropometry	blood pressure, cholesterol
Individual constitution	Biochemical markers, e.g. serum
	retinol, toe-nail selenium
	Disease state
	Anthropometry

aim is to address a clearly defined question, with due consideration to the potential effect other factors may have on the nature of the relationship. The development of a clear study question requires the researcher to have a sound knowledge of the literature already published in the area of interest. The research to be undertaken must offer a potential new insight into the nature of the relationship of interest or it must clarify (using better, more soundly based methods and study populations) the evidence already published. It may seem redundant to labour this point, but much research is undertaken without the researchers having a clear, simple, and relevant question to ask. As part of the formulation of this clear research question there must also be an assessment of whether the question can be addressed realistically, given the methods and the human and financial resources available.

It is important to form an idea of the magnitude of the effect expected from the exposure under investigation. The magnitude of the outcome that is considered relevant should be set down before the study is commenced. The sample size and accuracy of measurements should be such that an effect of the relevant magnitude can be established with required statistical confidence (see Chapter 2).

A research protocol develops a research aim into an effective study plan. Appendix 1 presents a summary of the factors to consider in preparing a grant application. A grant application must have an effective, achievable research plan and the project must be properly costed. It must also consider any ethical issues involved in the undertaking of the research. Any grant proposal should be drafted following the guidelines set out by the funding body. The research protocol should be the manual for the day to day conduct of the research, which, if properly followed, will lead to a sound study that adds new insight into the relationship under investigation. The protocol can also form the basis for writing the final report. The rest of this chapter focuses on issues that are essential to the development of this protocol and to the interpretation of the findings.

1.2 TYPES OF EPIDEMIOLOGICAL STUDIES

Broadly, epidemiological studies divide into experimental and observational investigations. The distinction between these types of study is that in experimental investigations exposures are assigned to subjects by the investigator, whereas in observational studies the investigator has no control over the way in which subjects are exposed. Practical and ethical issues may be important in determining which approach is used to address a particular question. In general, experimental studies provide strongest evidence for the effect of an exposure on an outcome. However, it is not ethical (or permissible) to do experimental studies where the exposure is known to be harmful. Under these circumstances non-experimental study designs must be used.

In observational studies, the investigator may be able to exploit 'natural experiments', where exposure is restricted in some groups of the community compared with other groups, for example, comparing groups of omnivores and groups of vegetarians who, as well as avoiding meat, show other dietary differences on investigation.

Another way of classifying investigations is according to whether measurements of exposure and outcome are made on populations or individuals (Table 1.2).

Table 1.2 Distinction between types of epidemiological studies

	Study group	
	Populations	Individuals
Experimental studies	Community trials	Clinical or field trials
Observational studies	Ecological studies	Cross-sectional studies Case-control studies Cohort studies

It is possible to have population-based experimental studies, such as community trials, and population-based observational investigations, such as ecological studies. Similarly, experimental and observational investigations can be conducted among individuals. Although population-based studies consist of data collected from individuals (e.g. death certificate diagnosis or household food consumption data), exposure measures are only related to outcome measures at the group level.

In an individual-based study it is possible to relate exposure and outcome measures more directly. Therefore, an advantage of individual-based studies over population-based studies is that they allow the direct estimation of the risk of disease in relation to exposure. For example, it is possible to assess whether individuals who eat more fat have higher rates of heart disease. With population-based methods it might be shown that populations that have a higher exposure of fat intake also have a higher rate of heart disease, but it would not necessarily follow that the excess of heart disease was occurring in the higher consumers of fat.

It is also possible in individual-based studies to measure and to take into account in the analysis the effects other factors may have on the relationship under investigation. In population-based studies it is usually only possible to consider the effects of a limited number of other factors, and it is therefore more likely that an association that is found could be due to the effects of other unmeasured factors.

The choice of a study method is often influenced by pragmatic issues such as cost and feasibility. However, this pragmatic approach should not be the sole determinant of the study design. It is optimal to clarify the aim of the study, and then to decide the best way to do the study. At this stage the investigator usually has to make decisions about how far he or she is prepared to deviate from the ideal, before a study protocol is so compromised that it is no longer viable. If a study cannot address the research question adequately, then it may be better not to do the study.

There follows a brief overview of each type of study and some comparisons are drawn between the different methods. For more details refer to Chapters 10 to 13 in this book and other texts.[2-7]

1.2.1 Experimental studies

Clinical or field trials These may be conducted on subjects who already have a disease (therapeutic or secondary prevention trials) or on subjects who, at the time of the study, are free from disease (primary prevention trials). It is also possible to select subjects who may be considered to be at high risk of developing a disease, such as people with high blood pressure, obesity, or high blood cholesterol levels. Irrespective of the type of subjects included, the principles governing the design and conduct of the investigation are the same.

Community trials These trials are conducted on groups of people. These groups may be communities, villages, towns or counties. The comparison in such trials is between communities, not between the individuals within the communities. For example, the effect of a mass education programme on reducing fat intake could be assessed by comparing communities that do and do not receive the programme. If, for example, television messages were used in the education package, the investigators would need to ensure that the control community did not also receive the same television stations and thereby also receive the treatment under investigation. The study would be analysed by comparing the group responses in the different communities. For example, if the study showed that the community that was exposed to mass education altered their behaviour and that this change, on average, led to a change in rates of ischaemic heart disease, it would not be possible to determine whether those who said they had altered their fat intake were the people who had lowered their risk of heart disease.

However, community trials sometimes do sample individuals from within the community to try to assess the association within individuals.

The general design of clinical or community trials is to allocate populations to different treatment or exposure groups and assess how this treatment or exposure affects the outcome of interest. It is best to compare the effect of a treatment relative to the effect of a control regime given at the same time and under the same conditions. Without a control group it is not possible to determine whether any change that is observed is due to the treatment or to some other factor that has also changed. It is also optimal that the allocation of populations to the treatment or control regime is by random allocation. This randomization ensures that any differences in other factors that occur between groups occur by chance. It is also desirable to measure other factors that may influence the outcome during the study, so that they can be considered in the analysis.

Other important issues (covered in more detail in Chapter 13) are how the study population is selected, length of observation, observer and subject blindness to the treatment allocation, maintenance and assessment of compliance, ascertainment of outcome, and statistical power. A clinical trial may provide an internally valid result but, because of the selected nature of the study group, the generalizability (or external validity) of the findings may be limited.

In all experimental studies, whatever the design, it is essential to have an idea of the magnitude of the effect the treatment is likely to have on outcome so that the number of subjects required in the treatment group can be estimated. In clinical trials, the nutritional exposure of interest needs to be measured with sufficient precision and validity to characterize the exposure of the individual. The relevant exposure must also be assessed during the study to determine both compliance with the treatment (dietary) regime and to assess change in other factors which might influence the outcome.

1.2.2 Observational studies

Ecological studies   The unit of study is not an individual but a group defined by time (calendar period, birth cohort), geography (country, province, or city), or by socio-demographic characteristics (ethnicity, religion, or socio-economic status). An example of this type of study is the plotting of fat consumption data by counties against breast cancer rates in the same counties in England. It is important to remember that the unit of study (or data point) is not an individual but a populaiton (in the above example it is a county). Therefore, there are generally relatively few data points and it is harder to disentangle the effects of multiple causes in these studies. Ecological studies use summary measures of exposure (assumed to be unbiased) that are likely to closely approximate the true estimate, although they may mask marked variation within the sample. Ecological studies are ideal for examining new, *a priori* hypotheses and may lead on to studies of individuals from which causality may be inferred with greater confidence.

Cohort studies   These are similar to field trials except that exposure is not randomly assigned by the investigator. The method begins with the supposed cause and seeks to determine the incidence of disease in those exposed and those not exposed to it. Each subject enters the cohort at a defined point in time, when exposure to suspected causative factors is measured; the cohort is followed over time and the rate of development of disease is observed in relation to exposure. The number of subjects included in the cohort, and the length of observation are determined by the expected rate of development of the disease and the statistical power required for the study (see Chapter 2).

Cohort studies can be conducted either prospectively (concurrently) or retrospectively (non-concurrently). A prospective cohort study defines a population in the present, measures relevant exposures and follows the subjects into the future to ascertain the development of disease. The disease status is then determined in different categories of the baseline and subsequent exposure. A retrospective cohort study uses measures of exposure from the past. The measures of exposure may have been collected prospectively in the past, or markers of past exposure (if available) may be collected in the present. For example, a cohort of men born in Hertfordshire between 1911 and 1921 was defined from health visitor records collected prospectively over those years. These men were subsequently followed up through the National Health Service Central Register to determine vital status. The mortality experience of these men was then related to birth weight and change in weight over the first year of life to determine if there was any association with rates of ischaemic heart disease.[8]

Case-control studies   Persons with an outcome or disease (referred to as cases) are compared with persons who do not have the disease (referent group or controls). The prevalence of past exposure to known or suspected risk factors is measured in each group and from this the risk ratio for the effect of each measured exposure can be estimated. In principle, a case-control study reconstructs (by sampling and with very much less effort) the outcome of the cohort study that would have given rise to the cases under study (Table 1.3). Information can be obtained on many exposure variables in a case-control study, although the validity of this information may be limited by the fact that the data were collected retrospectively. This is particularly a problem in dietary studies where food intake may have changed as a result of the disease process. Ideally, the measure of exposure should cover the period in time when the exposure is believed to cause the disease to develop. In a dietary study past diet, not the present diet, may therefore be the exposure of interest. If current diet is measured as a proxy for past diet it must be assumed that diet has remained stable over time. If

Table 1.3 Differences between types of cohort and case-control studies

	Time		
	Past	Present	Future
Prospective cohort		Define cohort measure exposure	Follow-up determine disease frequency
Retrospective cohort	Define cohort measure exposure	Determine disease frequency	
Case-control study	Exposure history recalled	Define cases and controls	

subjects are asked to recall their past diet it may be that their current diet influences their recollection of what they thought they ate in the past. For these reasons it is likely that the relevant measure of dietary exposure may be biased. This may be allowed for to some extent by the selection of appropriate study population groups. It is also important in case-control studies to define the population from which cases and controls are drawn. Miettinen refers to this as a dynamic population; each control is selected from a pool of eligible subjects in the defined sample.[9] It is an ongoing sampling procedure (defined at the beginning of the study) throughout the study. Cases should preferably be new cases arising over a specified period of time (incident cases). These and other issues are discussed in more detail in Chapter 11.

The usual aim in case-control studies is to measure risk across strata of exposure levels, for example, to determine whether risk of breast cancer increases across increasing categories of fat intake (often divided into thirds or fifths). As long as subjects are correctly classified as to whether they have high, medium, or low fat intake, the absolute level of intake does not affect the estimate of risk. It may, therefore, be possible to use a simpler method of measuring exposure than is required where an absolute measure of exposure is required as, for example, in cohort or some experimental studies. There is no disadvantage in using a more accurate method in a case-control study, but it may add considerable time and cost for relatively little benefit. It is desirable to have an indication of the measurement error of the method used and therefore some indication of the potential error in the diet–disease risk estimate.

Cross-sectional studies   These measure exposure and disease state at the same point in time. That is current, not past exposure (as in a case-control study) to the cause is documented in the population sample. Some writers may describe these as prevalence surveys.

It is difficult in cross-sectional studies to determine the nature of the relationship between the measured exposure and outcome. It is not possible to say whether the exposure caused the outcome or vice versa. If the exposure measure is elevated it is not possible to say whether the elevation was a result of the outcome but not in the causal pathway.

There are advantages and disadvantages in using either a case-control or cohort design and the choice of one or other method will depend on the balance between these after due consideration of the exposure and outcome measures of interest (Table 1.4).

Exposure in cohort studies is usually measured more accurately than in case-control studies and it is less likely that the outcome influences the measured exposure. A cohort study is less likely than a case-control study to have recall bias. If the disease of interest is rare, a cohort study will not be as efficient as a case-control study. If an exposure is rare a cohort study, where exposed and non-exposed can be preselected, may be more efficient than a case-control study. A case-control study is quick and less expensive than a cohort study, which may take many years and cost a great deal (unless the cohort is defined retrospectively). In an appropriately designed cohort study (with sufficient subjects) many different outcomes may be

Table 1.4 Advantages and disadvantages of cohort and case-control studies

	Case-control studies	Cohort studies
Advantages	Not so expensive and completed more quickly	Exposure measured more accurately
	More efficient for rare diseases	Outcome not influenced by measured exposure
	Multiple risk factors can be examined simultaneously	Less likely to have information bias
		Where exposure is rare, more efficient
		Able to relate different outcomes to exposure
		Provide absolute measure of risk
Disadvantages	Exposure not measured as accurately	Prospective cohort studies are expensive and time consuming
	Disease may influence exposure	Not very efficient for rare diseases
	Recall bias on past exposure	
	Only provide estimate of relative risk	

related to the exposures. A cohort study can provide absolute measures of risk whereas a case-control study can only provide estimates of relative risk (i.e. the ratio of risk in different exposure categories).

1.3 EPIDEMIOLOGICAL MEASUREMENTS

As mentioned in section 1.1 above, one of the major objectives of epidemiological research is to reduce the error of measuring exposure and outcome to an acceptable level. In this section the key issues in measuring exposure (with specific reference to dietary exposure) and outcome will be discussed. The measurement of disease frequency and effect is covered in Chapter 9. It is important to know whether a measured exposure or outcome variable is likely to reflect the true distribution. It is not possible to measure these factors with absolute accuracy and it is therefore an important part of epidemiological research to assess how inaccurate these measures are likely to be. One aspect of this issue, random and systematic error, will be discussed further in section 1.4 under the interpretation of epidemiological research. Here general issues related to validity and reliability will be discussed.

1.3.1 The assessment of validity and reliability

Validity   The term 'validity' is used in two ways. A study is considered to be valid if the findings can be taken as being a reasonable representation of the true situation. That is, if the study was repeated in the same population using the same methods, approximately the same results would be obtained. This is referred to as external validity, or generalizability, and involves some judgement because it is very unlikely that the true situation will be known. Another way in which the term validity is used is in the rather more narrow sense of whether a measure of exposure or outcome actually measures that exposure or outcome. This is referred to as internal validity. A study can not be valid (generalizable) unless the measures of exposure and outcome that are used are also valid (internally valid). It is this latter type of validity that will be discussed here. The former type of validity will be discussed in section 1.4 because it relates more to the interpretation of epidemiological findings.

A measure is valid if it measures what it purports to measure. This implies that there is an absolute measure of the variable against which the new or alternative measure is compared. In most situations it it not possible to have an absolute measure, and one method of measuring exposure is usually compared with another that is considered from previous research to be more accurate. This is referred to as relative validity (sometimes called concurrent validity). For example, for most nutrients there is no absolute measure of intake and researchers generally compare a new method of assessing the nutrient intake with a 7-day weighed record. If the new method measures the exposure in a similar way to the reference method, then the new method is considered to be valid.

If the new method consistently records higher or lower than the 'true' intake it may not affect the measure of association between exposure and outcome. For example, if a food frequency questionnaire estimate of fat intake differs on average from a 14-day weighed record estimate of fat intake, but it ranks subjects in the distribution of fat intake in exactly the same way then the measure of effect (e.g. relative risk) across rankings will be the same.

Measures of sensitivity and specificity relate to the validity of the measure. To be valid a measure should be both specific and sensitive. Sensitivity measures the proportion of truly exposed or diseased subjects who are correctly classified as such. Specificity measures the proportion of truly unexposed or non-diseased subjects who are correctly classified as such. Positive predictive value is the proportion of subjects measured to be exposed who are truly exposed. Negative predictive value is the proportion of subjects measured to be unexposed who are truly not exposed (Table 1.5).

In studies estimating the prevalence of an outcome, the proportion classified as diseased will be a function of the prevalence of the disease as

Table 1.5 Definition of sensitivity, specificity, and predictive value

		True Status		
		Diseased	Not diseased	Total
Measured	Positive	a	b	a + b
status	Negative	c	d	c + d
Total		a + c	b + d	a + b + c + d

Sensitivity $= \dfrac{a}{a + c}$

Specificity $= \dfrac{d}{b + d}$

Predictive value (positive) $\dfrac{a}{a + b}$

Predictive value (negative) $\dfrac{d}{c + d}$

The above are appropriate where there is a dichotomous variable.

well as the sensitivity and specificity of the measures used. Unless a measure is absolutely sensitive and specific, the measure of prevalence of the disease (or outcome) will be affected. If sensitivity and specificity are known it is possible to correct the prevalence measure. Any loss of validity in measuring either exposure or outcome will reduce the ability to determine risk accurately.

Repeatability   Repeatability (or some may prefer to use the terms precision, reliability, or reproducibility) refers to the consistency with which a measure of exposure measures that exposure. Is the same result obtained if a measure is repeated? Differences between repeat measures may be due either to true subject variation for that measure or to the effect of observer (measurement) variation. Subject variation may be either random or systematic. However, it is difficult to distinguish between the true subject variation and the effects of the repeated observation of that subject by an observer because it is difficult to have exactly the same conditions for the initial and repeat measures. It may therefore be difficult to actually assess the repeatability of a measure.

Lack of repeatability in a measure indicates that it is not valid and reduces the possibility of correctly identifying a causal relationship.

1.3.2 General issues in the measurement of exposure and outcome

The aim is to measure the variables of interest with required accuracy. Exposure and outcome variables can usually be measured in a variety of ways. The selection of an appropriate method to measure exposure and outcome and the correct use of that method must be considered at the design stage in any study. The way in which information is obtained should be the same regardless of the level of exposure or disease status.

Exposure and outcome are assessed in many studies by asking the subjects themselves. The basic issues in designing a questionnaire are covered in more detail in Appendix 2. A questionnaire can be either self-administered or administered by an interviewer.

If interviewers are used, they should be carefully trained so as to standardize the way information is collected from all study participants. As far as possible, the interviewer should be blinded as to the exact question being addressed by the research, so that there is less possibility that they lead the subject into giving particular answers.

It is essential that clear, written instructions accompany a self-administered questionnaire, so that subjects know how questions are to be answered.

There are advantages and disadvantages in using either approach (Table 1.6).

Where subjects complete the questionnaire themselves there is no way

Table 1.6 Advantages and disadvantages of different interview approaches

	Self-administered	Interviewer-administered
Advantages	Absence of interviewer bias Low cost	Ensures completion of all questions Allows complex questions and question sequences Misunderstandings can be clarified (but this may introduce bias) Facilitates cooperation
Disadvantages	Tendency to partial non-completion Complex questions and question sequences cannot be used Difficult to ensure questions understood Low response rate Restricts subjects (literacy)	Cost and time consuming Interviewer bias

that the researcher can influence their answers, provided the questions are framed properly. However, unless checked at completion, it is possible that some questions may not have been answered in a self-administered questionnaire; at interview this does not happen. Moreover, it is possible to clarify any confusion over what a question means. However, interviewing subjects is very time consuming and may not be practical for surveys with a large number of subjects, although the response rate may be better than that for self-administered questionnaires, particularly if these are sent to subjects in the post. It is also important to consider the subjects in deciding whether to use an interview or self administered approach. Obviously, if people cannot read it is not possible to use a self-administered approach.

Whether a questionnaire is self-administered or administered by interview, it is essential that the information obtained can be properly interpreted. The interviewer's perception of the meaning of the question may be different from the subject's, and it is important to try to assess the likely effect of this before the study has commenced. Careful attention must be given to the wording so as not to lead the subject into giving a particular answer. Any implication that a particular response is right or wrong should be avoided. As far as possible it is better to use closed rather than open questions because it is often difficult to analyse responses from open questions. For important measures of exposure, it may also be worthwhile including several questions that provide similar estimates of exposure. If the answers are similar for all questions then it is more likely that a correct measure has been obtained.

If a questionnaire is used to obtain information it should be carefully pretested and appropriately piloted before the study commences. The validity and reliability of the information obtained from the questionnaire should be assessed by reference to another measure of the variable and also by repeating the questionnaire on at least a subset of participants.

Exposure and outcome information about a subject can also be obtained from blood samples (serum cholesterol), urine samples (24-hour urinary nitrogen), or tissue samples (adipose fatty acids or toe-nail selenium). An exposure measure may also be measured on the subject, by weighing, or measuring blood pressure, for example. For either approach, the way the sample is obtained and processed, or the way the measure is taken, must be carefully standardized. It is also important to consider whether the measured variable is an appropriate representation of the exposure or outcome variable of interest.

1.3.3 Measuring dietary exposure

The appropriate approach to measuring dietary exposure is determined by the objective of the study. As already mentioned in section 1.2 above, the measurement of dietary exposure differs for different study designs. It is essential to have a clear idea as to the aspect of dietary exposure that is of interest. Dietary exposure is not the same as nutrient intake and, for some study questions, nutrient intake may not be the appropriate measure of exposure. In designing the study it is essential to have a good idea as to how the dietary exposure may affect the outcome of interest. It is important to assess exposure at the correct point in time, ideally at the time when the disease was being induced. If diet is measured at another point in time the investigator must then make some assumptions about whether exposure at that time is likely to be a reasonable estimate of the exposure at the critical time. This is a particular issue for case-control studies.

The following may need to be considered when deciding how to measure dietary exposure:

1. Food consists of many substances, not just nutrients. These other substances, such as additives, contaminants, chemicals formed in the preparation of foods, natural toxins, other naturally occurring compounds, and other as yet unknown compounds may all affect disease and may all, therefore, be important exposure measures. It is not adequate to equate nutrient intake with food intake. It is therefore essential to frame the objective of the assessment of dietary exposure as specifically as possible.

2. A food and its components (nutrients and other substances) is complex and may have different functions and physiological effects at different levels. Take vitamin A as an example. At one extreme of intake it may result in a deficiency state and at the other extreme it may result in toxicity. Somewhere in between is the amount at which optimal function occurs. Studying vitamin A intake at different points in this spectrum may give apparently different results. It may be important, therefore, to know prior to the study where in this spectrum the participants are likely to be and to consider whether this may be likely to affect the outcome.

3. If a component of diet is studied in isolation its effects may appear different to those seen when studied in conjunction with the other natural components of the food.

4. A nutrient may have more than one function and these functions may have different effects on the outcome of interest.

5. The requirements for nutrients may be quite different in growth, ageing, pregnancy or in states of infection. It is therefore essential to have a clear understanding of the physiological state of the population group of interest as the need for and use of nutrients may be quite different in these different groups.

6. The nutrient of interest may directly affect the outcome or it may have an indirect effect on some other factor which in turn affects the disease process.

7. The effect of one nutrient may be quite different at different levels of another nutrient. Protein intake may affect a disease process differently when total energy intake or levels of other essential nutrients are inadequate. The need for, and use of, nutrients may be quite different at different levels of total energy intake, and under different physiological states or under different physical stresses.

8. Food intake is not equivalent to biological availability. To be available for use, a nutrient must be ingested, separated from the rest of the components in the diet, absorbed across the gut wall and transported to its active site, and incorporated into its functional structure. This entire process is dependent on, and affected by, the availability and/or presence of many other factors. It may therefore be very misleading to assume that the level of a nutrient reported in a table of food composition represents the functionally available level. It may be important to study the effects that these other factors have on the measure of exposure and on the effect on the outcome and to consider the biological endpoint, rather than the dietary starting point.

9. Some nutrients have bioequivalence. For example, niacin can be synthesized from tryptophan. An experimental study undertaken to investigate the effect of depletion/repletion on niacin status will need to take account of the potential effect levels of tryptophan may have on niacin status.

10. There may be critical time periods in the development of an outcome where the level of intake of a nutrient may play a vital role. At other times, the same level of nutrient intake may have no effect on outcome. This may be the situation with folate and neural tube defects.

11. A specific level of a nutrient measured in blood or serum may not reflect the balance or status of that nutrient and may therefore be an inappropriate measure of exposure for that nutrient.

It should be clear from the above that diet is a very complex exposure to measure. It is important then, when interpreting the results from such studies, to consider the above factors. It is also desirable that the potential effects of the above factors are considered before commencing the study, to ensure that the most appropriate aspects of exposure are measured. Having an idea about the underlying mechanisms believed to be involved will help clarify some of these issues. It is also essential to consider the nutritional status of the subjects included in the study, as well as the effects such factors as age, gender, and general health may have on their exposure.

Various types of epidemiological study were described in section 1.2. Different measures of dietary exposure are required for these different types of epidemiological study. In an ecological study, where the unit of study is a group, the measure of dietary exposure is quite different from an experimental study, where it is essential to have an accurate measure of an individual's intake. In the former it is important only to characterize the group accurately.

Whatever study design is used, it is important that an appropriate measure of exposure is used. On the one hand it is a waste of time and money to have a very detailed assessment of diet when all that is required is a simple method. On the other hand, using a simple method when a more detailed method is required may introduce considerable error into the study, and mask a real effect. For example, in a case-control study the aim might be to assess the effect of calcium intake on bone density. The researcher may want to be able to divide the sample into thirds of the distribution and determine how risk varies across the thirds of calcium intake. It is not necessary to know exactly what each individual's actual calcium intake is, it is only important to ensure that the individual is correctly placed in the distribution (or that possible subject misclassification is minimized as far as possible, and is the same between cases and referent groups). For calcium it has been shown that this can be achieved using a ten-item food frequency questionnaire. A 7-day weighed inventory would give the same result but would cost a great deal more in time and money.

In summary, the aim should be to use the most appropriate method for the study. Because of the effect that misclassification of exposure may have on the interpretation of the research, it is desirable to have a measure of the misclassification occurring as a result of the method used. It is recommended that, whenever possible, a repeat measure of the exposure is incorporated in the study design, even if it is only on a numerically viable subsample. It may also be desirable to include different measures of the exposure of interest. This latter point needs careful thought. If there are two measures of the exposure, and after the study is analysed it emerges that the measures give different results, how will these differences be interpreted? Clearly established rules are required *a priori* for interpreting these differences. If the measure that disagreed with what was expected is ignored, why was it included in the first place? Ideally, before commencing the study the most appropriate methods should be selected, piloted, and pretested in a relevant group. A method may have been successfully used elsewhere in the past, but it is unlikely that all the conditions under which it is to be used in the present will be the same.

It is becoming more common to use biochemical and biological markers for assessing dietary and other exposures. Biochemical and biological markers can be used quantitatively to estimate the exposure of interest itself, or they might be used to reflect the body's response to such an exposure.[10] Researchers have turned to these markers because of the difficulties of measuring dietary intakes and obtaining information about what actually enters the body and affects the relevant processes under investigation. Biochemical markers of nutritional exposures are discussed in more detail in Chapter 7. It is commonly assumed that a blood or urine measure is more reliable and probably more meaningful than a dietary measure because it reflects what has actually been taken in. This may not always be true and careful thought must be given as to how the biochemical markers are used. It may be that a food frequency estimate of vitamin C intake at some relevant point in the past may be a more sensitive and specific measure of the exposure of interest than serum vitamin C. Recent research has also shown that serum zinc levels do not reflect the functional zinc status of an individual, and therefore relying on a serum measure may be misleading. Whether it is more or less misleading than a dietary measure of zinc, given the difficulties in estimating intake, as mentioned in Chapter 6, is a moot point, but these issues need to be considered. A urinary level of an electrolyte may reflect or be affected by a range of different processes. The disease state under investigation may affect the urinary excretion, rather than the urinary excretion reflecting an exposure that affects disease. Measurement error and misclassification are possible using any measure of exposure.

1.3.4 Measurement of outcome

This section considers problems of measuring outcome. In any aetiological study, classifying someone as not diseased when they are diseased will distort the estimates of risk. It is therefore essential in the planning stage to determine whether an outcome can be measured with sufficient validity (sensitivity and specificity).

Many cohort and experimental studies rely on death certificates for the ascertainment of outcome. For common diseases that may reasonably be expected to be included as a cause of death on the death certificate, the death certificate may provide a sensitive measure of outcome, but this is not always true. In several studies that have compared death certificate diagnosis with autopsy diagnosis there has not always been good agreement between the two measures.[11]

For diseases that may not be fatal, the diagnosis may be more likely to be omitted from the death certificate. For example, a recent follow-up study of elderly people in Britain determined whether diet (calcium intake) measured 15 years previously was related to risk of subsequently developing a hip fracture.[12] Subjects were followed up through the National Health Service Central Register. Death certificates were obtained for all participants who had died and only four of these mentioned fracture as an underlying cause of death. However, subsequent checking of general practitioner and hospital morbidity records revealed that considerably more subjects, who were now dead, had in fact sustained a fracture. If only the death certificate data were used to measure outcome, the rate of hip fractures would have been considerably underestimated.

If routinely collected data, like death certificates, hospital activity analysis, or mother and child health clinic attendances, are used to measure an outcome, some estimate needs to be made of the likely completeness of case ascertainment. It is also desirable to have an estimate of whether there is any sampling bias occurring in how subjects are eligible or included in the study. For example, rates of diarrhoea in children attending a clinic in a village in the Gambia may be quite different from rates obtained from a census of all the children living in the village. If the factors determining attendance at the clinic are related to the exposure of interest, a biased exposure–outcome relationship may occur.

If outcome is measured by the observer either by interview, medical examination, or mailed questionnaire, there is the potential for biased ascertainment of outcome. An observer interviewing a subject may lead the subject into answers that the subject feels the observer wants to hear.

A medical examination by a doctor in a white coat may evoke different responses from examination by a nurse who is perceived to be more friendly and approachable. Response rates to questionnaires sent in the post are generally lower than where the information is obtained by an interviewer. Those who respond are likely to be different in some ways from those who do not reply and it is therefore possible that the measured outcome (and exposure) does not reflect the distribution seen in the whole population. For outcome measures like blood pressure, the observer can have a considerable effect on the level of measurement. This effect alters over time as a subject becomes more familiar with the procedure. This error is in addition to any errors introduced in the way the observer measures the blood pressure.

1.4 INTERPRETATION OF EPIDEMIOLOGICAL RESEARCH

An investigator conducts a study and comes up with an association between a measure of exposure and a measure of outcome. What does this mean? There are several questions that need to be asked before it is reasonable to assume that the association can be interpreted as showing a cause–effect relationship. How likely is it that the finding did not occur by chance, or was not due to some bias or was the result of a confounding factor. In this section these issues will be discussed, followed by a discussion of causality.

1.4.1 The role of chance

In assessing the findings of a study the investigator needs to know whether the results obtained could have occurred by chance alone. This can be assessed by hypothesis testing or by reference to confidence intervals.

Hypothesis testing   This requires a clear statement of the hypothesis being tested (the null hypothesis). This usually states that there is no relationship between exposure and outcome; the alternative hypothesis states that an association is present. For example, in a case-control or cohort study the null hypothesis might be that the odds ratio (case-control study) or relative risk (cohort study) is equal to one (i.e. that there is no effect); the alternative hypothesis is that the effect is either greater or smaller than one. This hypothesis can then be addressed using an appropriate test of statistical significance. The principle of these tests of statistical significance is usually that there is a difference between groups (or observed and expected values) that can be measured and that the variance of the estimate of the difference can be estimated. The general form of the test (although this is not always the case) is the observed minus the expected divided by the square root of the variance. For a given variance, the bigger the difference between groups (or observed and expected values) the more likely that there will be a statistically significant result. For a given difference, the variance of the estimate will also affect the level of significance, the smaller the variance the more statistically significant the recorded difference. The standard error of the estimate is a function of the sample size. The larger the sample the smaller the standard error and therefore the greater the ability to detect a statistically significant result.

It is customary to express the level of statistical significance in terms of how likely it is that the result would have occurred by chance if there was no association (i.e. if the null hypothesis were true). The larger the value of the test of statistical significance (either positive or negative) the smaller the P-value, or the less likely that such a result would occur by chance alone. If the P-value is 0.05 it means that there is only a one in 20 chance that a result as extreme as that observed would have occurred by chance alone, if the null hypothesis were true. If this is the case it is conventional to reject the null hypothesis and accept the alternative hypothesis—that there is an association between exposure and outcome. If the P-value is greater than 0.05 it is customary to conclude that the result could have occurred by chance alone and that it is therefore not possible to reject the null hypothesis. If the null hypothesis is rejected it is possible that this is incorrect, and this type of error, incorrectly rejecting a null hypothesis is called a type I or alpha error. On the other hand, if the null hypothesis is false and is not rejected, this is referred to as a type II or beta error.

The P-value chosen as representing statistical significance is arbitrary and should only be used as a guide. For example, it does not make any sense to reject a P-value of 0.06, which is only just not considered statistically significant, if there is a clear notion as to how the exposure and outcome variables are related. This result may sensibly lead to another study that more specifically addresses that association.

In reporting P-values it is always preferable to present the exact P-value rather than to simply say that it was greater or less than 0.05. This enables readers to make their own judgements about whether a P-value of for example, 0.06 or 0.10 is a useful guide to a potentially important observation.

Unless there is a clear hypothesis as to the direction of the effect expected, it is better to use (where possible) a two-sided or two-tailed test of statistical significance. If a two-sided test is used there is no assumption made as to the direction of the effect. A one-sided test of statistical significance assumes that the effect is in a particular direction. The two-tailed test is more conservative statistically and therefore less likely to lead the researcher into assuming that a relationship is present when in fact one does not exist. However, the level of statistical significance should not be the sole arbiter of the importance of the results.

In some situations data are available on a whole range of variables that may have been included with no specific question in mind. If an investigator inspects the data and finds some comparisons to be different, but before the analysis began he or she had no idea that this comparison was important, care should be taken in the interpretation of the findings. If these variables are examined and some turn out to show statistically significant associations, it should be born in mind that even if no real associations exist, on average, one in 20 such associations will be statistically significant. Some would argue that it is not acceptable to do *post hoc* analyses, but if interpreted with caution they can often lead to new insights that can then be tested more formally in further research.

The major problem in using hypothesis testing is that it gives no direct indication of the size of the effect. For example, in a study assessing the effect of a change in diet on blood pressure, a *P*-value of 0.05 for the change in blood pressure gives no indication of the absolute change. If the sample size is very large, small differences will be statistically significant, but these differences may not have any biological importance. It may not be reasonable to equate statistical significance with the importance of the effect.

Confidence intervals   Another way of quantifying the possible contribution of chance to observed results is to derive confidence intervals. The confidence interval represents the range within which the variable (risk, prevalence, etc.) that is being estimated is likely to lie. The width of a confidence interval based on a sample statistic, such as the mean, depends on the standard deviation and the sample size.[13] The standard error, which is used to determine the confidence interval, is calculated from the sample size and standard deviation and represents the estimate of the uncertainty of the sample statistic. The larger the sample size, at a given mean and standard deviation, the smaller the standard error and therefore the narrower the confidence interval. The confidence interval also depends on the degree of confidence required for the interval. Separate formulae are available for calculating confidence intervals for means, proportions, and their differences. These formulae usually depend on the assumption that the data are normally distributed, but there are techniques for estimating a confidence interval about a median, for instance. The common underlying principle is the addition and subtraction of a multiple of the standard error to the sample statistic.

It is most common to use a 95 per cent confidence interval, but this is arbitrary and it is possible to use either a 90 or 99 per cent interval as required. In a recent study the effect of a vegetarian diet on blood pressure was assessed in a sample of mildly hypertensive subjects.[14] When subjects were on the vegetarian diet systolic blood pressure fell by, on average 3.5 mmHg. The 95 per cent confidence interval for this test statistic was −7.0–−0.1 mmHg. If the study were repeated on many different samples from the same population and the 95 per cent confidence intervals were calculated for each study, 95 per cent of these would include the population difference between means. It would be reasonable to assume from the above results that the effect of a vegetarian diet on blood pressure is therefore compatible with an effect as small as −0.1 mmHg and as great as −7.0 mmHg, although the best estimate is −3.5 mmHg, the difference between the sample means.

Wide confidence intervals, even if the result is statistically significant, indicate that the estimate is not very precise. That is, the data are compatible with a wide range of potential effects.

There is a relationship between the two-sided hypothesis test and confidence interval. For example, the 95 per cent confidence interval corresponds roughly to the 5 per cent level of statistical significance under the null hypothesis as assessed using an appropriate test of statistical significance. In the above cited study of the effects of a vegetarian diet on blood pressure, a zero difference in blood pressure between vegetarians and non-vegetarians corresponds to the null hypothesis. In the above study, however, zero was not included within the 95 per cent confidence interval and therefore the study could be considered statistically significant at the 5 per cent level. Had the zero value fallen within the 95 per cent confidence interval this would have indicated a non-significant result, that is, the probability of finding the mean difference obtained would have been greater than 5 per cent.

Where possible, both the P-value and confidence interval should be presented, although the latter is likely to be more useful in interpreting the results of the study. The confidence interval provides an indication of the likely magnitude of effect, while the P-value derived from a test of statistical significance does not.[13] Relying on tests of statistical significance incorrectly implies that the purpose of a study is to obtain 'statistical significance'.

Where no association has been found it is important to consider the possible reasons why this may be so. It is important to look at the design and conduct of the study before assuming that the results obtained are a reliable reflection of the true situation. It could be that the study was too small or that there was large random sampling variation in the particular study and that repetition of the study in a larger or different sample would give a statistically significant result. Irrespective of the width of the confidence intervals or level of statistical significance obtained, it is important to consider the effects that bias and confounding may have on the results obtained. These will be considered in the next two sections of this chapter.

1.4.2 Bias

Last defines bias as 'Any trend in the collection, analysis, interpretation, publication, or review of data that can lead to conclusions that are systematically different from the truth'. (p. 13).[15] This systematic error affects the validity of a study and can influence the estimate of effect in either direction.

Many different types of bias have been defined, but there are two main types of bias that can affect the validity of a study. These are selection bias and information bias. The effect these biases might have on the results of the study must be assessed before the study can be properly interpreted.

Selection bias Most epidemiological studies are concerned with comparing and contrasting two or more groups in some measure of their exposure or outcome frequency. The objective of drawing a sample from a population is to obtain a measure of effect such that the measure obtained in the sample is a reasonable reflection of the true effect in the population. A bias occurs if the relationship between exposure and effect for those who participate is different to that for those who are eligible to participate from the population but do not. Therefore, any factors that affect the inclusion of subjects at the beginning of a study might introduce a bias. It is then a matter of judgement as to how important this bias might be in interpreting the results of the study.

For example, in a retrospective cohort study of the relationship between infant feeding patterns and childhood diarrhoea, some subjects might be traced through health visitor records and some might be obtained through subjects contacting the investigators themselves; it is likely that the latter group might be different from the group obtained from the records. This may be termed self-selection bias.[2]

Another type of selection bias is diagnostic bias.[16] For example, if a case-control study uses as its case base only subjects who present to a particular hospital, and if the way subjects are drawn to that hospital is affected by their exposure then it is likely that a biased estimate of effect will be obtained. In case-control studies where cases are recruited as they present at hospital, consideration needs to be given as to the selection of appropriate control groups to represent the exposure in the dynamic population from which the cases are drawn.

A bias may also occur if the response rate is different in cases and controls. Cases, having recently been diagnosed may be more likely to participate because they may feel that they have a vested interest in finding out more about why they got the disease. Controls on the other hand, may not have the same concern, and those who participate may be more health conscious or behave differently from the dynamic population they are meant to represent.

In the design of the study some strategy should be considered as to how information on those people who refuse to participate, or who subsequently drop out could be obtained. Even if this information is only age, sex, and occupation it will allow an estimate of whether those who participate in the study reflect the population from which they are drawn. However, a non-representative sample may not affect the internal validity of the study.

Information bias   Information bias occurs when there are either random or systematic differences in the way exposure and outcome are measured in the study groups. The distinction between differential and non-differential bias is that in the former the information that is obtained is systematically different between different groups in the study whereas in the latter it is not. Differential misclassification may lead either to over- or under-estimation of an effect. Non-differential misclassification biases towards the null. As for selection bias, the likely effects this sort of bias might have on the interpretation of the study findings is a matter of judgement, and is influenced by whether the bias is likely to be different for cases and controls.

There are many potential sources of information bias, but two common ones are recall and interviewer bias.

Recall bias

Any studies attempting to obtain information from subjects about events in the past may be subject to recall bias.[17] Recall bias can be affected by the time interval since exposure, the degree of detail about the exposure that is required, personal characteristics of the subjects, the perceived social desirability of the exposure under investigation (for example, smokers might under-report their tobacco use), and the significance of the events under study. These biases may or may not be different for cases and controls.

There are several factors that might contribute to differential recall between cases and controls. The motivation to participate may be greater in cases than controls, where the former might be seeking an answer as to why they have got the disease. They might reflect on past exposures, or have been asked about the exposure under investigation by physicians responsible for their care, and they might therefore recall past exposure differently from controls who, before being recruited into the study, had not thought about the exposure under investigation. For example, in a case-control study of folate and neural tube defects, the mothers of the cases may be more likely to think back over events that occurred during their pregnancy to try to explain why their child has developed the defect. They may therefore, recall exposures differently from mothers of controls who have had not had the same incentive to think about exposures during their pregnancy. This effect may be reduced by the selection of appropriate controls as, for example, another group of congenital malformations with an aetiology unrelated to neural tube defects.

In case-control studies, where a measure of dietary exposure is required for some point in the distant past, it has generally been shown that the recalled exposure tends to be more like the current exposure. If current diet has changed from that consumed in the past, a bias may occur. This bias may lead to either differential or non-differential misclassification depending on whether it differs between cases and controls.

Interviewer bias

Interviewer bias may occur when there is any difference in the way information is obtained, recorded, processed, and interpreted in different groups in the study by the interviewer. If interviewers assess exposure in case-control studies and they know whether the subject is a case or a control, they may solicit the information differently. This is less likely to be a problem in a prospective cohort study where outcome is not known at the time of obtaining the exposure information.

The way subjects are followed, or the completeness of information obtained during follow-up within a cohort or experimental study, may also introduce a bias. If a distinct subset of subjects (the less healthy, the poorer, or those with high or low exposure status) are lost to follow-up, a biased result may occur.

A major consideration in epidemiological research is to reduce bias. The potential effect bias has on the measurement of cause–effect relationships needs to be assessed wherever possible in all studies. In practice this is often quite difficult. It is optimal to anticipate the likely sources of bias in a study at the design stage and to consider how to collect information in a way that is likely to reduce that bias to the required level. Consideration needs to be given as to how the choice of study population, methods of data collection and sources of exposure and outcome information may be obtained to reduce bias.

In a cohort or experimental study it may be better to select a group of subjects that can be followed up over a long period of time, even though they may not represent the general population. For example, the classic study of Doll and Hill[18] chose doctors as their cohort because they knew that they were an easy group to define and follow-up. It may be that the results from this study were not generalizable (although they probably were), but it was considered more important to have an internally valid study that provided information that could be reliably interpreted.

Interviewers should be blinded as to the nature of the question under investigation and they should be carefully trained so that they collect information in a standardized way throughout.

1.4.3 External validity

As already mentioned, there are two components of validity; one relating to the information obtained from the subjects in the study (internal validity) and the other relating to how the information obtained relates to people outside the study population (external validity or generalizability). A study cannot be externally valid unless it is internally valid.

In discussing generalizability it is important to consider what aspects of the sample are relevant when making a generalization about the findings. What factors about the sample will affect the generalizability of the findings? This requires an understanding of the likely mechanism of the effect on the outcome. In some situations it may be reasonable to generalize, say from a study of men to women, but in others it may not, for example, where female sex hormones are believed to play a key role in the causal process.

There are two broad views about the importance of external validity or generalization. One view considers that the study sample should be representative of the population from which it was drawn and that it is, therefore, important to assess how the study sample differs from the population from which it was drawn. Thus, for example, data on age, sex, and other socio-economic factors would be compared between the sample and the population from which the sample was drawn. If they are similar it would be considered reasonable to generalize from the sample to the population. However, it may be that the variables for which comparable information has been obtained, or is available, are irrelevant to the causal process under investigation. For example, generalizing from middle-aged people to children may not always be appropriate.

The other point of view argues that the generalizability of a study is not assessed by such simple comparisons of the study sample to the population from which it was drawn. This view argues that generalization is from the experience of the actual study to the abstract and is founded on judgement rather than statistical sampling and technical sample-to-population inference.

In reality, both views are similar in that they rely on the investigator making a sensible judgement about whether the results obtained in the present study are likely to be the same in another study in a different sample. The objective of the research should be to increase understanding about a particular process. This understanding requires going from the information that is available to the abstract formulation of a particular theory that subsequently can be tested and redefined. In terms of trying to understand the causal process, it may therefore be that the selection of a particular sample that can better address the question under test is more important than how far the results can be generalized.

1.4.4 Confounding

The third major issue to consider in interpreting epidemiological research is the possibility that variables (confounders) other than the exposure of interest have influenced the estimate of effect of the exposure on outcome.

In one sense confounding may be considered as another form of bias in the interpretation of epidemiological research.

Confounding has been defined in a number of different ways. For consistency we have used that definition used by Coggon in Chapter 11. A confounding factor is one that is associated with the risk factor (exposure) under study *and* that independently determines the risk of developing the disease (or outcome). Failure to consider the effect that potential confounders may have on an exposure–outcome relationship may give rise to spurious associations. The estimate of effect may be either increased or decreased by the effect of a confounding factor.

For a variable to be a confounder it:

(1) must be associated with, but not causally dependent upon, the exposure of interest;
(2) must be a risk factor for disease, independent of its association with the exposure of interest.

The above must apply within the study population at issue. It is important to consider the effect of implying that a factor is a confounder when it is actually in the causal pathway. Adjusting for this factor will reduce the risk estimate with the exposure and thereby may, falsely, lead an investigator to discard the exposure variable under investigation as not being important. It is therefore important to consider how a variable may influence the exposure–outcome relationship before assuming that it is a confounder.

A study should be designed to minimize, as far as possible, the effects of confounding variables. However, it is never possible to eliminate all confounders, and it is therefore important to measure known or suspected confounders so that they can be considered in the analysis. Where variables are known to be confounders, the investigator can control for them by randomization, restriction, or matching.

Randomization

This is only applicable in experimental studies where the allocation of exposure categories is determined by the investigator. Randomly allocating subjects to different treatment (exposure) groups ensures that any differences that arise between groups do so by chance alone. Randomization provides a mechanism for subject allocation that is not able to be affected, deliberately or otherwise, by manipulation. If the investigator wants to make sure that groups are exactly alike for certain key variables, it is possible to block on these variables. For example, sex and age are often potential confounders and subjects can be allocated to groups such that they contain the same numbers of men and women at different ages. Subjects are grouped into the appropriate age and sex blocks and, within each block, they are randomly allocated to treatment groups. For studies with small samples, if allocation is not blocked it is possible that by chance alone all the older men may be allocated to one treatment group. By blocking, the investigator is assured that there will be equal numbers of old men or young women in each treatment group. While it is possible to determine the age and sex composition of each treatment group in the study after randomization, if the sample size is small, there may not be sufficient subjects to do an appropriate subgroups analysis to determine, for example, whether the effect is similar in old men and young women.

It is important to measure the variables of interest during the experiment to determine whether there is any change occurring during the study; if there is change it may be possible to adjust the measure of effect for it. For example, in one of our studies on the effect of changing to a vegetarian diet on blood pressure, even though we asked subjects not to change their physical activity and alcohol intake during the study, a number did in fact change other factors. By measuring these factors at baseline and during the study we were able, at least in theory, to adjust the diet–blood pressure relationship for these factors.

Restriction

If a variable is believed to be a confounder it is possible to restrict the inclusion of subjects into the study so that, for that variable, all subjects are effectively the same. This variable cannot then confound the relationship of interest. For example, the researcher may restrict subjects to be men aged between 55 and 59 years. The width of the age band in this example should be such that the response to the effect under consideration is not affected by age. Similar criteria could apply for other factors such as body weight or blood pressure.

The restriction criteria are set down in the study design and recruitment of subjects simply follows these criteria. Where the number of eligible subjects is limited it may be a disadvantage to restrict the number of people who can be included. Where participation is restricted, the generalizability of the findings may be similarly restricted.

Matching

The objective of matching is to ensure that potentially confounding factors are identically distributed in each group in the study. Unlike restriction, where only selected levels of the factor are included, matching admits all levels of the potential confounder to the study and subjects are then distributed between the groups so that groups are identical for that factor. In a matched case-control study, controls are selected so as to have the same distribution for the required matching variables as occurs in the unrestricted case series. The same criteria could be used in a cohort study, where the distribution of the unexposed group is matched to that in the exposed group; although matching is not commonly used in these types of studies.

When matching is used it is often limited to age and sex, as any more specific matching makes it much more difficult to find appropriate controls.

Analysing for confounding   It is important that the potential effects of a confounder can also be allowed for in the analysis of the study. This means that the confounding variable of interest must be measured during the study and is therefore subject to the same potential sources of error and misclassification as any other measure taken in the study. If a confounding variable is measured poorly, with considerable misclassification, it is likely that, when that measure is included in the analysis, an incorrect estimate of the effect of the confounder on the exposure–outcome measure of interest will be obtained. The potential effect of a confounder can either be assessed by stratification or by using multiple logistic regression.

To assess whether a variable is confounding the relationship between exposure and outcome of interest it is possible to analyse the association in appropriate strata of the confounding variable. For example, if sex is believed to be a confounder the estimate of effect is measured in the whole sample and for men and women separately. The estimate in each sex group is then unconfounded by sex. The stratum-specific estimates can also be combined to give a single estimate of the association between exposure and outcome once the confounding factor has been taken into account (adjusted for). The magnitude of the effect of a confounding factor can then be assessed by comparing the unadjusted with the adjusted measure of effect. The greater the effect on the risk estimate of adjusting for the confounder, the larger the effect of the confounder.

If the stratum-specific estimates of the effect are similar then there is no effect modification (or interaction). If, on the other hand, the stratum specific estimates are different, then it is more likely that the suspected confounder is an effect-modifier. Stratification is used to control confounding and to describe effect modification. The exploration of effect modification is an important part of epidemiological research.

Confounding can also be controlled by multiple logistic regression. An advantage of this over stratification is that the effects of many different variables can be controlled for at the same time. However, it is often difficult to interpret the results from these analyses. Some workers argue that if all potential confounders are included in the regression model, the best possible estimate of the association between the exposure and outcome measure will be obtained. This may not always be logical and the criteria listed above as to whether a variable is a confounder should always be considered before including a variable in an analysis. There are also a number of statistical assumptions that need to be satisfied before it is appropriate to use multiple logistic regression. A discussion of these and other issues in the use of multiple logistic regression is beyond the scope of this chapter; other texts are recommended for further reading.[2]

1.4.5 Causal inference

Once the researcher has considered the effects of chance, bias and confounding, the final step in the interpretation of epidemiological research is to draw inferences about the nature of any possible cause–effect relationship. A detailed discussion of the philosophy behind causal inference is beyond the scope of this chapter.

The aim of epidemiological research is to uncover the causal relationships between exposures and outcomes. In our general use of the word 'cause' it is implicit that we are talking about the role that some process plays in producing a particular event. The notion that some exposure causes a disease can only make sense if another level of exposure does not. Eating a high fat diet causes heart disease only makes sense if eating a low fat diet can be said to prevent it.

The understanding of causation can be developed a little further by way of a simple example. To start a car the driver puts his or her key into the ignition switch and turns the key, which 'causes' the car to start. The chain of events activated by the process of turning the key is complicated and unless the driver is a mechanic he or she may know nothing of the events in this causal pathway. More may be discovered about the process when the car will not start and the driver needs to find out why (if a rescue service is not available!). The driver then may discover that to start the car a battery, starter motor, alternator, and connections between these various parts of the process are required and that without all of these factors operating, turning the key will not 'cause' the car to start. Several points emerge from this simple example. The effect of turning the key will only cause the car to start if all the other components operate—that is, if there is a sufficient cause. All of the above mentioned components are necessary for the car to start. Remove any one of them and the car will not start; a sufficient cause no longer exists. This is irrespective of how important each part may be considered to be. It may be that a simple connection is loose, but this will be enough to break the chain and the act of turning the key will not cause the car to start.

To illustrate the above a real example recently used by Kok and van't Veer will suffice.[19] Many studies have shown that children with rickets have lower exposure to sunlight than children without rickets. On further investigation, however, it is apparent that the outcome 'rickets' only occurs when several components are acting (or not) to complete a sufficient cause. If one of the component causes is missing the child does not get rickets. The child has to be deficient in dietary intake of vitamin D and has to be growing, as well as not being exposed to sunshine. If the child is not growing, the disease does not occur, irrespective of the presence of poor diet and lack of sunshine.

In other situations it might be that there are several sufficient causes that enable the disease to develop, and that not all the component causes are necessary in all situations for the disease to occur. All that is required is that a sufficient cause be satisfied and the disease occurs.[2]

The above examples are relatively simple. Most often, particularly in complex diseases like coronary heart disease and cancer, there may be several sufficient causes for a disease. This implies that different combinations of component causes may result in the presence of disease. It also implies that disease may occur without the presence of a component cause which, in previous research, was considered 'causal'; because there may be enough other component causes to make up a sufficient cause. Thus, there may be three or four sufficient causes with substantially different component causes, except for one essential or necessary cause, that can result in disease occurrence.

The onset of disease using the above terminology is equivalent to the completion of a sufficient cause. Not all men who smoke get lung cancer, other component causes need to be acting to complete a sufficient cause leading to lung cancer. It may be that a factor that is measured to have only a weak effect on risk is a necessary component cause. In fact, the strength of any measured association may not give a true indication of the importance of that factor in causing the disease. It is also possible that, if there is more than one sufficient cause of a disease, adding together all the estimates of the size of the effect of various exposures on outcome (for example, per cent variance accounted for in a regression model), may total to more than 100 per cent.

A combination of circumstances needs to be present or acting for disease to occur. For a sufficient cause to arise, the required component causes need to have time to be brought into effect. This is defined as the induction time. The latent period is the time between the induction of disease and the clinical manifestation leading to the diagnosis of the disease. If we are interested in causality we need to be able to distinguish between these two periods, at least if the relevant exposure is likely to vary after the disease process has started. The investigation of causal inference needs to focus on the time when the disease is being induced. Exposure outside the potential induction period will be irrelevant to causation.

Some may criticize the use of inductive arguments to infer causality. Nevertheless, criteria have been used to draw such inferences. Some of these are discussed below.

Strength of association   The larger the measure of effect (either increased or decreased risk estimate), after appropriate consideration of confounders, the more likely it is that there is a cause–effect relationship between the exposure and outcome. Weak associations are more likely, but not necessarily, to be explained by undetected bias and are less likely to be causative. However, it is not possible to say with certainty that a weak association is not causal.

Consistency in the research findings is often used to imply causality If several different research groups, using different study populations and research methods, show similar results then it would seem reasonable that there is a causal relationship. A lack of consistency should perhaps lead to caution about drawing causal inferences.

Dose–response relationship If the association between exposure and outcome is consistent across a range of exposures, or the estimate of risk increases as the exposure increases, then it might be considered more likely that a causal relationship exists. For example, if the exposure measure is divided into thirds and the risk increases in a step-wise manner from the lowest to the highest level of exposure, it might be reasonable to assume a causal relationship.

It might also be that a step-wise increase in risk is not the appropriate model for the effect of exposure under investigation. There may be a threshold effect, above which no further effect is apparent. In this situation a dose–response relationship would not be expected, and the lack of a dose–response relationship would not imply a lack of causality.

Temporality To infer causality, it is logical that the disease only occurs after the exposure. There may be some diseases (or outcomes) where the disease affects exposure, for example, stomach cancer, colorectal cancer, or the effect of chronic malnutrition and diarrhoea on dietary intake. In these cases a non-causal relationship is indicated because 'exposure' has followed the onset of disease.

Plausibility A strong association between an exposure variable and an outcome is more plausible if there is a known or postulated biological mechanism by which exposure is likely to alter the risk of developing the disease. However, the lack of a known plausible mechanism does not preclude the existence of a causal relationship, it may be more a reflection of the lack of current knowledge.

1.5 SUMMARY

The purpose of this chapter has been to outline the basic principles in the design and interpretation of epidemiological research. The aim has been to delineate the major problems and where appropriate, to offer some guidance as to how to avoid or handle the problems. Several key points should be restated.

1. The first step in designing an epidemiological study is to ensure that an appropriate research question has been framed. The researcher has to have a good idea as to how the exposure to be measured is likely to effect the outcome to ensure that both are measured appropriately and with required accuracy.

2. The study design that is used should be appropriate to address the study question.

3. The study should be set up and conducted in accordance with a research protocol that has been developed to ensure that appropriate measures of exposure, outcome and other variables of interest are measured with required accuracy.

4. When it comes to analysing the study, the effects that chance, bias, and confounding may have on the exposure–outcome relationship of interest should be carefully assessed.

APPENDIX 1: WRITING A RESEARCH GRANT APPLICATION

Every research grant application should include the following components:

1.1 A statement of the aims or objectives

This should be a brief, clear, and specific statement of the research question.

In developing a specific research question the following steps may be followed:

1. State the general research questions.
2. Define the population available, or of interest, in which it can be studied.
3. Define the period of time for the study.
4. Select the variables to be measured.
5. Change non-specific variables into specific variables that can be measured.
6. Determine how to measure each variable.
7. Estimate the resources required to measure each variable.
8. Estimate the feasibility of conducting the study by comparing the resources needed with those available or likely to be provided by the funding body.
9. Restate the research question in a refined form that can be studied with available resources.
10. State the hypothesis arising from the research question.
11. Describe the aims of the study.

1.2 A review of relevant existing knowledge and justification of the proposed research

The review of existing knowledge should establish the relevance and need for the proposed research and show how it will extend existing knowledge. The following should be considered:

1. Represent all relevant points of view fairly and assess the strengths and limitations of previous research.
2. Establish the *unique* contribution that your project will make to knowledge.

3. Identify and justify aspects of your research that duplicate previous research.
4. If the study is a pilot study, state why a pilot study is necessary.

1.3 A description of the research plan

The following questions should be addressed in the research plan:
1. What is the basic study design (e.g. case-control study, cohort study, controlled trial, etc.)?
2. From what population do the study subjects come and how will they be selected?
3. How many subjects will be selected, giving justification for the number selected?
4. Where relevant, how long will subjects be observed?
5. What data are to be collected and why (mention should be made of exposure, confounding, and outcome variables)?
6. What are the details of any planned interventions?
7. How are the data to be collected and the measurements made (raise questions of reliability, validity, sensitivity, and specificity and whether or not they will be explicitly addressed in the study)? Consider the need for blinded observations.
8. How will the data be processed and analysed?
9. What is the expected timetable for study?

(A timetable flowsheet is desirable—don't forget time for development and pilot testing of study instruments).

1.4 A consideration of any ethical issues raised by the research

The application should consider:
(1) the possible risks, inconveniences, and benefits to the subjects involved in the study;
(2) the nature of the information that will be provided to subjects in seeking their consent for participation in the study (include a consent form where relevant);
(3) special incentives may be offered to participating subjects (e.g. reimbursement of travel costs, payment, etc.);
(4) steps that will be taken to preserve the confidentiality of all subjects records;
(5) compliance with local government regulations about subject access to personal data stored on computer;

(6) the nature of ethical review and approval that is provided by the institution in which the research will be conducted. The approval of an ethics committee does not absolve the applicant from specifying the ethical safeguards implied above.

1.5 A statement of the resources required to conduct the study

This statement should indicate:

1. The resources already available to the investigator (personal time, other participants or consultants, staff, space, equipment, other funds) must be stated to inform the funding body about the research environment into which their investment will be placed.

2. A statement of resources requested of the funding body, with some detail as to the justification of the amount requested. Break the request down into; staffing costs (with salaries, salary scale and oncosts such as national insurance), travel, equipment, consumable, and other relevant categories. It is important that what is requested is realistic (in terms of amounts normally granted to single projects by this body); sufficient, given other resources available for the project; and correct in detail.

APPENDIX 2: PREPARING A QUESTIONNAIRE

Questionnaires are used in all forms of epidemiological studies to document exposure levels both to possible causal agents and to interacting or confounding variables, and occasionally in cross-sectional studies, to determine the presence or absence of disease (measure outcome).

2.1 Objectives of questionnaire design

1. Valid measurement of the variables under study.
2. Ease of completion by the interviewer and/or subject.
3. Ease of processing and analysis.

2.2 Principles of questionnaire design

1. *Content*: the questionnaire should be designed to investigate the minimal amount of an individual's total experience to provide sufficient information concerning the problem under investigation.

The questionnaire should be as brief as possible, with every question being carefully justified in terms of the objectives of the study.

2. *Types of question*:
(a) open—these allow the respondents to answer in their own terms;
(b) closed—these specify in detail the alternative answers possible.

Epidemiological questionnaires usually contain a majority of closed questions to reduce the possibility of interviewer, response, interpretation, and/or coding bias, and to facilitate processing.

The following points should be considered:

(a) open questions should be used for non-categorical data (for example, age, date of birth);
(b) with multiple alternative answers, a final alternative 'Other, please specify . . .', should be provided unless it is certain that all possible answers have been provided for;
(c) when using mainly closed questions, respondents should be invited to make additional comments either in writing or to the interviewer.

3. *Wording of questions*: questions must be written in simple, non-technical language, avoiding the use of jargon. The wording should avoid any suggestion that a particular answer is preferred. In particular, leading questions and 'loaded' words should be avoided.

Each question should contain only one idea.

4. *Question sequence*: questions should follow a logical sequence resembling, as far as possible, the sequence that the respondents might expect to follow. On each subject, questions should proceed from the general to the particular. When a response to a general question makes further responses in that subject irrelevant (e.g. a life-time non-drinker need not answer questions about present and past drinking) a branching of the question sequence may be introduced. This should be as simple as possible.

5. *Questionnaire layout*: is important in both self- and interviewer-administered questionnaires, to arouse interest and ensure correct completion. An introduction, explanatory notes, and instructions should be brief, and precede and occupy a separate page from the first question. Different type faces may be used for different components of each question.

6. *Method of administration*: can be either self-administered or interviewer-administered (see Table 1.6 for the advantages and disadvantages of each type). Generally, self-administered questionnaires must be simpler and much more carefully designed than those intended for use by interviewers.

7. *Recording of responses*: the relevant objective is to obtain clear and unambiguous answers to each question, which are both easy for the respondent to provide and easy to process. From the processing point of view, self-coded questions are highly desirable.

8. *Coding*: most questionnaires will be prepared to allow numerical coding of all responses for processing by computer.

2.3 Evaluation of questionnaire

Questionnaires should be subject to two forms of evaluation:

1. *Pretesting*: is an essential part of the development of any questionnaire, it involves administration of drafts of the questionnaire to samples of subjects similar to those to be studied. Its purpose is to identify questions that are poorly understood, ambiguous, or which evoke hostile or other undesirable responses. Pretests should be carried out in the way that the questionnaire will be finally administered. Multiple pretests will usually be necessary before the final form of a questionnaire is obtained.

2. *Assessment of validity*: the main concern will usually be with validity of the questionnaire as a measure of the variables about which information is sought. Independent, valid measures of the variables will be necessary.

Validation is usually difficult, often expensive, and sometimes impossible. It is often undertaken as a preliminary step with a sample of subjects.

2.4 Use of standard questionnaires

Where a standard questionnaire exists for measurement of a particular exposure it will be desirable to use it for the following reasons:

1. It will usually have been used extensively and proved satisfactory in use.
2. It may have been validated (although validity in one population may not ensure validity in another).
3. It will permit comparison of your data with that collected by other workers.
4. It will expedite questionnaire design.

Any change in the format of standard questionnaires may affect the nature of response to them and therefore their validity and comparability. A modification can, of course, be tested for validity against the original questionnaire.

REFERENCES

1. Alderson, M. (1983). *An introduction to epidemiology*, second edn. Macmillan, London.
2. Rothman K. J. (1986). *Modern epidemiology*. Little, Brown and Co., Boston.
3. Hennekens, C. H. and Buring, J. E. (1987). *Epidemiology in medicine*. Little, Brown and Co., Boston.
4. Kelsey, J. L., Thompson, W. D., and Evans, A. S. (1986). *Methods in observational epidemiology*. Oxford University Press, New York.
5. Mienert, C. L. (1986). *Clinical trials: design, conduct, and analysis*. Oxford University Press, New York.
6. Schlesselman, J. J. (1982). *Case-control studies: design, conduct, analysis*. Oxford University Press, New York.
7. Breslow, N. E. and Day, N. E. (1987). *Statistical methods in cancer research. Volume II—the design and analysis of cohort studies*. IARC Scientific Publications No. 82. International Agency for Research on Cancer, Lyon.
8. Barker, D. J. P., Winter, P. D., Osmond, C., Margetts, B., and Simmonds, S. J. (1989). Weight in infancy and death from ischaemic heart disease. *Lancet*, ii: 577–80.
9. Miettinen, O. S. (1985). *Theoretical epidemiology*. Wiley, New York.
10. Griffith, J., Duncan, R. C., and Hulka, B. S. (1987). Biochemical markers: implications for epidemiological studies. *Arch. Environ. Health*, **44**: 375–81.
11. Barker, D. J. P. and Rose, G. (1984). *Epidemiology in medical practice*, third edn. Churchill Livingstone, Edinburgh.
12. Wickham, C. A. C., Walsh, K., Cooper, C., Barker, D. J. P., Margetts, B., Morris, J., and Bruce, S. A. (1989). Dietary calcium, physical activity and risk of hip fracture: a prospective study. *Br. Med. J.*, **299**: 889–92.
13. Gardner, M. J. and Altman, D. G. (1986). Confidence interval rather than *P*-values: estimation rather than hypothesis testing. *Br. Med. J.*, **292**: 746–50.
14. Margetts, B. M., Beilin, L. J., Vandongen, R., and Armstrong, B. K. (1986). Vegetarian diet in mild hypertension: a randomised controlled trial. *Br. Med. J.*, **293**: 1468–71.
15. Last, J. M., (ed.). (1988). *A dictionary of epidemiology*, second edn. Oxford University Press, New York.
16. Sacket, D. L. (1979). Bias in analytic research. *J. Chron. Dis.*, **32**: 51–63.
17. Coughlan, S. S. (1990). Recall bias in epidemiological studies. *J. Clin. Epidemiol.*, **43**: 87–91.
18. Doll, R. and Hill, A. B. (1950). Smoking and carcinoma of the lung: preliminary report. *Br. Med. J.*, **3**: 739–48.
19. Kok, F. J. and Van't Veer, P. (1989). The strength of relationships which can be detected between diet and disease. In L. Kohlmeier, and E. Helsing, (eds) *Epidemiology, nutrition and health*, 19–29. Smith-Gordon and Co., London.

2. Sampling, study size, and power

T. J. Cole

2.1 SAMPLING

2.1.1 Populations

After deciding on the research question to be investigated, the next most important decision to make is the population to be studied. There are many possible populations of individuals identifiable by their place of residence or occupation and personal characteristics, for example inner-city families, vegans, hospital patients, or nuns. Imaginative choice of population can make the difference between a dull study that just reiterates known facts and an interesting study providing a useful extension to knowledge.[1]

The choice of population inevitably depends to a large extent on the nature of the research question. However, it is important that the results found can be extrapolated confidently to the broader population of which the study population is a part. There is no point in studying, say, hospital patients with a peptic ulcer and presuming that the results will automatically apply to people with the condition in the community. The very fact of their being in hospital makes them different from those in the community, and care should be taken to be aware of, and avoid, biases in interpretation due to selection.

It is important then to specify very precisely what the population is, where it comes from and how the sampling frame (see section 2.1.2) is constructed. This will then make clear to which population the conclusions of the study refer. For example, a population might be defined as 'pregnant mothers recruited in the district maternity hospital during the last trimester of pregnancy, and living within five miles of the hospital'. This population might then be further qualified in terms of race, parity, or recent morbidity, say, allowing almost unlimited scope for defining different subpopulations of the broader population of urban pregnant women. The more clearly the population is defined at the outset, the easier subsequent recruitment, data collection and writing up will be.

It is necessary to define two populations in case-control studies (Chapter 11), the cases and the controls. Here the population of controls should match the population of cases with respect to major potential confounders such as sex and age, the principle being that the controls and cases should have equal chances of being exposed to the agent being investigated. Thus, when the cases ascertained are hospital in-patients, it is common practice to obtain as controls in-patients from other departments of the same hospital, where their condition is unrelated to the exposure. This ensures that the cases and controls come from the same catchment area (that of the hospital), which matches roughly for social and occupational conditions; these might affect exposure.

An alternative to hospital controls is a control group obtained from the community. This usually involves some form of sampling from population registers, but can be much simpler, being based on friends or neighbours of the cases. Community controls tend to be more expensive to obtain than hospital controls because the sampling and visiting is more extensive, so that hospital controls are very commonly used.

2.1.2 Sampling

Once defined, the target population is usually too large to investigate in its entirety. To produce a workable number of subjects, some form of sampling procedure is necessary. In the simplest case (for example, subjects presenting to hospital or their GP clinic) all suitable cases identified between two points in time are sampled. The sampling period is assumed not to be atypical, so that any conclusions drawn apply to patients presenting to the hospital or clinic at other times. This assumption may actually be invalid; if there is an infectious epidemic, say flu, current at the time, this would obviously influence the pattern of cases seen, and might make the conclusions relevant only to cases seen during flu epidemics.

In cross-sectional or prospective studies, the sample is likely to be obtained from the target population by selection based on criteria other than time. It has already been stressed that the results obtained from the sample must be applicable to the target population. This will not be the case if the sample is not representative of the population, i.e. if any selection effects operate. The correct way to avoid selection in the drawing up of the sample is to make use of randomization. This ensures that no biases, conscious or unconscious on the part of the researchers, influence the choice of subjects. The other major benefit of randomization is that standard statistical methods can be applied to the sample data to obtain population estimates, and the estimates can be given confidence intervals.

This latter point is crucial. It may be much easier and cheaper to go out into the street and recruit the first 100 people that pass by, but there is no way of knowing how closely their results reflect those of the target population (unless of course, the target population happens to be people in that particular street at that particular time).

There are a variety of different forms of random sampling, of increasing complexity. The purpose of having different forms is to provide a trade-off between the precision of the population estimate (i.e. the width of its confidence interval) and the complexity of the sampling design. It is possible to shrink the confidence interval substantially while keeping the total cost of sampling fixed, by choosing a sampling design that exploits the structure of the population appropriately.

Formulae to derive estimates of the population mean and standard deviation for many of the simpler sampling designs are given by Kelsey, Thompson, and Evans.[2]

Sampling units and sampling frames   The items that are to be sampled are called *sampling units*. Sampling units are usually subjects, but in more complex, multistage designs they may be GP clinics in a town, or schools in a county, or counties in a country.

All forms of sampling require a *sampling frame*, a real or imaginary list of the sampling units eligible to be sampled. In some cases the list actually exists, e.g. electoral registers or school registers; in others it exists only notionally, e.g. the filing cabinets of case notes in a GP surgery; in others still it does not exist at all, e.g. the patients attending a hospital clinic— here the actual sampling frame can only be known retrospectively, although the rule for its construction must of course be defined at the outset of the sampling procedure.

Simple random sampling   Simple random sampling requires a pre-existing sampling frame, where the sampling units are numbered sequentially. Random numbers (from random number tables) are then drawn to identify the sampling units to be sampled according to their position in the sampling frame. This ensures that every unit in the frame has an equal probability of being sampled, and this probability is known as the *sampling fraction*. For example it might be a 1 in 10 sample, with a sampling fraction of 0.1.

The disadvantage of simple random sampling is the requirement for an existing and numbered sampling frame. Even where the sampling frame actually exists it is often unnumbered, so that a form of sampling that avoids these two requirements is far more practical.

Systematic sampling   Systematic sampling is a version of simple random sampling that avoids the need for a sampling frame at the outset, and so simplifies the randomization procedure.

Like simple random sampling, it ensures the same sampling fraction for each sampling unit, but in practice only the first unit sampled is randomly selected. If the required sampling fraction is say 1 in k, then the first unit is randomly selected from the first k in the sampling frame, and thereafter every kth unit is drawn.

It is clear that if the first k units have an equal chance of being drawn, then this also applies to all subsequent units. On this basis, systematic sampling is equivalent to simple random sampling, and the same formulae apply. The one occasion in which the two are not equivalent is when there is some form of cyclical pattern within the sampling frame with a wavelength close to a simple multiple of k. Examples of this would be school classes, or households, where the individuals are clustered into groups.

Stratified sampling　The measurement made in each sampling unit may differ substantially in magnitude from one subgroup (or stratum) to another within the sampling frame. Obvious examples are weight, or other measures of body size, in children of different ages or in men versus women. If each stratum is sampled separately and the results are combined appropriately, this gives a population estimate with a tighter confidence interval than simple random sampling.

Another advantage is that separate estimates are available for each stratum, ensuring that each is adequately sampled. The results for the different strata can be combined using suitable weighting coefficients, thus adjusting for the distribution of units between strata within the population.

Cluster sampling　Stratified sampling splits the sampling frame into more homogeneous groups (strata). In contrast, cluster sampling splits it into groups that are in general less homogeneous (clusters), but which are administratively linked in some way. All the units within each cluster are then sampled.

Households are an example of clusters. Although they are more heterogeneous than the population at large, they are very cheap to sample. Thus, for a given total cost more clusters can be sampled, and the population estimate is more precise than the equivalent under simple random sampling.

Multistage sampling　It is quite possible to combine the different forms of sampling so as to work from larger to progressively smaller sampling frames. The sampling units at one level then provide the sampling frame for the next level down. This is a form of extended cluster sampling where the clusters are sampled rather than included in their entirety.

The British National Food Survey, discussed in Chapter 5, is a good example of a multistage sample.

2.1.3 Non-response

All surveys have a degree of non-response. Subjects refuse to take part, or do only some of the questions or tests they are supposed to complete. It has been widely observed that non-responders as a group are different from responders, so that the effect of non-response is to make the sample unrepresentative of the sampling frame and the target population.

The level of non-response varies widely, according to the amount of commitment required of the subjects taking part. In nutritional studies involving the measurement of food intake over several days, the degree of non-response can be 30 per cent or more. In simpler studies the figure ought to be less.

This is a perennial problem with nutritional surveys, as it seriously weakens the value of the study. Indeed the high level of non-response is often implicitly recognized by workers who restrict studies to volunteers, where the drop-out rate is, by definition, much smaller. Unfortunately, in most epidemiological studies, the results for a survey of volunteers cannot be extrapolated to any larger population, and the study may be of less value for that reason. An exception is certain types of intervention study where the endpoint is a measure of metabolic change within individuals; here the use of volunteers, if well described, may be acceptable.

To minimize the effects of non-response, it is important first of all to encourage all the subjects to take part in the study, and to keep on encouraging them as it progresses. Secondly, as much information as possible should be obtained from a sample of the non-responders, for example age, sex, and occupation as a minimum. This provides the opportunity to adjust the results to take account of the non-responders, and to come up with a less biased result.

Another effect of non-response is that the final sample size is smaller than originally planned. It is important to include a scaling-up factor in the calculation of sample size to cover this. So if a sample size is calculated as 100, but the response rate is expected to be only 70 per cent, then 100/0.7 or 143 is the number to be sampled altogether.

2.2 VARIABILITY

Designing an epidemiological study requires an understanding of the nature of variability, the different sources of variability, and how they can be controlled for. Central to the concept of variability is the idea that measurements come from a hypothetical population of such measurements, whose mean needs to be estimated. This population is effectively the same as the target population discussed in the previous section, except that in this context it is usually assumed to be infinitely large.

The quantity to be measured may be a continuous variable (like weight or energy intake) or it may be grouped (like blood group or sex). An important special case of grouped data is where the quantity is either present or absent. This is particularly relevant for studies of disease where the cases have the disease and the controls do not, and some of the subjects are exposed to the agent of interest while others are not.

For continuous variables, the population mean and variance are estimated from the sample mean and variance. For binary and categorical variables, the population proportions in each category are estimated from the sample proportions. If σ^2 is the variance for a continuous variable, then the standard error of the mean based on a sample of size n is given by $\sigma/\sqrt{n}$, and the variance of the mean is σ^2/n.

The variance of a proportion derived from a binary variable differs from that for a continuous variable in that it can be estimated directly from the proportion. If the proportion is p, based on a sample size n, then the variance of p is given by $p(1-p)/n$. This shows that proportions near to zero or unity have a small variance, and the largest variance occurs when $p = 0.5$.

There are two particular aspects of the process of data collection that adversely affect the quality of the data. The first of these is bias—the name given to a consistent discrepancy between the sample mean and the population mean. It is inevitable that the two means will not be exactly the same, but in theory, with large enough sample size, the difference between the two should be very small. In situations where this does not happen, bias is said to be present.

The other aspect of the data that reflects the quality of data collection is its variance. All data are, by their nature, variable, but the variance can be increased by the way the data are measured.

2.2.1 Bias

Bias is a very real problem in dietary intake studies, but one that nutritionists have in the past tended to ignore. Two particular factors have conspired in this, one being the plethora of different methods that are available to measure dietary intake, the other the absence of a 'gold standard' or accurate and unbiased estimate of dietary intake against which other methods can be validated. Nutritionists have felt that if one method of intake assessment is similar to another, then this provides the validation, when in fact both methods may be equally biased.

The precise mechanism for bias in dietary intake assessment depends on the particular method used (Chapter 6). Many of the methods have an inbuilt tendency to be biased downwards, in that subjects are more likely to forget a food they ate than to invent a food they did not eat. Diary or weighed intake methods, where the eating and the recording of food eaten occur largely concurrently, ought to be less prone to this than recall methods. However, there is ample opportunity, by any method, for subjects to consciously or subconsciously distort their apparent eating pattern to better suit their self-image. This distortion has been shown to generate under-reporting of up to 30 per cent in the energy intakes of obese women.[3]

Modern objective methods of determining nutrient intake (see Chapter 7) at last provide the opportunity to validate some aspects of dietary assessment properly. Even so, they are unlikely to remove the possibility of bias in existing methods, rather, they quantify and perhaps reduce the bias. Nutritionists need to be aware of the importance of bias, and its ability to devalue otherwise well designed studies.

That said, bias is not always a problem. There are situations where the non-differential bias may cancel itself out, for example, a sample surveyed on two separate occasions or a correlation study. If the bias in the method is systematic, and tends to reduce the estimate of intake for every observation by some fixed amount, say 10 per cent, then the comparison in the two examples, i.e. the change in intake between surveys or the size of the correlation, will be unaffected.

The situation where bias is very serious is when it affects only a subset of the sample (differential misclassification), so that relationships between intake and other health measures become distorted. In this situation genuine relationships can be hidden and spurious relationships generated. An obvious example is the one cited above where obese subjects underrecorded their energy intake, so disguising the strong association between obesity and raised energy intake. Normal controls in the same study did not show a bias, so that there was no apparent difference in intake between them and the cases.

2.2.2 Variance

There are many different factors that contribute to the variance of a quantity. Three factors in particular can be identified, and these can be subdivided in a variety of ways. The first and perhaps most important source of variability is between-subject or interindividual variance, denoted by s_b^2. This assumes that each individual in the population has some fixed, but unknown, constant value for the measurement that is appropriate to them. In terms of nutrient intake, for example, this might be called their usual or habitual intake. The between-subject variance is then the population variance of these true means. As a quantity it cannot be measured directly because the true means cannot be measured without error, but it can be obtained by calculation.

The second source of variation is within-subject or intraindividual variance, denoted by s_w^2. This represents the variation of individuals around their true mean value when measured repeatedly by a valid measurement instrument.

The third category of variability is measurement error. This is the difference between the observed value and the corresponding true but unknown value, for a particular observation. It is also called reproducibility. The term 'measurement error' is confusing because it implies that an error has occurred in taking the measurement. Errors of measurement do occur, e.g.

writing down the wrong figure or failing to calibrate the instrument properly; however, if the error is large enough it can be identified as an outlier from the main body of data. So, gross errors like these are assumed to have been identified and dealt with, and measurement error as used here describes the combined variability of all the factors influencing the measurements.

In some circumstances the measurement error is included with the within-subject error, where the two cannot easily be separated. Nutrient intake provides an example; the variance of daily intake as obtained by weighed inventory in a single individual combines the day to day variability about the true mean and the measurement error of the weighed inventory method.

The magnitude of the within-subject variance may depend on how frequently the measurements are made. The weight of a child measured every few minutes has a relatively small variance, whereas the variance of daily or weekly measurement is progressively larger. The minute to minute variance represents measurement error, because it is known from physiological considerations that true weight does not change on this timescale. However, daily and weekly variances are larger because they include within-subject variance and also because the true weights of individuals themselves change. When quantifying within-subject variance it is useful to define the frequency with which measurements are taken, so as to standardize for the time component in the variance.

Of the three sources of variation: between-subject, within-subject, and measurement variance, the first is the most important in the calculation of sample size and power. The other two are nuisance variables which, by their presence, weaken associations and obscure differences. For this reason it is important to minimize their impact on the power calculations.

Measurement error, unlike within-subject variance, is affected by the quality of the data collection. It is often a good idea to design a pilot study specifically to investigate the size of the measurement error, and to split it up into its component parts. What the components are will depend on the measurements being made; for example, height is influenced by the observer, the time of day and the type of measuring scale used. The relative contributions of the separate factors to the reproducibility of the measurement can be obtained by analysis of variance from a suitably designed study. For details of the design and analysis of such studies see Snedecor and Cochran.[4]

The results of such a pilot study can then be used to reduce the measurement error, for example, by retraining outlying observers or by recalibrating aberrant instruments.

Minimizing the impact of within-subject variance on the power calculations is less easy because the variance cannot be manipulated by the observer. It is a property of the individuals being studied and is a fixed quantity. However, one way of keeping it small is to study subjects whose within-subject variance is likely to be relatively small. The usual assumption in epidemiological studies is that subjects all have the same within-subject variance, but in practice it may be possible to identify in advance subjects whose variability is greater or less than average. Nurses as a group are likely to be more variable than housewives or nuns in their eating habits, so that a given dietary study would need to be slightly larger if based on nurses than if housewives or nuns were used.

A second and more important strategy for dealing with within-subject variation is to take several measurements for each subject, and to work with the mean. If the within-subject variance for a single measurement is s_w^2 and k measurements are averaged, then the variance of the mean is s_w^2/k. In principle, if k is large enough, the effect of the within-subject variance can be reduced almost to zero. In practice, though, there is no sense in making k too large because beyond a certain point the cost of each extra measurement outweighs its benefit.

There is a substantial literature addressed to the question of the number of days of dietary intake required to distinguish adequately between individuals. Consider a particular nutrient, energy or vitamin C say, and assume that the between-subject variance is s_b^2. If the intake is measured over k days, then the within-subject variance is s_w^2/k. The total variance of an individual's intake is therefore $s_b^2 + s_w^2/k$, obtained by adding the two variances together, and the standard error is $\sqrt{(s_b^2 + s_w^2/k)}$.

Extending this to a sample of n individuals from the population, the variance of the mean intake for the sample is $(s_b^2 + s_w^2/k)/n$ or $(s_b^2/n + s_w^2/kn)$, and the standard error is $\sqrt{(s_b^2/n + s_w^2/kn)}$. The standard error of the sample mean in the absence of within-subject variance would be $s_b/\sqrt{n}$, so the ratio of standard errors is:

$$\frac{s_b/\sqrt{n}}{\sqrt{(s_b^2/n + s_w^2/kn)}}$$

or

$$\frac{1}{\sqrt{(1 + s_w^2/ks_b^2)}}. \tag{2.1}$$

This, or more correctly its square, is a measure of the efficiency of the estimate of the mean, a statistical term indicating how much the variance of the estimate is increased because of within-subject variance.

The presence of within-subject error also means that individual means are measured with error, so that there is an imperfect correlation between the true intakes of individuals and their intakes as measured. This correlation is given by $s_b/\sqrt{(s_b^2 + s_w^2/k)}$, which is the same as eqn 2.1 above. This term (2.1) can be referred to as the coefficient of attenuation. As well as being the correlation of the true versus the observed intake, it also measures the extent to which the correlation of the intake with other factors is reduced (i.e. attenuated). The factor might be some disease marker, e.g. serum cholesterol or blood pressure.[5,6]

If the number of days, k, is sufficiently large, then the coefficient can be made very close to unity. However the crucial issue is the ratio of s_w^2 to s_b^2, the within- to between-subject variance. If this is small, i.e. subjects in the population are widely spaced relative to the standard errors of individual means, then the attenuation is not too important. Conversely, if the ratio is large, so that subject means are relatively close together, then the effect of within-subject error can be large and serious. As well as weakening correlations, it also leads to gross misclassification when the population is split into groups, e.g. thirds or fifths, on the basis of intake. Gross misclassification means that individuals with true intakes in the lowest group are classified into the highest, and vice versa. So a comparison of high versus low intake groups is weakened due to a fraction of the individuals being allocated to the wrong group.

For the special case of weighed intakes, many studies have documented the ratio s_w^2/s_b^2 for different nutrients in a variety of populations (see Nelson et al.[7] for a recent summary). The results show that for the coefficient of attenuation to be 0.9 or greater, less than 7 days of weighed intake are adequate for many nutrients, but that for certain vitamins and minerals, several weeks of intake need to be measured (Chapter 6). It is clear that for the latter class of nutrients, the detection of a correlation or a difference between groups requires a much increased sample size, to compensate for the attenuation due to the large s_w^2/s_b^2 ratio. This topic is discussed in more detail in later sections.

2.3. SAMPLE SIZE

2.3.1 Null hypothesis

The calculation of sample size and power is closely tied up with the concept of the significance test. A significance test involves a test statistic, that is, a statistical quantity with known distribution whose value is to be tested, and a null hypothesis. The null hypothesis states that the mean of the test statistic is equal to some predefined value. The purpose of the significance test is to decide whether to accept or reject the null hypothesis. This decision involves a preset error rate that specifies how often the null hypothesis should be rejected when it is true. The error rate is called the Type I error, α, or the significance level.

A typical example of a significance test is the comparison of two group means. Here the test statistic is the difference between the two means, and the null hypothesis is that this mean difference is zero.

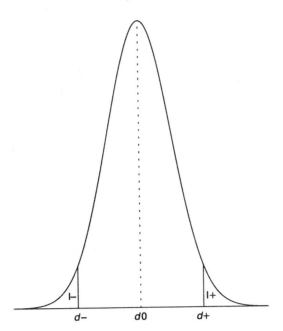

Fig. 2.1 A two-tailed test of the null hypothesis that the variable d is distributed with mean d0. The size of the type I error is set at 5 per cent, shown by the areas marked in the two tails of the distribution.

Figure 2.1 illustrates the distribution of a test statistic that is to be tested for significance, and the null hypothesis is that the mean of the statistic has value d0. The uncertainty about the mean, i.e. its standard error, is represented by the area under the distribution. The total area sums to unity, so that the statistic has a probability one (i.e. certainty) of taking a value somewhere under the distribution.

The distribution shows that, even when the true mean is d0, the observed statistic may lie anywhere over a wide range of values. In particular, there is a small probability that the statistic will fall beyond one or other of the two cut-offs marked d− and d+. These cut-offs define areas in each tail of the distribution of size $\alpha/2$ (marked I− and I+ in Fig. 2.1), a total area (or probability) of α.

The basis of the significance test is that if the null hypothesis is true, the observed value ought to be near d0. Conversely, if the null hypothesis is false, the value ought *not* to be near d0. Thus, the further away from d0 the value is, the less likely the null hypothesis is to be true. The arbitrary probability α determines at what point we cease to accept the null hypothesis, and instead reject it. By doing this we run a small risk α of rejecting the null hypothesis when it is actually true, and this is the Type I error.

Figure 2.1 illustrates two cut-offs (d− and d+), each of size $\alpha/2$. This form of significance test is called a two-tailed test, because the null hypothesis can be rejected by values of the test statistic in either tail of the distribution. When testing two group means, this means that either can be significantly larger (or smaller) than the other.

In certain circumstances it is permissible to use a one-tailed test instead of a two-tailed test. In this case the area α is all in one tail. This means that the null hypothesis can only be rejected for values of the statistic in one direction, and even very large values in the other direction are ignored. There are situations where this can be justified, e.g. the testing of a new treatment against a conventional treatment where the new treatment has to be an improvement—if it is the same or worse then it is of no value. Nevertheless, such situations are relatively unusual, and one-tailed tests should in general be avoided.

A one-tailed test of size α has its cut-off at the same point as a two-tailed test of size 2α, so that if the probability of the observed statistic is between α and 2α, then it is significant by the one-tailed test but not by the two-tailed test. This allows marginal levels of significance to be exaggerated because the use of a one-tailed test is often not made clear to the reader.

2.3.2 Alternative hypothesis

A significance test is used to test whether or not there is a difference between groups. However, when the hypothesis is rejected there is no information about the size of the difference, only that it is non-zero. When epidemiological studies are planned it is very important to know in advance what difference is being looked for, as this determines how big the study should be.

Figure 2.2 is an extension of Figure 2.1 and includes information about the magnitude of the difference between groups that is to be sought. This difference is termed d*. Like Figure 2.1, Figure 2.2 shows the distribution of the observed difference under the null hypothesis, centred on d0, and a second distribution, centred on d*, which shows the distribution of the difference if it is actually present. This is known as the alternative hypothesis, that the true difference between groups is d*.

Figure 2.2 shows the two tails for the null hypothesis (marked I− and I+) plus a single tail for the alternative hypothesis (marked II). The area of this latter tail represents the Type II error, which is the probability of accepting the null hypothesis when the alternative hypothesis is true. So areas I− and I+ (probability α) on the one hand, and II (probability β) on the other, are the misclassification errors in deciding which hypothesis is appropriate. The quantity $(1-\beta)$, known as the power of the experiment, is the probability of accepting the alternative hypothesis when it is true. In a well designed experiment the power to detect the desired effect should be set to 80 per cent ($\beta = 0.2$), 90 per cent ($\beta = 0.1$) or even 95 per cent

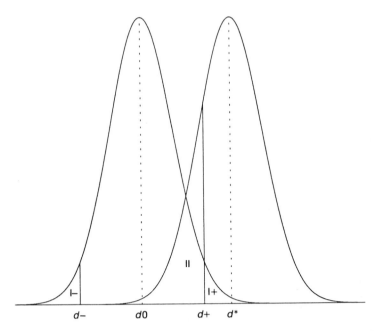

Fig. 2.2. A two-tailed test of the null hypothesis that the variable d is distributed with mean d0, versus the alternative hypothesis that the mean is d^*. The type I error is set at 5 per cent as in Figure 2.1, while the type II error is 20 per cent, shown by the area in the left tail of the right distribution.

($\beta = 0.05$). This ensures that there is little chance of a negative result when the effect is actually present. Figure 2.2 is drawn with Type I and Type II errors of 0.05 and 0.2 respectively, i.e. a power of 80 per cent.

In planning a study, the choice of d^* is of paramount importance. It must not be too large, or there is a risk of failing to detect the effect. Moreover, if d^* is too large, the estimated size of sample required will be too small, and the power to detect a smaller effect will be low. Pocock points out that this is a weakness of many experimental studies.[8]

Conversely, if d^* is too small, implying a very large sample size, the effect may not in practical terms be worth having. To demonstrate that mortality from some disease is reduced from, say, 10 to 9 per cent as a result of some treatment would require several thousand subjects, and yet many would feel that the improvement was not sufficiently striking to be worth the effort.

2.3.3 Power and sample size

Figure 2.2 shows the probability of observing particular values of the test statistic under the null hypothesis and the alternative hypothesis. Three values of d are particularly important; the mean under the null hypothesis (d0), the mean under the alternative hypothesis (d*), and the value at the cut-off point between the two distributions (d+). If the distribution of d is known, in particular its standard error, the value of d+ can be defined simply from α. Assuming a normal distribution, then the value of d+ is such that it is $Z_{\alpha/2}$ standard errors away from d0, where $Z_{\alpha/2}$ indicates the point on the normal distribution defining area $\alpha/2$ in the tail. So:

$$d+ = d0 + Z_{\alpha/2}\ SE(d) \qquad (2.2)$$

where SE(d) is the standard error of d. However d+ is also defined from d0, d* and β, i.e.:

$$d+ = d* - Z_{\beta}\ SE(d) \qquad (2.3)$$

where Z_{β} is the point on the normal distribution defining the cut-off d+ relative to d*. Note that eqns 2.2 and 2.3 assume that the standard error of d is the same under the two distributions, although this is not always the case. Substituting for d+ in eqn 2.3 and rearranging gives:

$$d* - d0 = Z_{\alpha/2}\ SE(d) + Z_{\beta}\ SE(d)$$
$$= SE(d)\ (Z_{\alpha/2} + Z_{\beta}) \qquad (2.4)$$

In general the standard error of d decreases inversely as the square root of the sample size n, so that as n increases the power to detect d* increases.

Equation 2.4 shows that the power $(1-\beta)$ is determined by d0, d*, α and n (which affects the standard error). Of these, d0 and α are fixed, because they constitute the significance test (Fig. 2.1). Thus, to change the power, only d* or n can be changed. If, for example, d* is made larger, this has the effect of shifting the distribution of d* in Figure 2.2 to the right, while leaving d0 and d+ where they are. As a result, the left tail of the d* distribution, the type II error, is reduced in size, and the power increases. Reducing d* has the opposite effect—the distribution shifts to the left, the size of the left tail increases, and the power is reduced.

The power can also be changed by altering n, the sample size. If n is doubled, say, then the standard errors (i.e. the widths of the distributions) of both d0 and d* shrink by 30 per cent. In particular the cut-offs d− and d+ move 30 per cent closer to d0. Thus, if d* remains unchanged, the distance between it and d+ increases, so that the tail defining the type II error gets smaller and the power is increased. This is illustrated in Figure 2.3, where doubling n reduces the type II error from 20 per cent (in Fig. 2.2) to half the type I error, i.e. about 2.5 per cent.

Equation 2.4 is the fundamental equation linking n, d0, d*, α and β, and all

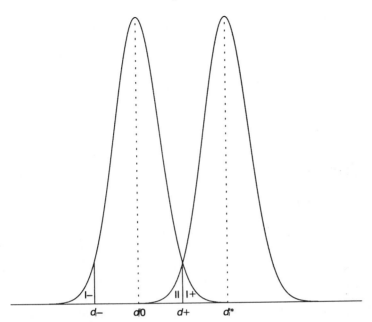

Fig. 2.3. A two-tailed test of the null hypothesis that the variable d is distributed with mean d0, versus the alternative hypothesis that the mean is d*. The sample size is twice that shown in Figure 2.2, so that although the type I error is unchanged at 5 per cent, the type II error is reduced from 20 to 2.3 per cent.

the formulae that appear in section 2.4 are derived from it. The value of d0 is always zero in practice, and does not usually appear in the formulae. Kelsey *et al.*[2] provide a summary of the formulae, with examples, for all except the correlation formulae, which are developed here. Table 2.1 gives, for a series of values for α and β, the corresponding values of $Z_{\alpha/2}$, Z_β, and $(Z_{\alpha/2}+Z_\beta)^2$ —the latter term appears in many of the formulae in section 2.4.

2.3.4 Types of hypothesis

The derivation of eqn 2.4 uses as its test statistic d, the difference between two group means. There are actually three different forms of test statistic as they affect eqn 2.4, and they need to be distinguished. The first is relevant for continuous measurements, such as cholesterol intake or systolic blood pressure. Here the standard error of d is obtained from the standard deviation of the measurement, and two different forms of SE(d) apply according to whether or not the measurements in the two groups are paired (matched).

A slightly different situation arises when the quantities being compared in the two groups are rates or proportions, e.g. the colon cancer incidence

Table 2.1 Values of $(Z_{\alpha/2} + Z_\beta)^2$ for various $Z_{\alpha/2}$ and Z_β. The corresponding values of $Z_{\alpha/2}$ and Z_β and the power are also shown. The value $(Z_{\alpha/2} + Z_\beta)^2$ is required in equations (2.5), (2.8), (2.9), and (2.10) of section 2.4

Type I error α	$Z_{\alpha/2}$	Type II error β Power Z_β	0.5 50% 0.00	0.2 80% 0.84	0.1 90% 1.28	0.05 95% 1.64
0.1	1.64		2.7	6.2	8.6	10.8
0.05	1.96		3.8	7.8	10.5	13.0
0.02	2.33		5.4	10.0	13.0	15.8
0.01	2.58		6.6	11.7	14.9	17.8

rate or the proportion with brown eyes. As explained earlier, the standard error of a proportion depends on the magnitude of the proportion, so that SE(d) in eqn 2.4 takes a different form.

The third case is the testing of a correlation between two variables, and here d is the correlation to be detected. The null hypothesis, that $d = 0$, is equivalent to the absence of a correlation between the two variables. The standard error of d in this case is a function of the correlation to be detected.

Each of these three forms of alternative hypothesis is considered in turn in section 2.4.

2.3.5 Transformations

The calculation of power in eqn 2.4 assumes a normal distribution for d. If d is based on a continuous variable then it is important for the variable to be (at least reasonably) normally distributed. If it is not, then the distribution of d may not be normal either, and in addition (and more importantly) the standard error of d may be inflated. This has the effect of increasing the size of sample required.

For this reason it is worthwhile checking that the variable is reasonably normal, and if not, transforming it to a new scale which is. This is particularly relevant for many of the nutrients commonly investigated in nutritional epidemiology, whose distributions tend to be skew to the right. For example Nelson et al.[7] found that in up to half of the 30 nutrients they studied (depending on the sex and age of the subjects), a logarithmic transformation improved the efficiency of the comparison.

A logarithmic transformation is very commonly used to remove right skewness, but there are other alternatives that may be more suitable in particular situations. If X is the variable as measured, then four possible convenient transformations of X can be considered, arranged here in order of increasing adjustment; $\sqrt{X}$, $\log_e X$, $1/\sqrt{X}$, and $1/X$. Each transformation stretches the left tail of the distribution and shortens the right, so that if X has a right skew distribution, one of these transformations will be best for removing the skewness.

There is a simple way of seeing which transformation reduces the skewness most, as follows: first calculate the mean and standard deviation (SD) of X and its four transformations. Then antilog the mean of log X to obtain the geometric mean of X; call it $\dot{X}$. Now scale the standard deviations of the five forms of X using $\dot{X}$, as follows: $SD(X)/\dot{X}$; $2\,SD(\sqrt{X})/\sqrt{\dot{X}}$; $SD(\log X)$; $2\sqrt{\dot{X}}\,SD(1/\sqrt{X})$; $\dot{X}\,SD(1/X)$. These five quantities all represent the coefficient of variation (CV) of X, and can be multiplied by 100 to give percentages. The smallest value among the five CVs indicates the transformation that best removes the skewness in X. It may be that the CVs are all very similar, in which case the choice of transformation is not critical. Nevertheless, it gives an indication of where skewness is present and how best it can be removed.

It should be noted that three of the four transformations cannot be used for data that are zero or negative (as log 0 and 1/0 are infinitely large). If there are data with zero values they must be made positive. This is best done by adding a small amount, ε, to all the data, perhaps trying more than one value of ε to ensure that the result is not too sensitive to its precise choice.

2.3.6 Non-response and drop-out

Virtually all studies are less than 100 per cent successful in recruiting subjects. Also, longitudinal studies tend to lose subjects as they progress. All the calculations for sample size given in the next section assume a 100 per cent response rate, so that the numbers given need to be scaled up to cater for non-response. If, for example, a response rate of 80 per cent is expected, then the number obtained should be divided by 80/100, increasing it by 25 per cent. A further adjustment may also be advisable for longitudinal studies, to cover drop-out.

2.4. TYPES OF STUDY

2.4.1 Ecological studies

Ecological studies are distinct from other forms of epidemiological study in that the unit of measurement is a group rather than an individual (see Chapter 10). For discussions of power and sample size it is the number of groups, not the numbers of individuals in each group, which is important.

The basis of the grouping may be geographical, e.g. by country, state, or county; it may be temporal, e.g. by year of birth, age group, or month of the year; or it may be cultural, e.g. by religion, migrant status, or social class. Ecological studies often represent an early stage in the pursuit of a causal relationship, so that the data are routinely collected statistics obtained for other purposes, which are then linked together. For example Barker and Osmond[1] demonstrated a strong correlation between infant mortality rates in the 1920s and coronary heart disease rates in the 1970s across 212 local authority areas in the UK, using published data.

Many ecological studies have correlated national or regional cause-specific incidence rates or mortality rates with the corresponding intakes of specified foods or nutrients to look for an association. If a certain correlation, d^* is to be detected at level α (two-tailed) with power $(1-\beta)$, then the number of groups (i.e. countries or regions) required to ensure this is given by:

$$n = (Z_{\alpha/2} + Z_\beta)^2 \, (1 - d^{*2})/d^{*2} + 5. \qquad (2.5)$$

As an example, set the type I error α to 0.05, the type II error β to 0.1 and assume we want to detect a correlation d^* of 0.5. This gives $(Z_{\alpha/2} + Z_\beta)^2 = 10.5$ from Table 2.1, from which $n = 36.5$ or 37, rounded up to the nearest whole number. Thus, to detect a correlation of 0.5 with 90 per cent power at 5 per cent significance requires at least 37 distinct groups.

An alternative question might be: what correlation is likely to be detectable for given α and β if n points are available? Equation (2.5) can be rearranged as:

$$d^* = (Z_{\alpha/2} + Z_\beta)/\sqrt{[(Z_{\alpha/2} + Z_\beta)^2 + n - 5]}. \qquad (2.6)$$

If just 20 points are available, what correlation can be detected for the same α and β? The answer from (2.6) is $d^* = 0.64$.

Finally, it may be that with α and n known, the question is: 'What is the power of the study to detect a correlation of d^* or greater?' Rearranging (2.5) again gives:

$$Z_\beta = d^* \, \sqrt{[(n - 5)/(1 - d^{*2})]} - Z_{\alpha/2}. \qquad (2.7)$$

Then Z_β can be converted to probability β and hence the power $(1-\beta)$ using normal distribution tables. Table 2.1 includes some values for Z_β, which can be interpolated or extrapolated.

By their very nature, ecological studies often use existing data, so that the power calculation to determine sample size (eqn 2.5) may be irrelevant if n is already fixed. Equation 2.7 is probably of greater value because it shows how likely the study is to detect a specified association.

Other forms of ecological study may involve a comparison between one set of groups (or clusters) and another, the aggregated version of the comparison of two groups of individuals. The formulae for this are given in the next section. Note that for ecological studies the sample size should be interpreted as being the number of clusters, not the number of individuals, in each half of the comparison.

2.4.2 Cross-sectional studies

Cross-sectional studies are the simplest form of epidemiological study involving individuals and they investigate relationships at a single point in time (see Chapter 11). Because they lack a temporal element they are generally unable to provide evidence of causality, so that subsequent retrospective or prospective studies and/or experimental studies are required to demonstrate that relationships are causal.

There are three general forms of relationship that might be looked for in a cross-sectional study—a difference between groups in the level of some variable, a difference between groups in the *rate* of a condition, and an association (correlation) between two variables in the sample.

In addition to the question of sample size, there is also (in nutritional epidemiology) the important question of what type of dietary intake assessment to use. The existence of within-subject variance in dietary intake means that assessments based on 1 day or only a few days may be poor at categorizing individual intakes. However, the number of subjects can be increased to compensate for this. There is a trade-off between the number of subjects, n and the number of days per subject, k.

To decide on the optimal choice of n and k, three distinct types of study need to be identified—group comparisons, ranking of individuals, and assessing an individual's usual intake.[7] In the simplest case of group comparisons, the best form of assessment is a cheap 1-day method (i.e. $k = 1$), allowing the number of subjects, n, to be maximized.[10]

The second type of study involves the ranking of individuals for dietary intake, where the aim is to make the coefficient of attenuation (section 2.2) sufficiently near unity to ensure that subjects in the extremes of the distribution are correctly identified. Nelson *et al.*[7] show that 7 days of weighed intake are adequate for some nutrients, but other nutrients require substantially more than 7 days, and for others a weighed intake is not appropriate at all.

The third type of study, assessing an individual's usual intake, is irrelevant in an epidemiological context and is not considered further here.

Nutritional epidemiologists are insufficiently aware of the distinction that needs to be drawn between studies comparing group means and studies ranking individuals. There is no benefit in using an expensive method of assessment to compare group means because a cheap method applied to a larger number of subjects is more efficient. Conversely, studies that relate the intakes of individuals to other variables should ideally use a

7-day (or more) weighed intake, or some other validated form of dietary assessment (see Chapters 6 and 8).

The sample size required to compare the means of two groups involves four quantities; α and β (the type I and type II error levels), σ (the standard deviation of the variable), and d* (the difference between the groups to be detected). The sample size n required *for each group* is then given by

$$n = 2\sigma^2 (Z_{\alpha/2} + Z_\beta)^2 / d^{*2} \tag{2.8}$$

A study is set up to determine whether nutritionists (being fitter) have a higher energy intake than epidemiologists. To be sure of detecting a difference of 840 kJ with 90 per cent power at 5 per cent significance requires:

$$n = 2 \times 2205^2 \times 10.5 / 840^2$$

$$= 145$$

subjects in each group, or 290 altogether. The figure of 2205 kJ for σ is taken from Hall,[11] and the 10.5 is obtained from Table 2.1.

It may be that subjects in one group are easier or cheaper to recruit than in the other. In cross-sectional studies the two groups are unlikely to be the same size anyway, unless they are sampled stratified. Assume that, for each subject in one group, there are r subjects in the other group. Equation 2.8 then generalizes to:

$$n = (r+1)\sigma^2 (Z_{\alpha/2} + Z_\beta)^2 / rd^{*2} \tag{2.9}$$

where n is the number of subjects in the smaller group and the larger group contains $r \cdot n$ (r times n) subjects. Note that when $r = 1$, i.e. equal numbers in the groups, eqn 2.9 is equivalent to eqn 2.8.

On the assumption that nutritionists are cheaper to recruit than epidemiologists, twice as many nutritionists as epidemiologists are to be recruited (i.e. $r = 2$). From eqn 2.9 the required numbers of epidemiologists and nutritionists are 109 and 218 respectively. Thus, the total sample is 327 as compared to 290 for equal numbers in the groups, with the increase in numbers offset by the cost saving.

Equation 2.9 applies with little modification to the comparison of proportions. The variance of the proportion p is known to be $p(1-p)$, so this replaces σ^2 in eqn 2.9. Also, because the value of p differs under the null hypothesis and the alternative hypothesis, there are two separate variances to consider. Schlesselman[12] suggested using the average of the two proportions to calculate the variance. Let $p0$ be the proportion in one group and

$p1$ the other, so that the difference d^* in proportion is given by $d^* = p1 - p0$. Also let the average proportion $\bar{p}$ be $(p0 + p1)/2$ and the average proportion $\bar{q} = 1 - \bar{p}$. Then the required sample size, n, for given α and β is given by:

$$n = (r + 1)\,\bar{p}\bar{q}\,(Z_{\alpha/2} + Z_\beta)^2/rd^{*2} \qquad (2.10)$$

This, like eqn 2.9, allows for unequal group sizes, so that the group sizes are n and $r \cdot n$ respectively.

The proportions, or rates, in the two groups can be related in terms of the *relative risk*. In cross-sectional studies this is simply the ratio of the proportion in one group to that in the other, i.e. $p1 = p0$ RR. So if the required relative risk, RR, to be detected is known, and the proportion in the baseline $p0$ is also known, then $p1$ can be calculated and substituted into eqn 2.10.

A study is set up to determine the relative risk of achilles tendon rupture in squash players as compared to badminton players. If the lifetime risk of rupture is known to be 1 per cent in badminton players and a relative risk of 5 is to be detected, how many ex-players from each sport need to be questioned? The baseline risk $p0$ is 0.01, so that $p1 = 0.01 \times 5 = 0.05$. This makes $\bar{p}$ 0.03, $\bar{q}$ 0.97 and d^* 0.04. If α is set to 5 per cent with power 95 per cent, giving the value 13.0 for $(Z_{\alpha/2} + Z_\beta)^2$ from Table 2.1, then:

$$n = 2 \times 0.03 \times 0.97 \times 13.0/0.04^2$$

$$= 473$$

To look for correlations in cross-sectional studies, the formulae in the previous section are applicable (eqns 2.5, 2.6 and 2.7), where n represents the number of individuals to be sampled in the whole group, and d^* is the correlation to be detected.

If one of the variables being correlated is a nutrient intake, then the true correlation will be attenuated due to the presence of within-subject error in the nutrient intake estimate (section 2.2.2). Thus, if the true correlation to be detected is 0.5, and the coefficient of attenuation is 0.8, then the correlation likely to be observed is $0.5 \times 0.8 = 0.4$. In this case the attenuated correlation should be used in the formula, to scale up the required sample size appropriately.

2.4.3 Case-control studies

To investigate causality in epidemiological studies it is important to include a temporal element relating the cause and the effect. The case-control study is a relatively cheap way of doing this and works backwards in time from the effect to the cause (see Chapter 11). Cases with the disease are identified (the effect) and controls are obtained for comparison. The exposures of the cases and controls to the agent under investigation (the putative cause) are then compared, and if the exposures are sufficiently different then this supports the case for a causal link.

In addition, the controls may be matched to the cases, either on an individual or group basis. For more details of the design and analysis of case-control studies see Chapter 11.

An important deficiency of case-control studies is that they cannot compare directly the rates of disease in the cases and controls, and so cannot estimate the relative risk. This is because the two groups are sampled from the population using different sampling fractions[13]. However they do allow the odds ratio to be calculated, which is the ratio of the odds of cases being exposed to the agent and the equivalent odds for controls. In situations where the disease is rare, the odds ratio is a reasonable estimate of the relative risk.

The simplest form of case-control study is one where the cases and controls are either exposed or unexposed. The proportions of controls and cases so exposed are denoted by $p0$ and $p1$ respectively, and to calculate sample size $p0$ needs to be estimated from previously published data. The value for $p1$ can then be obtained from $p0$ and the odds ratio (OR) to be detected, using the formula:

$$p1 = p0 \text{ OR}/[1 + p0(\text{OR} - 1)] \qquad (2.11)$$

For generality, assume that r is the number of controls chosen per case, analogous to eqns 2.9 and 2.10. Then given $p0$ and $p1$ the weighted mean proportion is calculated as:

$$\bar{p} = (p1 + rp0)/(1 + r) \qquad (2.12)$$

and as before $\bar{q} = 1 - \bar{p}$ and $d^* = p1 - p0$. Equation 2.10 is then used to calculate the required sample size.

Suppose that in an unmatched case-control study, $p0 = 0.25$, $r = 1$ and an odds ratio of 2 is to be detected with 90 per cent power at 5 per cent significance. The value of $p1$ from eqn 2.11 is:

$$p1 = 0.25 \times 2/(1 + 0.25 \times 1)$$

$$= 0.4$$

so that $\bar{p} = 0.325$, $\bar{q} = 0.675$ and $d^* = 0.15$. Then, from eqn 2.10 and Table 2.1:

$$n = 2 \times 0.325 \times 0.675 \times 10.5/0.15^2$$

$$= 205$$

is the number of cases required, together with an equal number of controls.

There will be situations where the number of cases is restricted, perhaps due to the rarity of the disease. In this case it is useful to know the power available to detect a given odds ratio when the sample size n is known. This is obtained by rearranging eqn 2.10:

$$Z_\beta = d^* \sqrt{\left(\frac{nr}{\bar{p}\bar{q}(r+1)}\right)} - Z_{\alpha/2} \qquad (2.13)$$

And Z_β can be converted to a probability with normal distribution tables.

Another alternative is that both the power and the sample size are known, and the question then is 'What size of odds ratio can be detected?' This is known as the smallest detectable risk, and is discussed in detail by Schlesselman[13]. The relevant formulae are too complicated to include here, but an equivalent effect can be obtained by substituting a series of different values for the odds ratio into eqn 2.11, and seeing which gives a sample size close to the known value.

The discussion so far has assumed that the cases and controls are unmatched. If they are matched on an individual basis, then they need to be analysed in terms of concordant and discordant matched pairs, and the calculation of sample size should take this into account. The proportion P is defined as:

$$P = OR/(1 + OR)$$

and $Q = 1 - P$, while $p0$ and $p1$ are as previously defined. Then n, the sample size for each group (and hence the number of matched pairs), is given by:

$$n = \frac{(Z_{\alpha/2}/2 + Z_\beta\sqrt{PQ})^2}{(p0q1 + p1q0)\ (P - 0.5)^2} \qquad (2.14)$$

Using the same example as before, find the number of subjects needed to detect an odds ratio of 2 when $p0 = 0.25$. As before, $p1 = 0.4$ and $P = 2/(1+2) = 0.67$. Assuming 5 per cent significance (two-tailed) and 90 per cent power gives:

$$n = \frac{(1.96/2 + 1.28\sqrt{(0.67 \times 0.33)})^2}{(0.25 \times 0.6 + 0.4 \times 0.75)(0.67 - 0.5)^2}$$
$$= 193$$

This compares with the figure of 205 obtained using eqn 2.10 for unmatched cases and controls, so that the matching reduces the number of subjects required by some 6 per cent.

Schlesselman[13] discusses the issue of matched pairs in more detail, and gives formulae for the situation of multiple controls per case.

2.4.4 Cohort studies

The main difference between a cohort study and a case-control study is that a cohort study moves in time from the cause to the effect, rather than the other way round (see Chapter 12). A sample of a population is drawn and data about exposure to the agent of interest are collected. Then the sample is followed up for a sufficiently long time for cases of disease to occur in the sample. These cases can then be compared either with *all* the non-cases (i.e. controls) or else a sample of them, as regards their exposure.

Unlike a case-control study, a cohort study is able to estimate relative risk, because the sampling fractions of the cases and controls are known. If $p0$ is the proportion of unexposed subjects that get the disease and $p1$ is the corresponding proportion for exposed subjects, then $p1 = p0$ RR, where RR is the relative risk. Also required is r, the ratio of the number of unexposed subjects to exposed subjects in the population. In contrast to case-control studies, the value of r in cohort studies is predetermined and cannot be selected. The only other requirement then is to define $\bar{p}$, the mean proportion of subjects getting the disease, from eqn 2.12.

With these changes in definition, eqns 2.10 and 2.13 can be applied to cohort studies. In general r is rather greater than 1, so that the total sample size required, $n + r \cdot n$, is larger than for a case-control study. For example, consider a 10-year prospective study to measure the protective effect of a high fibre diet on colon cancer. Note here that the relative risk to be detected is less, rather than greater, than 1, because a protective effect is sought. A high fibre diet is defined as being in the top fifth of intake, so that $r = 4:1$, and assume the 10-year colon cancer incidence rate $\bar{p}$ is 0.01. The relative risk to be detected is $\frac{1}{3}$, with a power of 80 per cent at 5 per cent significance. From this and eqn (2.12) $p0$ can be calculated as:

$$p0 = \bar{p}(1 + r)/(\text{RR} + r) \qquad (2.15)$$

so that $p0 = 0.0115$, $p1 = 0.0038$ and $d^* = 0.0077$. From eqn 2.10 and Table 2.1:

$$n = (4 + 1) \times 0.01 \times 0.99 \times 7.8/4/0.0077^2$$

$$= 1629$$

and the total sample required, $n + r \cdot n$, is over 8000 subjects.

2.4.5 Experimental studies

Experimental studies, unlike the other types of epidemiological study discussed so far, involve an *intervention* (see Chapter 13). Subjects at risk of some disease are allocated, usually randomly, to receive either a live treatment or a placebo treatment, and their subsequent progress over a period of time is monitored. Chapter 13 discusses experimental studies in more detail.

Subjects are either exposed (treated) or unexposed (placebo), and they either succumb to the disease (cases) or they do not (controls). In this sense the design is similar to a case-control study, except that the selection is by exposure rather than outcome. The sampling fraction used to obtain the two treatment groups is by definition the same because they have an equal chance of being assigned to the two groups. Thus, the proportion developing the disease can be estimated, and the relative risk as well.

As before, eqn 2.10 can be applied, where $p0$ is the proportion of placebo subjects succumbing to the disease, and $p1 = p0\,RR$ (where RR is the relative risk).

A vitamin A supplement is to be tested to see if it will reduce mortality in lung cancer patients by 10 per cent (i.e. $RR = 0.9$) for 5 per cent significance and 95 per cent power. The proportion of deaths $p0$ over a year is known to be 50 per cent, so that $p1 = 0.45$ and:

$$n = 2 \times 0.475 \times 0.525 \times 13.0/0.05^2$$

$$= 2594$$

subjects are required in each arm of the study.

Of course, the outcome measure need not be a binary response, it could be, say, blood pressure after treatment or birth weight after supplementation. In this case eqn 2.9 rather than eqn 2.10 is appropriate, and the number of subjects required is likely to be smaller.

These are the very simplest designs of experimental study. More complex designs may have more than two treatment arms, or they may be group sequential designs which allow for the study to be stopped before the end point if a clear treatment effect has emerged early. See Pocock[8] for practical details concerning the design and conduct of experimental studies.

REFERENCES

1. Abramson, J. H. (1984). *Survey methods in community medicine*. Churchill Livingstone, Edinburgh.
2. Kelsey, J. L., Thompson, W. D., and Evans, A. S. (1986). *Methods in observational epidemiology*. Oxford University Press, New York.

3. Prentice, A. M., Black, A. E., Coward, W. A., Davies, H. L., Goldberg, G. R., Murgatroyd, P. R., Ashford, J., Sawyer M., and Whitehead, R. G. (1986). High levels of energy expenditure in obese women. *Br. Med. J.* **292:** 983–7.
4. Snedecor, G. W. and Cochran, W. (1980). *Statistical methods*, seventh edn. Ames, Iowa.
5. Liu, K., Stamler, J., Dyer, A., McKeever, J., and McKeever, P. (1978). Statistical methods to assess and minimize the role of intra-individual variability in obscuring the relationship between dietary lipids and serum cholesterol. *J. Chron. Dis.*, **31**: 399–418.
6. Liu, K., Cooper, R., McKeever, J., McKeever, P., Byington, R. Soltero, I., Stamler, R., Gosch, F., Stevens, E., and Stamler, J. (1979). Assessment of the association between habitual salt intake and high blood pressure: methodological problems. *Am. J. Epidemiol.* **110**: 219–26.
7. Nelson, M., Black, A. E., Morris, J. A., and Cole, T. J. (1989). Between- and within-subject variation in nutrient intake from infancy to old age: estimating the number of days required to rank dietary intakes with desired precision. *Am. J. Clin. Nutr.*, **50**: 155–67.
8. Pocock, S. J. (1983) *Clinical trials: a practical approach*. Wiley, Chichester.
9. Barker, D. J. P. and Osmond, C. (1986). Infant mortality, childhood nutrition, and ischaemic heart disease in England and Wales. *Lancet*, **i**: 1077–81.
10. Cole, T. J. and Black, A. E. (1983). Statistical aspects in the design of dietary surveys. In *The dietary assessment of populations*. MRC Environmental Epidemiology Unit Scientific Report; **4**: 5–7.
11. Hall, J. C. (1983). A method for the rapid assessment of sample size in dietary studies. *Am. J. Clin. Nutr.* **37**: 473–7.
12. Schlesselman, J. J. (1974). Sample size requirements in cohort and case-control studies of disease. *Am. J. Epidemiol.*, **99**: 381–4.
13. Schlesselman, J. J. (1982). Case-control studies: design, conduct, analysis. Oxford University Press, New York.

3. Covariate measurement errors in nutritional epidemiology: effects and remedies

David Clayton and Caroline Gill

3.1 THE PROBLEM AND SOME TERMINOLOGY

This chapter reviews the implications for dietary epidemiology of the inaccuracy of measurements in this field. It discusses the effects of measurement error and the extent to which these can be offset by appropriate statistical methods. Finally, the implications for the design of studies are discussed.

Figure 3.1 illustrates the problem we face in chronic disease epidemiology. A series of variables which are possibly related to a disease process are denoted by $z(t)$, this notation indicating that these will usually vary over time, t. In statistics these variables are simply called *covariates*, while in epidemiology they are called exposures or confounders, depending on their status in the analysis. The distinction between exposure and confounder may be understood most clearly by analogy with experimental science: an exposure is a factor which one would wish to vary in a systematic experiment, while a confounder is a factor which one would prefer to have held constant in the experiment. The fact that epidemiology relies, for the most part, on observational studies in which confounders cannot be held constant, necessitates statistical analyses which seek to re-create the ideal experiment. Since, in the natural experiment observed, several (even many) influences may vary simultaneously, the 'experiment of nature' is a factorial experiment—one in which several factors of interest are studied at the same time.

In dietary epidemiology, the difficulties of estimating the separate effects of different foods and nutrients is particularly challenging. There are many possibly relevant variables and these are often strongly interrelated. A topical example is the separation of the effect of fat intake from the total caloric intake, since people with more 'fatty' diets also tend to have higher total energy intakes.

The classification of a covariate as either an exposure or confounder is not a stable one. When two factors, z_1 and z_2, are related to disease and to

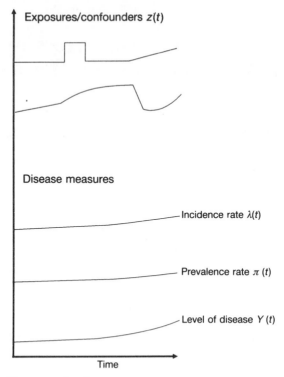

Fig. 3.1. The disease–exposure process over time.

each other and z_1 is of primary interest, z_1 is the exposure and z_2 the confounder. In another analysis, their roles may be reversed.

It may also not be clear when a variable should be considered as a confounder and corrected for in the analysis, and when it should be ignored. Here the decision is dictated by the ideal experiment which the statistical analysis seeks to mimic. In the example of fat consumption and total energy intake, it may be appropriate to carry out an analysis in which energy intake is treated as a confounder and fat intake is regarded as the exposure of interest. This analysis simulates an experiment in which total energy intake is held constant and fat intake is varied. Such an experiment would be difficult to carry out in practice—the calories lost from reducing fat intake would have to be replaced by increasing intake of some other nutrient. When interpreting statistical analyses of multifactorial problems it is important to bear such considerations in mind. The problems are rendered particularly acute in dietary epidemiology by the difficulty of making accurate measurements of diet.

All analytical approaches to the problem of confounding require, either implicitly or explicitly, a model for the joint effect of two or more exposures or confounders upon disease. The nature of this model, and the methods for drawing inferences about it, depend upon the outcome measure of the disease process. Outcome measures are usually of three types:

(1) the observation of an event, usually the first clinical sign of a disease (incidence);
(2) the recording of presence or absence of disease at a point in time (prevalence);
(3) the measurement of level of disease on a metric scale.

The arguments for preferring incidence to prevalence data are well known. The most serious limitation of prevalence data is that they may be influenced by a relationship between the presence of disease and subsequent mortality and migration. Studies which record a metric measure of the disease level (for example, blood pressure) suffer the same difficulties of interpretation, unless the disease level is measured repeatedly in a longitudinal study.

Modern epidemiology is largely concerned with processes for which it is impossible to build deterministic models or theories. Instead we must rely on models which relate covariate levels to the probability of outcome. For event data the most useful probability measure of the disease process is the probability per unit time, or 'hazard rate', of event occurrence. This is a function of time and is often denoted in the statistical literature by $\lambda(t)$ (see Fig. 3.1). For first occurrence of disease this is an incidence rate, while with mortality endpoints it is a mortality rate. In prevalence studies, the corresponding measure is the probability of disease presence, $\pi(t)$. For metric measures, statistical models allow for random errors of measurement of the level of disease, usually by assuming that the observed measurement has a probability distribution with mean equal to the true level but with variability (error) around this value. In Fig. 3.1 the mean level is denoted by $Y(t)$.

3.2 MODELLING DISEASE–COVARIATE RELATIONSHIPS

Most elementary treatments of epidemiological theory concentrate upon simple binary comparisons of exposed versus non-exposed groups. Dietary intakes, however, represent a continuum of exposure and in this chapter we shall concentrate upon models for a smooth dose–response relationship between intake and disease.

At some time of observation, t_{OBS}, the disease measure—$\lambda(t_{OBS})$, $\pi(t_{OBS})$, or $Y(t_{OBS})$—depends upon the entire history of exposure up to t_{OBS}. This is referred to as the *covariate history*. Only certain aspects of the covariate history will be relevant to later disease, although we often do not know which aspect is directly relevant. For example, a disease may be affected by nutrition in childhood with later diet being largely irrelevant. In the case of cancer, considerations of latency would suggest that exposure in the period immediately before the incidence of disease must be irrelevant and that analysis should concentrate upon earlier exposure.

If sufficient knowledge (or, at least, a working hypothesis) is available, it is possible to define a summary measure of the relevant exposure history at t_{OBS}. This shall be denoted by z^* (t_{OBS}). In nutritional epidemiology this is that summary measure of the dietary history which is relevant to the incidence of disease at t_{OBS}. The asterisk serves to remind us that this may differ considerably from the corresponding true intake at t_{OBS}. This in turn may differ substantially from the measured intake. For this reason, observed relationships between measured intakes and disease will reflect the underlying causal relationships rather imperfectly.

In statistical analysis we adopt a mathematical model for the relationship between $z^*(t_{OBS})$ and the measure of disease. Such models involve unknown constants, or parameters which control the strength and form of the relationship. Usually available data do not justify other than rather simple models, such as:

(1) linear dose–response relationships between level of exposure and outcome;
(2) additive or multiplicative models for joint effect of two factors.

These are the relationships implied by multiple regression models and this chapter will consider only models of this general form. If biological knowledge were to suggest other dose–response relationships, the same principles would apply, if not some of the detailed results. Correct analysis requires careful examination as to whether the data support the model assumed for the dose–response relationship.

The statistical theory surrounding regression models has become highly developed in recent years. Although developed originally for the case of metric outcome measures, the modern theory includes variants for binary outcomes (logistic regression), ordered categorical measures of outcome (ordinal regression), and event occurrence over time (proportional hazards, or 'Cox' regression).

A widespread misconception is that these methods represent a philosophically different approach to the analysis of epidemiological data from that of older methods based upon the idea of stratification. In fact these older methods are special cases of the modern modelling approach. The greater generality of the regression modelling approach lends itself particularly to computer implementation, and software is widely available. In the epidemiological literature progressively more complex analyses are being performed and reported.

A limitation with this methodology, only widely appreciated quite recently, is that regression models only allow for random influences or errors on the disease side of the equation. The fact that exposures and confounders are subject to measurement error is ignored. In these circumstances the regression model is a mathematical model for the relationship between the measurements of the covariate history and the disease outcome. While this is quite appropriate for actuarial prediction of future disease from measured characteristics of individuals, the fitted model may be a serious distortion of the causal relationship between true covariate history and disease. One aim of this chapter is to urge some caution in the interpretation of statistical analyses in these circumstances. We shall also discuss the possibilities for inferring the true causal relationship from epidemiological studies, and explore the implications of these considerations for their design.

3.3 MEASUREMENT ERRORS AND BIAS IN EPIDEMIOLOGICAL STUDIES

Figure 3.2 illustrates the possible influences upon the relationship between observed exposure and observed disease status in epidemiological studies.

Path 1 represents the true relationship between relevant exposure and disease. In the absence of confounding, this will reflect the causal relationship.

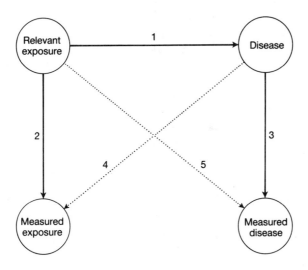

Fig. 3.2. Path diagram showing the possible influences on the observed disease–exposure relationship.

Path 2 represents the relationship between true relevant exposure and the observed surrogate.

Path 3 allows for measurement error of disease status or onset time.

The remaining paths allow for the major sources of bias which have been widely recognized to distort epidemiological findings:

Path 4 represents influences of disease status upon the measurement of exposure. This leads to information bias, the most widespread example of which is recall bias in case-control studies. Such influences present serious problems in dietary epidemiology; for example early disease may influence diet or, at least, the reporting of diet.

Path 5 allows the exposure to influence the recording of disease status. Examples include referral or investigation bias arising because certain groups may be more likely to be diagnosed than others, and bias arising from direct effects of early disease on physiology or behaviour. In dietary epidemiology, such paths are most likely to arise out of indirect relationships with socioeconomic status—more affluent groups may be better investigated and diagnosed and their diet differs from that of the less wealthy. This could induce a spurious relationship between diet and disease which would disappear if it were possible to correct for the confounding effect of socioeconomic status.

Paths 4 and 5 represent *differential misclassification*. They have been widely recognized as having the potential to lead to seriously erroneous findings. In particular, they may create an apparent relationship when no true relationship exists (i.e. when path 1 is truly absent). For this reason, in the design of any study, the epidemiologist must take every possible step to exclude such influences. If attempts are unsuccessful, it is unlikely that any degree of sophistication of analysis will salvage useful results.

The realization that epidemiological studies may yield biased results even in the absence of differential misclassification has come more recently. In particular, *symmetric misclassification* (errors of measurement of exposure unrelated to disease state indicated by path 2), although incapable of introducing spurious relationships where no true relationships exist, may distort the true causal relationship. The most frequently occurring distortion arising from exposure measurement error is attenuation of effect—the observed relationship is weaker than the underlying true relationship. This has implications for the design, analysis, and interpretation of studies.

More serious distortion may be caused by an inability to accurately measure strong confounders. A statistical analysis which attempts to control for confounding by stratification according to the observed level of the confounding variable will be misleading, since the stratification will fail to achieve its goal of holding the true confounder constant within strata. Two forms of distortion may occur:

(1) *residual confounding*, in which the inability to measure accurately the confounder means that the correction for confounding is incomplete;

(2) *spurious or exaggerated confounding*, in which the relationship between exposure and confounder is exaggerated by the measuring instrument.

An example of exaggerated confounding could be the relationship between fat intake and total energy intake. If this relationship is exaggerated by errors of measurement, a naïve correction of the relationship between fat intake and disease for the confounding effect of energy intake may be misleading.

Since there is no likelihood that such measurement errors can be excluded from epidemiological studies, the question is raised of whether one should only report relationships between observed quantities and discuss their implications for underlying causal models informally, or follow statisticians in social science in attempting to model underlying causal pathways. The remainder of this chapter discusses some possibilities and associated problems of the latter approach.

3.4 COVARIATE MEASUREMENT ERROR IN LINEAR REGRESSION

We have discussed above how regression methods allow for random influences or recording errors on outcome measures. In epidemiology, an equally serious problem is the discrepancy between the true value of the relevant history, $z^*(t_{OBS})$, and an imperfect measure, $x(t_{OBS})$, say. The difficulty is particularly acute since we are often unsure what aspect of the covariate history is relevant—if fat intake is implicated in breast cancer, should we be interested in lifetime intake, recent intake, childhood intake …?

This section briefly reviews the problem of exposure measurement error in the simple case of a linear regression relationship between covariate z^* and metrically measured disease outcome y. The observed relationship is between y and x, but the causal relationship between y and z^* is of more interest to the epidemiologist. These are not usually the same! The results outlined below are well known in the statistical literature, but their implications for epidemiology have only recently been widely discussed.

Consider first the case where we assume a linear relationship between level of disease and true relevant exposure. Since all quantities now refer to the time of observation, t_{OBS}, this may be omitted from the notation. The (causal) model for the relationship between relevant exposure and measured disease outcome must allow for random error of measurement of disease level. We assume the recorded level to have some probability distribution (perhaps a normal distribution) with expected (E) (mean) value determined by relevant exposure according to the linear dose–response relationship:

$$E(y) = Y = \alpha + \beta z^* \qquad (3.1)$$

and with variance$(y) = \sigma^2$. The parameter β determines the slope of the line and, therefore, the strength of the dose–response relationship.

Unfortunately this model cannot be fitted directly since the true exposure, z^*, is unknown except for the flawed measure, x. To progress further we need to model the process of exposure measurement. This measurement error model specifies the conditional probabilities of observations x given true exposures z^*, Prob$(x|z^*)$. This model specifies the distribution of measured exposures amongst individuals who share the same true relevant exposure.

Figure 3.3 represents the problem as an influence diagram. The disease outcome, y, and the measured exposure, x, are both causally related to the true relevant exposure, z^*. We only directly observe the relationship between x and y. To understand why this is not the same as the relationship between z^* and y gives insight into the potential for more accurate inference.

A simple analysis of the data is to plot disease level, y, against measured exposure, x. How would we expect this plot to appear given the model

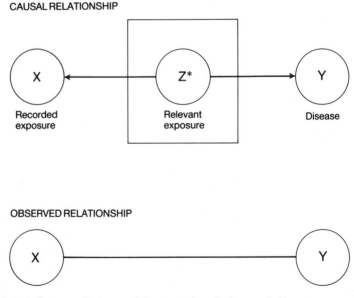

Fig. 3.3. Influence diagram of the causal and observed disease–exposure relationship.

outlined above? Since y is not causally related to x, but only to z^*, it follows that the mean value of y for persons with the same measured exposure, x, depends on the mean true exposure in that group. Naïvely we might think that this is simply x, but more usually it is not! The measurement error model gives the probability distribution of measured exposure given true exposure, $Prob(x|z^*)$, but we need the distribution of true exposure amongst people with the given measured exposure, $Prob(z^*|x)$. The shape of this distribution is given by a fundamental theorem of probability theory—Bayes theorem:

$$Prob(z^*|x) \propto Prob(x|z^*)Prob(z^*) \tag{3.2}$$

$Probs(x|z^*)$ is the measurement error model and $Prob(z^*)$ is the overall distribution of true exposure in the study group. If both these distributions are known (or can be estimated), Bayes theorem allows estimation of the distribution of true exposure for people with given measured exposure. The mean or expected value of this distribution is written as $E(z^*|x)$, and is referred to as the *Bayes estimate* of z^* (the true exposure) given x (the measured exposure).

The Bayes estimate is usually 'shrunk' towards the population mean exposure; i.e. the mean true exposure is less extreme than the measured exposure. When the measured exposure is high the mean true exposure is rather lower and when the measured value is low the mean true exposure is rather higher. The reason for this is the same as for the well-known phenomenon of *regression to the mean*. We will discuss this and the important special cases in which it does *not* occur below. For the present, we will examine its effect upon the observed relationship. Figure 3.4 illustrates this in a plot of outcome versus exposure for four points. The crosses represent measured exposure while the circles represent mean true exposures. A line fitted to the circles estimates the correct disease–exposure relationship, and this is stronger than the relationship between disease and measured exposure, corresponding to the line through the crosses.

The regression to the mean which leads to the discrepancy between the observed relationship and the true relationship arises as follows. The group of people who share the same measured exposure, x, are a mixture of persons whose true exposure was more extreme than x and persons whose true exposure was closer to the population mean than x. However, if the distribution of true exposure is bellshaped, so that there are progressively fewer individuals in each band of exposure as we depart from the mean, it follows that individuals with true exposures less extreme than x will predominate. Thus, the mean true exposure will be intermediate between the measured exposure and the population mean exposure. Note that the effect is crucially dependent on the shape of the distributions of exposure and of measurement error.

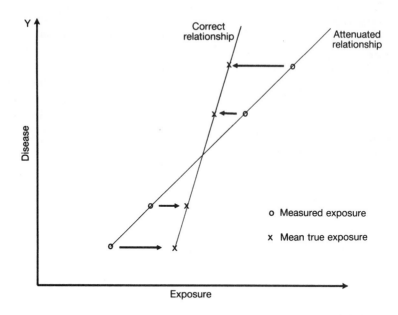

Fig. 3.4. Graph showing the attenuated disease–exposure relationship resulting from 'regression to the mean'.

Sometimes errors of measurement do not lead to this effect. In such cases, the measurement errors are referred to as Berksonian after a paper by Berkson[1] which pointed out these results. One case is when the measurement error and the measured value are uncorrelated, and the distribution of measurement errors is symmetric. This case is sometimes referred to as control knob error since it would arise if the experimenter sets the control knob of some apparatus to deliver some level of stimulus (the measured value), but the true stimulus delivered differs from the nominal value by a random error, symmetrically distributed above and below zero. In these circumstances, the mean stimulus delivered, $E(z^*|x)$, is identical to the nominal stimulus, x. In epidemiology, two examples of this situation are as follows:

1. Prentice[2] suggested that the estimates of radiation dose received by atom bomb survivors are subject to Berksonian errors. The dose is calculated from information concerning the location of the individual at the time of the explosion. While these estimates are subject to considerable error, it remains likely that the mean dose for individuals with the same measured dose will not be too far wrong.

2. Of more relevance to nutritional epidemiology is the case of 'ecological' studies of diet and disease. Plotting community disease rates against

estimated mean intake yields the same regression relationship as would be obtained from individual data, if each individual's intake were estimated by the community mean. Although this strategy clearly leads to very considerable exposure measurement error, the errors are Berksonian and do not lead to distortion of the relationship. (Ecological studies, however, have other difficulties!)

Berksonian errors occur when the measurement error is uncorrelated with the measured exposure. More commonly in analytical epidemiological studies exposure measurement errors are not Berksonian. It would more often be reasonable to assume that measurement error is uncorrelated with true exposure. The next section explores the possibility of correcting for the resultant distortion of the relationship in the statistical analysis.

3.5 CORRECTING FOR MEASUREMENT ERROR

When measurement errors are uncorrelated with true exposure, we have shown that the correct relationship may still be estimated providing we can calculate the Bayes estimate of the true exposure, $E(z^*|x)$. This can be calculated if we know (or reliably estimate) both the distribution of true exposure and the distribution of measurement error.

This is particularly easy when both these distributions can be assumed to be normal. Let the true exposures, z^*, be normally distributed with mean μ and variance σ^2, and let the measurement errors be normally distributed (independently of z^*) with mean 0 and variance τ^2. In these circumstances there is a simple linear shrinkage of the Bayes estimates of exposure towards the mean—the distance between the expected true exposure and μ is a constant proportion, ρ, of the distance between the measured exposure and μ. Algebraically,

$$E(z^*|x) - \mu = \rho(x - \mu) \tag{3.3}$$

The 'shrinkage factor', ρ is determined by the relative magnitudes of true variability of exposure, σ^2, and of measurement error, τ^2:

$$\rho = \frac{\sigma^2}{\sigma^2 + \tau^2} \tag{3.4}$$

The square root of ρ is the coefficient of correlation between the measured exposure and the true exposure and ρ is the correlation between two independent measurements of the same underlying exposure.

It follows that the induced relationship between y and x remains a straight line relationship, but the slope is reduced by the factor ρ. If ρ is known, the regression coefficient in the underlying causal model may be estimated, either by calculation of the regression coefficient of y on x and subsequently scaling it up by division by ρ, or by regression of y on Bayes estimates of the true exposure, z^*. These two approaches will yield identical results.

In practice ρ is rarely known, although in some circumstances it may be estimable from test–retest reliability data. If repeated measures are taken on the same individual, and it may be assumed that the measurement errors on the different occasions are uncorrelated with each other, then ρ is simply the coefficient of intra-class correlation between different measurements on the same individual. In nutritional epidemiology, however, the independent errors assumption is unlikely to hold and the intra-class correlation coefficient will overestimate ρ.

When validation studies are available which use several methods on several spaced occasions, it is possible to obtain estimates of measurement variances and covariance by, for example, assuming that different methods on different occasions do not have correlated errors.

When it is believed that the relevant exposure is the average of the dietary intake of some nutrient over many years, then test–retest studies carried out over a relatively short period may underestimate measurement error, and it may only be possible to informally estimate ρ. As an aid to this, Table 3.1 relates ρ to the percentage of individuals who could be classified in the correct third of the distribution of true exposure using the measured exposure.

When we cannot assume normal distributions, the problem is more difficult although, if the relevant distributions are known, the correct relationship is always estimable. In practice the difficulty will be lack of good data concerning these distributions.

Table 3.1 Correct classification by thirds of the exposure distribution

ρ	% Correctly classified
0.1	42.8
0.2	46.5
0.3	51.4
0.4	54.8
0.5	59.2
0.6	63.2
0.7	67.9
0.8	73.4
0.9	81.0

An interesting possibility is to attack the problem empirically by allowing regression to the mean to occur. The study group can be classified into, say, deciles on an initial measure of exposure and mean true exposure in subgroups may be estimated by the mean of a second measure. An 'ecological' analysis relating this estimate of group exposure to the mean disease level in the subgroups will yield the correct relationship, providing that the errors in the second measurement are unrelated to the errors in the first. If the errors are correlated, then the regression to the mean is not complete and some distortion of the relationship will remain. This approach was used by McMahon et al.[3] in studying the relationship between blood-pressure and cardiovascular disease. Table 3.2 shows

Table 3.2 Diastolic Blood Pressure (DBP) in 5 categories.[3]

Baseline DBP	Number of subjects	Mean DBP in category		
		At baseline	At 2 years	At 4 years
−79	1719	70.8	75.7	76.2
80−89	1213	83.6	83.0	83.9
90−99	566	93.5	90.2	90.3
100−109	186	103.4	99.2	98.5
110−	92	116.4	107.3	104.7
Range:		47.7	31.6	28.5

blood-pressure for groups classified according to an initial, or baseline, measurement. Regression of disease rates for these groups against the mean baseline blood-pressure would yield an incorrect slope since the range of variation of long-term average blood-pressure is overestimated. Use of a further measure 2–4 years later will lead to a much improved estimate. In nutritional epidemiology, however, the assumption of uncorrelated measurement errors may not be justified and regression-to-the-mean estimated from repeated measurements in this way may not correctly estimate long-term intakes. For example, habitual underreporting of energy intake by some subjects is often reported.

3.6 REGRESSION MODELS FOR INCIDENCE AND PREVALENCE DATA

The results set out in the last section have been known for many years. More recently similar results have been shown to hold for relative risk regression models for the occurrence of events in time[2,4] and for logistic regression models for prevalence studies and case-control studies.[5] This section briefly reviews the results for regression analyses of incidence data. Similar results hold for logistic regression analyses of prevalence data.

In recent years, the analysis of event data has been dominated by the relative risk regression model introduced by Cox[6]. In the present notation this may be written:

$$\text{Incidence Rate}(t_{OBS}) = \lambda_0(t_{OBS})\theta(z^*(t_{OBS});\beta) \qquad (3.5)$$

The incidence rate at t_{OBS} is expressed as the product of a 'baseline' incidence rate, $\lambda_0(t_{OBS})$, and a relative risk term, $\theta()$ which is a function of the relevant exposure history. Again, regression coefficients, β, express the strength of the relationship between exposure(s) and risk of disease occurrence. The most convenient relative risk function, and that most frequently available in current computer software, is the log-linear function:

$$\theta(z^*;\beta) = \exp \beta z^* \qquad (3.6)$$

or

$$\log \theta(z^*;\beta) = \beta z^* \qquad (3.7)$$

This model implies that a one-unit change in exposure confers a relative risk of $\exp \beta$ at every point on the scale. As in the case of a metric disease measure, if the measure of the relevant exposure history is flawed, there will be an induced relationship between the measured exposure, x, and subsequent incidence of events. In the same way as a linear regression relationship between true exposure, z^*, and disease level, y, induces a (rather weaker) relationship between measured exposure, x, and y, the relative risk model for the effect of exposure upon incidence induces an attenuated relative risk relationship between measured exposure and incidence. The derivation of the degree of attenuation follows very similar lines as before. A group of persons with the same measured exposure, x, will in fact have had varying true exposures, z^*, and so will experience varying relative risks, $\theta(z^*;\beta)$. The average relative risk for such persons is *not* $\theta(x;\beta)$ but a rather less extreme value. The size and pattern of discrepancy between the observed relationship and the underlying causal relationship depends on the magnitude of measurement error in relation to the true variability of exposure. Again one special case leads to simple equations; if true exposure and measurement error are both normally distributed with variances σ^2 and τ^2 respectively, and incidence is related to true exposure in the log-linear manner discussed above, the relationship between incidence and measured exposure follows exactly the same log-

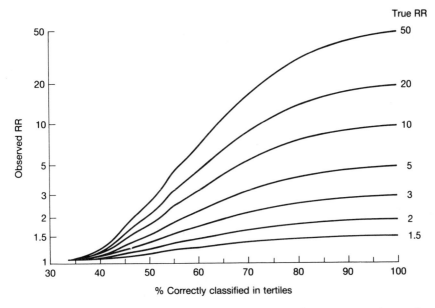

Fig. 3.5. Graph showing the effect of exposure misclassification upon observed relative risk.

linear relationship, but with a regression coefficient which is reduced by the factor ρ.

Since many epidemiologists do not find regression coefficients and correlation coefficients very intuitive, these relationships are explored in terms of comparisons between tertiles of the exposure distribution in Fig. 3.5. Each curve shows, for a causal relationship of given strength, the rate ratio for the top versus the bottom thirds of the distribution of measured exposure plotted against the accuracy of the measurement, expressed in terms of our ability to correctly classify subjects into thirds of the exposure distribution. The 7 curves shown represent underlying true rate ratios of 1.5, 2, 3, 5, 10, 20, and 50. It would appear that the attenuation is not too serious when we can correctly classify at least 75 per cent of subjects into thirds of the distribution.

3.7 CONFOUNDER MEASUREMENT ERRORS

The relationships set out in sections 4, 5, and 6 between regression models in z^* and regression models in x may be extended to the case where there are multiple exposures (confounders). However, the situation becomes more complex. Even in the case of a single exposure and a single confounder, the discrepancy between the exposure effect as estimated by conventional methods and the true 'causal' effect depends upon:

(1) size of the effect of the confounder;
(2) strength of association between exposure and confounder;
(3) measurement error for the exposure;
(4) range of variation of exposure in the study group;
(5) measurement error for the confounder;
(6) range of variation of the confounder;
(7) correlation between measurement errors of exposure and confounder.

If a confounder is measured with error, any control for confounding in the analysis is flawed. If confounder measurement error is independent of exposure measurement error, then we have the phenomenon of *residual confounding*. The coefficient of the exposure variable is adjusted in the correct direction but by an insufficient amount.

If confounder measurement error is correlated with exposure measurement error, then the bias may go in either direction. In particular we may overestimate the correlation between exposure and confounder and, as a result, overcorrect for the effect of the confounder. The potential for this type of error has not been widely recognized, yet it remains a strong possibility in nutritional epidemiology—the methods of measuring diet are very likely to lead to strongly correlated measurement errors, as is the use of current diet as a surrogate for diet during the period relevant to the development of disease.

Further difficulties arise if the error variance is related to the level of true exposure. It has been shown that this may lead to spurious curvature of dose–response relationships and spurious interaction (effect modification).

In principle, and given sufficient data, these distortions may be corrected in the analysis. However this would require extra modelling assumptions and extra data. The final section discusses the implications for the design of epidemiological studies.

3.8 DISCUSSION

For the sake of clarity this chapter has oversimplified some of the statistical problems, and there is need for more research in this area. We have shown that correct estimation of exposure/disease relationships requires us to have knowledge of:

1. The probability distribution of measurement errors.
2. The distribution of true exposures and confounders in the population studied.

We have also shown that both distributions may be multivariate. Then it will be necessary to consider not only the variability of each component but also their interrelationship. While simple results are available if the distributions are multivariate normal, the development of statistical methods based on weaker assumptions is a considerable challenge. For the present the multivariate normal results serve as a yardstick for gauging the seriousness of the measurement error problem.

Even the simplest model requires knowledge of its parameters and the estimation of the magnitude of measurement errors presents serious problems to the nutritional epidemiologist. Ideally this requires validation studies to be carried out on subsamples of the study population, but this is not possible in a field in which no error-free 'gold standard' measurement is available. To some extent this lack can be redressed by reliability studies in which several different measuring instruments are used on several occasions. Inference from such studies depends upon the validity of assumptions made in modelling measurement errors. While these may be checked to some extent, there is considerable danger in extrapolation. For example, results of a reliability study with repeated measures over a 1-year period could not be applied with any confidence to inference concerning the relationship between disease and dietary intakes over 20 years or more. This problem is particularly acute when it is not possible *a priori* to identify the relevant exposure.

Conventional concerns over information bias ensure that case-control studies are not the method of choice in nutritional epidemiology. The need to study measurement error whilst simultaneously studying diet/disease relationships provides additional rationale for advocating long-term prospective studies with repeated measures of diet. To minimize the intercorrelation between measurement errors on different occasions, the repeated measurements should be well separated in time. The use of more than one measuring instrument is essential.

Although, for estimation in the measurement error model, detailed reliability studies need only be carried out on a subsample, measurement errors cause a loss of power in the study as a whole, and some repetition of dietary measurements will be desirable for all subjects. The efficient analysis of such studies will best be achieved by the use of 'nested' case-control studies. Statistical analysis which attempts to allow for measurement error effects will not be easy and further methodological research is needed.

3.9 REFERENCES

1. Berkson, J. (1950). Are there two regressions? *J. American Statistical Assoc.*, **45**: 164.
2. Prentice, R. L. (1982). Covariate measurement errors and parameter estimation in a failure time regression model. *Biometrika*, **69**: 331–42.

3. McMahon, S., Peto, R., Cutler, J., Collins, R., Sorlie, P., Neaton, J., Abbott, R., Godwin, J., Dyer, A., and Stamler, J. (1990). Blood pressure, stroke, and coronary heart disease. *Lancet*, **335**: 765–74.

4. Armstrong, B. G. and Oakes, D. (1982). The effects of approximation in exposure assessment on estimates of exposure response relationships. *Scandinavian Journal of Work, Environment and Health*, **8** suppl. 1: 20–3.

5. Armstrong, B. G., Whittemore, A. S., and Howe, G. R. (1989). Analysis of case-control data with covariate measurement error: application to diet and colon cancer. *Statistics in Medicine*, **8**: 1151–63.

6. Cox, D. R. (1972). Regression models and life tables. *J. Royal Statistical Soc. Series B*, **33**: 187–202.

PART B

The measurement of exposure and outcome

Introduction

At the core of any nutritional epidemiological study, no matter how well designed or cleverly analysed, is the matter of measurement of exposure and outcome. Inappropriate or inaccurate measurements will lead to spurious conclusions. The focus of this part of the book is therefore to consider how best such measurements can be made, and how the errors associated with the measurements of exposure can themselves be measured and taken into account during analysis.

Table B.1 shows the measures of exposure and outcome that are likely to be of major interest in nutritional epidemiological studies. The term 'diet' includes food, drink, and non-food items (such as clay in picophagia), and the components of food, both nutritional and non-nutritional (including additives and contaminants). Data may be available at national, house-hold, or individual level, and the nature of the investigation will dictate the type of data required. For instance, ecological studies, in which groups of people are compared, may utilize existing data at national or regional level, or may require the specific collection of data to characterize the groups (Chapters 5 and 10). Alternatively, if it is important to measure diet in individuals for case-control, cohort, or experimental studies, then

Table B.1 Measures of exposure and outcome in nutritional epidemiological studies

Exposure	Outcome
Diet	Death
national	Morbidity
household	Anthropometry
individual	Per cent of standard
Biochemical markers	(Recommended daily allowances
Anthropometry	anthropometric, biochemical, clinical)
Clinical measures	Physiological measures
Vital statistics	
Individual characteristics	

techniques appropriate both to the nature of the dietary exposure and the hypothesis being tested must be utilized (Chapter 6). A persistent problem in all dietary measurements is the lack of validity due to measurement error that leads to differential and non-differential misclassification. This arises in part because of the need to translate food consumption data into estimates of nutrient intake using food composition tables (Chapter 4), and in part because of weaknesses inherent in the measurements themselves. Further to the matters raised in Chapter 3, a major emphasis in Part B is the ascertainment of measurement error as a key component of any measurement, be it at national, household, or individual level. In particular, the use of questionnaires is widespread in nutritional epidemiological studies, and Chapter 8 is devoted to the validation of questionnaires and a consideration of how to assess and cope in analysis with the likely errors associated with their use.

An appreciation of the need to use biochemical markers rather than direct measurements of diet in the assessment of nutritional status has enhanced the objectivity of some measurements. For instance, the use of urinary sodium as a measure of sodium intake, or the use of leucocyte ascorbic acid levels to assess medium term vitamin C intake, helps to overcome some of the difficulties inherent in direct measurements of diet. However, while biochemical markers offer considerable scope in epidemiology, they are not without their limitations, and Chapter 7 looks in detail at both the range of possible measurements available and the nature of the problems associated with their use.

Anthropometry, clinical measures, and vital statistics can provide useful summary measures of nutritional status. For instance, the distribution of per cent height for age in children may be a good reflection of the availability of energy, and changes in weight in individuals in experimental studies may reflect compliance. Some clinical measures are highly specific in relation to nutrient intake (e.g. goitre and the availability of iodine), although the majority of clinical signs relate to deficiency and do not, therefore, cover the whole spectrum of nutrient status, which is often required for epidemiological studies. Vital statistics such as neonatal mortality again provide a useful starting point for the investigation of group status (Chapter 9). All of these types of measurement are more straightforward in their assessment and yet more complex in their interpretation than dietary or biochemical assessments.

Measures of outcome are equally subject to error and the same attention must be paid to error in the measurement of outcome as in the measurement of exposure. The use of mortality and morbidity data and their associated measurement errors are discussed in Chapter 9. There is also a range of outcome measurements expressed in terms of accepted international standards. These are sometimes the same as those used as a measure of exposure, but their interpretation is different. For example, risk of anaemia might be assessed by looking at the distribution of the population in relation to the Recommended Daily Amount (RDA) for iron (assuming that a valid measure of intake had been obtained) rather than by a direct measurement of haemoglobin levels in blood. Measures of physiological status (e.g. blood pressure, treadmill ergometer performance) or biochemistry (e.g. change in erythrocyte glutathione peroxidase activity in an intervention trial with selenium) are also effective measures of outcome that have known associations with risk of morbidity from other diseases. The principles of measurement described throughout this section primarily in relation to measurement of exposure apply equally to measurements of outcome.

4. Food consumption, nutrient intake, and the use of food composition tables

C. E. West and W. A. van Staveren

4.1 INTRODUCTION

Food consumption data are collected for a variety of purposes. The most relevant to this chapter are:

(1) estimation of adequacy of the dietary intake of population groups;

(2) investigation of relationships between diet and health and to nutritional status;

(3) evaluation of nutrition education, nutrition intervention, and food fortification programmes.

In general, data obtained on food intake by individuals or groups of individuals is converted to consumption of nutrients. This conversion process can be achieved either by analysing the foods consumed directly or by using food composition tables. Table 4.1 classifies the most commonly used dietary survey methods on the basis of whether chemical analysis of food samples or food tables are used to estimate nutrient intake.

The methods using direct analysis are considered to be the most accurate and most appropriate for examining the effect of changes in nutrient intake on parameters of nutritional status over a period of time. However, for observational studies of large populations, these methods are too cumbersome, costly, and time consuming. Methods based on the use of food composition tables are more often used.

Food composition tables, or nutrient databases, which are their electronic/magnetic equivalent, are available in many countries. However, there may still be a need to carry out food analyses under a number of circumstances, including:

(1) when the content of a nutrient or other food component is not available in an existing food table;

(2) when there is no information available on which foods are important sources of a nutrient/other food component of interest;

Table 4.1 Classification of the most commonly used methods for measuring nutrient intake[40]

Use of chemical analysis	Characteristics of method		
	Use of food composition tables		
	Record methods	Interview methods	Short-cut methods
Duplicate portion technique	Precise weighing	Recall	Record
Aliquot sampling technique	Weighed inventory	Dietary history	Recall
Equivalent composite technique	Present intake recorded in household measures		

(3) when there is no information on the loss or gain of nutrients in foods during preparation by the methods being used by the population under investigation;

(4) when it is necessary to check the comparability of the various food composition tables being used in a multicentre study.

4.2. THE USE OF FOOD ANALYSIS IN DETERMINING FOOD INTAKE

Of all the dietary survey methods available, the duplicate portion technique method is regarded as the most accurate, although its accuracy depends on being able to obtain a sample that is identical to the food consumed by the subject under study. This is probably more difficult when composite foods such as a stew or a food with a lot of free fat is being consumed.[1] In addition, an observer may not be able to include small items in the duplicate portion[2] either because he or she is unaware that they have been eaten, such as snacks between meals, or because they are not available. Often the cook may not have prepared sufficient for a complete duplicate portion and the food prepared for the subject under study would be consumed in its entirety by the subject or shared with the duplicate portion thus resulting in reduced food intake by the subject.

In the aliquot sampling technique, the weights of all foods eaten and all beverages drunk, usually with the exception of water, are recorded and aliquot samples, e.g. one-tenth of all foods and beverages consumed, are collected daily. Subsequently, the combined aliquot samples collected over the survey period are chemically analysed. Errors can arise in this method, in addition to those inherent in the duplicate portion method, from the recording of weights and volumes. However, the method is often preferred to the duplicate portion technique because less food is required and only one analysis is required for the entire survey period.

In the equivalent composite technique, which is hardly ever used, the weights of all foods eaten and all beverages drunk are recorded, as for the aliquot sampling technique. At the end of the survey period, a sample of raw foods equivalent to the mean daily amounts of food eaten by an individual during the survey period is taken for analysis. Errors over and above those experienced with the aliquot sampling technique arise from the analysis of raw foods as opposed to foods as consumed (see section 4.3.7) and from qualitative differences between foods in the composite and those eaten. The method is cheaper than the duplicate portion and aliquot sampling techniques and it is relatively easy to collect the food samples, although this process cannot commence until the average consumption of foods over the whole period of study has been calculated.

There are two additional problems with all three of these techniques. The first is that the techniques are very difficult to validate in an absolute way, and differential misclassification may occur in the collection of samples in free-living populations. Nevertheless the duplicate portion technique is the method to which all other methods should be compared. Secondly, the accuracy of the results will depend on the accuracy of the analyses, in the same way as the accuracy of results based on the use of food composition tables. Thus, good laboratory practice is essential in order to obtain satisfactory results (see section 4.3.5).

4.3 FOOD COMPOSITION TABLES AND NUTRIENT DATABASES

National epidemiological studies may want to look at nutrient intake as well as food consumption data. It is necessary, therefore, to be able to convert information on food consumption into intake of nutrients. Thus, the needs of the nutritional epidemiologist are not always identical with other users of the tables, such as medical practitioners and dietitians involved in giving dietary advice, or those involved in food production and preparation at various levels. Therefore, it is essential that the needs of epidemiologist are taken into account when food composition tables/ nutrient databases are being constructed. Guidelines for the preparation of food composition tables have been prepared by Southgate[3] and by Greenfield and Southgate[4]. The requirements of food composition tables, particularly relevant to the nutritional epidemiologist, include:

4.3.1 Foods included in the table

To be able to calculate nutrient intake, the foods delivering the nutrients of interest should be included in the table. If the foods are not included, information on their nutrient content could be obtained from other sources, including other tables or by analysing foods especially for the study. However, if the number of foods on which information was not available was very large, methods based on direct analysis could be considered (see section 4.2). The number and nature of foods required will depend not only on the population or individuals under study, but also on the information being sought. A study of the energy intake of a group of farm workers in a traditional rural area would require fewer foods than an international case-control study of cancer at a particular site aimed at estimating the intake of 13 vitamins. First, because the range of foods consumed by the farm workers would be much narrower than that consumed by those in the international study. Secondly, because information on fewer foods would be required for measuring energy intake only, than for measuring energy and vitamin intake. In addition, more detailed descriptions of the foods would be required for the study on vitamin intake because foods differ more markedly in their content of individual vitamins than in their energy value. The vitamin content of plants, for example, is more dependent than the energy value on variety, degree of maturity, part of the plant, method of food preparation, and the method and duration of storage. Indeed, the naming and general description of foods is a very important aspect of constructing a food composition table, not only for epidemiological purposes.

It is important that a food is labelled unequivocally and that all those involved in a study understand what is meant by the food described. For international studies, a thesaurus can be used to relate the locally used name to that by which the food is known in other countries. For unprocessed plants and animals, the scientific name will assist in identification while for plants, the variety should also be given. Prepared foods are more difficult to name because some proprietary names have restricted use while some describe products with different formulations. The problem is even more complicated for cooked dishes because the composition of a named dish varies between countries, regions, and even households. Thus, the name on its own is quite often not sufficient to characterize and identify a cooked dish. Another approach to studying foods from different countries has been developed by EUROFOODS and involves grouping foods together on the basis of their similarities. A food coding system based on 14 major food groups has been agreed upon by representatives from 17 countries. The 14 groups were subdivided into 2500 subcategories and the system so developed has been revised a total of five times. The result is called EUROCODE 2 and is part of a food coding and descriptor system.[5]

4.3.2. Nutrients included in the table

The nutrients to be included in the food composition table will depend on the purpose of the study. It should also be remembered that it is sometimes better to estimate the intake of nutrients not from food intake, but indirectly using biological markers. Thus, sodium and chloride intake are often measured more readily by measuring excretion in the urine, but such estimates can be subject to large errors. More sodium chloride is lost through perspiration in a hot climate or during physical exertion than during sedentary work in a temperate climate and there is increased loss of water and electrolytes during fever, vomiting, and diarrhoea. Even though intake can be estimated from excretion, it is still necessary to estimate intake of electrolytes using food tables to be able to determine which foods in the diet are sources of such electrolytes. The use of biological markers for estimating nutrient intake is discussed further in Chapter 7.

4.3.3 Methods of expression of nutrients

It probably does not matter how nutrients are expressed for many epidemiological studies, as long as the method is generally accepted by the scientific community. However, for certain studies, it may be important. For example, a study on the role of vitamin A and carotenoids in lung cancer would require more information than the vitamin A activity expressed in retinol equivalents. At the very least, vitamin A and provitamin A activity would be required separately. Perhaps information on provitamin A should be divided into the various provitamin A carotenoids, and it may also be desirable to have information on other carotenoids present. Unfortunately, much of the information desired may not be available. Thus, the original study design may have to be re-examined or more analytical work carried out before the study can proceed. Other problems related to the method of expression of nutrients may arise from the long-standing convention of using protein values derived by applying a factor to measured total nitrogen values and from the calculation of energy values using energy conversion factors.[6]

4.3.4. Methods used for the estimation of nutrients

The basic principle is that the method used should provide information that is nutritionally appropriate. Traditionally, carbohydrate was estimated by difference: that is, by directly measuring the percentage of protein (from the nitrogen content), fat, ash, and water, and deducting these from 100 to give the percentage of carbohydrate. This method is clearly inadequate for all nutritional purposes because it combines in one value all the different carbohydrate species: sugars, starch, and components of dietary fibre, together with all the errors in the other determinations. Nutritionists require much more detailed information, because the metabolic effects of all the components are quite different.[7] The biological action of related nutrients was referred to above with respect to vitamin A and carotenoids (section 4.3.3) because the method of expression of a nutrient is often related to the analytical method used to obtain the data. This is also so for the vitamers of other vitamins including vitamin B_6 (pyridoxal, pyridoxal phosphate and pyridoxamine), folic acid (with a side chain with one, three, or seven glutamic acid residues), vitamin D (D_2 or D_3), vitamin E (various tocopherols and tocotrienols), and vitamin K (with various numbers of saturated and unsaturated isoprene units in the side chain). The problem of biological availability is addressed in section 4.3.8.

4.3.5. Data quality

If you ask someone whether they want to use high quality food composition data for their epidemiological study, the answer will invariably be 'yes'. Thus, the question is really whether the data are of sufficient quality to answer the question being asked; and a number of specific aspects need to be addressed.

Naming and description of foods   The question that has to be addressed is whether the food being consumed is similar to that described in the food composition table (see section 4.3.1). Describing foods precisely is a difficult task and much is required to ensure that foods are described adequately.[8]

Origin of foods   A plant food being consumed and the same plant food in the table should be sufficiently similar with respect to soil type, method of husbandry, fertilizer treatment, harvesting, and post-harvesting treatment. Animal products should take into account locality, methods of husbandry, and methods of slaughter. Such differences may not be important for many studies, but sometimes they may be significant.

Sampling framework of food on which data are included in the food table   If information is available on data in the food composition table with respect to a description of the sampling process, place and time of sampling, number of samples, origin of samples and state of sample when purchased, it should be possible to judge whether the sample is representative of the food as a whole, of a subset of the food, or whether the data apply merely to the food analysed. With cooked foods, the cooking procedures and recipe should be known (see section 4.3.7). Some data in food composition tables are based on analyses on pooled samples and this may influence the value of the data obtained. In addition, information on treatment of samples before analysis may be important. Before analysis, inedible material is usually removed and details of the portion taken for analysis should be known. For example, a Frenchman would never think of eating brie with the hard outside coat, but many people from other countries do. This type of difference may mean that the food analysed is not the same as that being consumed in your epidemiological study.

Quality of food analysis   Differences in sampling techniques and the quality of the analytical work *per se* are usually the most important reasons for differences in analytical data in food composition tables. Differences in the methods used can be important (see section 4.3.4), but this is usually over-emphasized. When compared with the traditional methods of titrimetry and gravimetry, modern methods of instrumental analysis, such as high performance liquid chromatography and atomic absorption spectrometry, are more convenient and allow more samples to be analysed but are not necessarily intrinsically more accurate. The problem of the quality of food analysis as a source of variation between data in different food composition tables was recognized by EUROFOODS, who organized an interlaboratory trial in 1985 in which 20 leading laboratories in Europe and the USA participated.[9] Each laboratory received a well homogenized dried sample of six foods and was requested to perform analyses of dried weight by a prescribed vacuum method, and of protein, fat, available carbohydrates, total dietary fibre, and ash by its own routine method. The results obtained were far from satisfactory. There were large between-laboratory coefficients of variation (CV) for dietary fibre (ranging from 23 per cent for French beans to 84 per cent for biscuits), which could be explained by the use of different methods. The CV for protein ranged from 2.8 per cent for egg to 6.4 per cent for wheat and rye but recalculation of these values using uniform Kjeldahl factors reduced these CVs to 2.7, 4.7, and 5.2 per cent, respectively. It could be concluded that leading laboratories in different countries may produce widely different values for proximate constituents in common foods. Thus, there is a need for better standardization of methods and for the essential elements of good laboratory practice to be followed. These include:

(1) replicate analyses carried out as a matter of course;
(2) analysis of reference materials such as those provided by the Association of Official Analytical Chemists in the United States and by the Community Bureau of Reference of the European Commission;
(3) regular use of standards;
(4) recovery of added standards;
(5) analysis of concealed replicates;

(6) exchange of samples between laboratories;

(7) collaborative tests of methodological protocols;

(8) comparison of values obtained with literature values.[7]

Information on sources of data   It is important to have information on the source of the data in a food composition table to be able to check its appropriateness for the study and to confirm its authenticity. Data in food composition tables can be original analytical values, imputed, calculated or borrowed.[10] Original analytical values are those taken from published literature or unpublished laboratory reports. This latter category includes original calculated values, such as protein values derived by multiplying the nitrogen content by the required factor and 'logical' values, such as the content of cholesterol in vegetable products, which can be assumed to be zero. Imputed values are estimates derived from analytical values for a similar food or another form of the same food. This category includes those data derived by difference, such as moisture and, in some cases, carbohydrate and values for chloride calculated from the sodium content. Calculated values are those derived from recipes by calculation from the nutrient content of the ingredients corrected by the application of preparation factors. Such factors take into account losses or gain in weight of the food or of specific nutrients during preparation of the food (see section 4.3.7). Borrowed values are those derived from other tables or databases without referring to the original source. When a value for the content of a specific nutrient in a food is not included, there is an 'absent' value and, when a table has no values for a particular nutrient, the value is regarded as being 'not included'. The proportion of the various types of data differs between tables and for different nutrients.[11] In some tables, such as the McCance and Widdowson tables in the United Kingdom[12] and the tables in the United States,[13] most data are based on analyses that have been carried out especially for inclusion in the tables. In other tables, such as those in the Netherlands, where sources of the data are given in the references,[14] information on how the data have been obtained can also be obtained. However, this is not the case for all tables of food composition.

4.3.6 Missing values in food composition tables

In general, original analytical data provides information of the highest quality for inclusion in a food composition table or nutrient database. However, it is not always feasible to construct a food composition table with only such data. Thus, tables often have missing values, which are usually represented by zeros. It is important to realize that missing values in a food table can lead to an under-estimate of the intake of a nutrient, especially when there are no values for a nutrient in those foods that make a significant contribution to the supply of that nutrient in the diet. If it is not possible to arrange for foods to be analysed, data can be sought in the literature, imputed, sought from other tables or estimated as outlined in section 4.3.5. Alternatively, the intake of a particular nutrient could be estimated by direct analysis (section 4.3.2), excretion (section 4.3.2), or by the use of biological markers (Chapter 7).

4.3.7 Nutrient losses and gains during the preparation of foods

The content of nutrients per unit weight of food changes when foods are prepared; such losses and gains can be classified in two ways. The first is related to yield, when the primary ingredients at the precooking stage are compared with the prepared food at the cooking stage and also with the food as consumed at the postcooking stage. The second is related to changes in the amount of specific nutrients when foods are prepared. In a perfect world, original analytical data would be available for foods at all stages of preparation. However, it is often necessary to make estimates based on the use of factors for calculating the nutrient content of prepared foods from raw ingredients.[15]

4.3.8 Bioavailability

The concept of bioavailability has developed from observations that have shown that measurements of the amount of a nutrient consumed do not necessarily provide a good index of the amount of a nutrient that can be utilized by the body. The bioavailability of a nutrient can be defined as the proportion of that nutrient that is available for utilization by the body.[16] This is not simply the proportion of a nutrient absorbed, and cannot be equated with solubility or diffusibility in *in vitro*-simulated physiological systems. Bioavailability is not a property of a food nor of a diet *per se*, but is the result of the interaction between the nutrient in question with other components of the diet and with the individual consuming the diet. Because of the many factors influencing bioavailability, tables of food composition cannot give a single value for a nutrient's bioavailability. Most research up until now has centred upon inorganic constituents, particularly iron, but the concept is applicable to virtually all nutrients. Iron incorporated into haem is more readily absorbed than non-haem iron, and these two forms of iron are sometimes listed separately in food composition tables. But such information does not take into account, for example, the effect of ascorbic acid on iron absorption. In the coming years, it can be expected that much more work will be carried out on bioavailability than in the past, because of its key role in relating functional nutritional status to nutrient intake.

4.3.9 Ease of use of food composition tables

As well as possessing the attributes outlined above, a food composition table is easier to use if the format allows ready access to the information available. This is not only true for tables in the written form but also for those in a magnetic/electronic form. For the latter, the format in which the data are made available to a user depends more on the database access software available (see section 4.4) than on the way data are stored. Although there is not one correct way of constructing a food table or nutrient database, those contemplating constructing such a table or database are urged to consult the guidelines prepared by Greenfield and Southgate.[4]

4.3.10 Food composition and nutrient databases available

When planning a nutritional epidemiology study, a decision needs to be made as to which table or database will be used. In the first instance, consideration will be given to using national tables/databases because these are more likely to include data on the foods available in the country. However, for international studies, or for those in which it is planned to compare the data with that obtained in another study, consideration may be given to using international tables/databases.

National food composition tables and nutrient data banks   Most people are aware of the tables/databases available in their own countries but are less aware of those available in other countries. A bibliography of food composition tables was published by FAO.[17] To allow people in Europe to know what information is available, a series of inventories of food composition tables and nutrient databases has been prepared by EURO-FOODS.[18,19] Details of the major food composition tables in Europe with English translations of the introductions, where appropriate, have also been prepared under the auspices of EUROFOODS.[5] The INFOODS Secretariat has prepared an international directory of food composition tables which lists tables published throughout the world.[20]

International food composition tables   At the present time, the main sources of international data on food composition are the tables published by FAO for various regions including Africa,[21] East Asia,[22] and the Near East,[23] and for amino acids.[24] A table for use in tropical countries was prepared by Platt.[25] In addition, there are regional tables such as that prepared by the Caribbean Food and Nutrition Institute[26] for use in the English-speaking Caribbean, by INCAP and ICNND for use in Central America,[27] and by West, Pepping and Temalilwa[28] for East Africa.

However, a number of initiatives are under way to make data on food composition more internationally available. In 1985, EUROFOODS carried out a study to investigate the feasibility and methodology of developing an easily accessible database of food consumption data derived from tables and databases currently existing in various European countries. The construction of such a merged database was found to be technically feasible. The problems encountered were tedious but not difficult and were related mostly to language and terminology. There are also questions related to copyright, but these are not insurmountable. Proposals for resolving the remaining issues of comparability of the different national data sets have been made and, if funds become available, it is planned to construct a series of nutrient databases for use at different levels. The first will allow food supply data at the national level to be converted to data on nutrient supply, the second will allow the same for household food consumption data, while the third is an extension of the EUROFOODS study on the feasibility of merging databases and the development of compatibility and interchangeability between national databases. It is proposed to use the EUROCODE system developed by EUROFOODS (see section 3.3.2) and the interchange proposals from INFOODS to establish compatibility between the national databases. INFOODS, the International Food Data Systems Organization, was established in 1983 under the aegis of the United Nations University to promote international cooperation in the acquisition, quality improvement, and exchange of data on the nutrient composition of foods.[29] It has convened a number of working groups, which have prepared a series of guidelines on the preparation of food composition tables and nutrient databases,[4] on compiling data for food composition databases,[30] on identifying food components in data interchange,[31] for describing foods,[8] and for exchanging data between nutrient databases,[32] and on the needs of those who use food composition tables.[33] EUROFOODS has also produced a number of documents including several which have been referred to earlier.[5,9,11,18,19,34,35,36]

Databases for non-nutrients Databases for non-nutrients have not been developed to the high degree of sophistication found with those for nutrients. Non-nutrients are a diverse group of substances including 'pseudo-nutrients', such as cholesterol, taurine, and choline; innate natural toxins, such as cyanogenic glycosides; toxins of microbial origin, such as aflatoxin; contaminants, such as polychlorinated biphenyls; and food additives, including emulsifiers, colouring agents, and flavours. As yet, few epidemiological studies have used non-nutrient databases but it can be expected that, as the number and diversity of such databases increase in the coming years, so will the number of studies based on them. There is no readily available inventory of non-nutrient databases.

4.4. CALCULATION OF NUTRIENT INTAKE FROM DATA ON FOOD INTAKE AND ON THE COMPOSITION OF FOODS

Up until about 30 years ago, the conversion of food consumption into nutrient intake had to be done manually—a laborious and time consuming task. With the advent of mainframe computers, much of the work, especially for larger surveys, could be and in fact has been done on such machines. As with many applications previously confined to mainframe computers, much of the work has now passed on to microcomputers, because of their ready accessibility and ease of use. Data on food and nutrient intake is often subsequently transferred to a mainframe computer where it can be combined with other survey data for further analysis.

4.4.1 Entry and checking of data

Before proceeding to calculate nutrient intake from data on food consumption, it is necessary to ensure that mistakes that have crept into the data set during collection, coding, aggregation, transcription, and storage, are reduced to an acceptable level. Errors associated with the collection of data on food consumption are discussed in other chapters in this book, and those associated with food composition data are discussed earlier in this chapter. Such problems will therefore not be discussed further here. Regardless of the method used for the collection of data on food consumption, consideration should be given to how the data will be entered into the computer. Suitable forms should be designed for the collection of data. These can be on paper or in a personal computer-based program that can save time and eliminate errors associated with transcription of data from paper to the computer. The use of carefully prepared forms, with information to guide those collecting the data, can reduce the chance of error during the collection of data and, if a separate process, during entry into the computer. Common errors associated with the collection of data include:

(1) recording of data on the wrong subject's form, or incorrect assignment of subject's identification number;

(2) incorrect identification of food;

(3) recording of wrong (sometimes improbable) amounts of food;

(4) omission of data on parts of meals, entire meals, or entire days.

Common errors associated with the entry of data include:

(1) reading errors, which are sometimes associated with illegible handwriting or data that have been altered at the time of collection;

(2) wrong identification numbers being assigned to subjects and entered;

(3) transcription errors often arising from inversion of digits, transposition of amount and food code or addition/omission of zero values, which give rise to incorrect amounts or food codes;

(4) omission or double entry of data on parts of meals, entire meals, or entire days;

(5) lines or segments of data are shifted, resulting in misreading of data in the data file;

(6) data are erased or lost once entered into the computer.

Because the collection and entry of data are subject to both human and machine error, procedures need to be developed to ensure that the quality of data is as high as possible. Editing and error-checking routines should be incorporated in the data entry process and subsets of data entered into the computer should be compared with the original written records. Where mistakes are found, the extent of the error should be determined, because it could involve data of the previous (or next) subject or day, or that previously (or subsequently) entered by the operator involved. In addition to such checks, frequency distributions of all amounts of food and food codes should be carried out.

4.4.2 Calculation of nutrient intake

The conversion of food consumption to nutrient intake requires computer software and a nutrient database. Great care should be taken to ensure that the software chosen meets the needs of the study adequately. There has been an explosion in the number of software packages available in recent years and there are many to choose from[37] but it is often difficult to make a choice. Apart from the usual criteria that are used to select a computer program, such as compatibility with the computer(s) available, user-friendliness, speed of operation, etc. it is necessary that the program can accept the type of data that are being collected and can produce the type of output required.

An example of how the problem can be approached is provided by the procedures we adopted in selecting a program for an international study coordinated from our laboratory. We sought a program that could accept data from dietary histories. Information on the meal when each food was eaten was required because we were interested in the interaction between various foods and nutrients. It was also necessary for the program to be able to accept and work with nutrient databases from a number of countries. As far as output was concerned, data on food groups were required, so it was necessary to have the ability to amalgamate frequencies of eating various foods into frequencies of eating groups of foods. The output of the program should also be capable of being read into statistical programs such as SPSS and SAS. Many of the centres did not have access to mainframe computers and therefore a microcomputer program operating under the most common microcomputer operating system at the time (MSDOS) was required. Up until that time, most of our experience was with mainframe computers and microcomputers operating under P/OS. Thus, it was necessary for us to choose a program that could meet our requirements and we made a decision for MicroNAP (Northern Technical Data Inc., Box 386, 905 Corydon Avenue, Winnipeg, Manitoba R3M 3V3, Canada).

Other nutritional epidemiologists will have similar problems that will need to be approached in a similar way. Sometimes it may be necessary to develop new software. If this is necessary, there must be close cooperation between the users and the developers of the software. As time goes on, the collection of dietary information will become more automated, as outlined by Arab.[38] With such automation the need for coding foods is unnecessary. It is hoped that further automation will lead to reduced costs and increased quality of the data.

4.5. FOOD GROUPS AND FOOD SCORES

Foods may be categorized into groups, based on biological characteristics, function in meals or the daily food pattern, or based on their nutrient value. In food composition tables, categorization is based mainly on biological charactristics and/or function within a meal in order to facilitate food identification and the retrieval of comparative foods. For this reason, each food group is allocated a specific code, thus allowing the amount of food in these food groups and the contribution of each food group to the intake of a specific nutrient to be assessed. In the EUROCODE (see section 4.3.1), there are 14 main food groups and there are subgroups based on species for animal foods and variety for plant foods, plus data on methods of food preparation. In some tables, particularly those for educational purposes, there are subgroups based on the content of specific nutrients such as high fat and low fat dairy products.

Some methods for assessing food consumption, in particular the dietary history and food frequency methods, enquire about the consumption of groups of foods, and not about individual foods. For example, questions on vegetable consumption are directed towards the consumption of dark green leafy vegtables, carrots and pumpkins, and other vegetables. Division of vegetables into these groups is, to some extent, based on their carotene content. Generally, foods are not classified in such a way in food composition tables or nutrient databases. Therefore, specific entries have to be created in the nutrient database to provide appropriate food composition data on such food groups. Values of food composition can be calculated from the weighted mean of the most commonly eaten foods in the food groups. This method has the disadvantage that it is less accurate and, if at a later date there is interest in other nutrients, such as trace elements, the grouping of foods used may not be appropriate. Thus, for this reason and in order to be able to repeat a study, it is important that the method of compiling the food groups is clearly documented.

When assessing nutrient intake, two types of nutrient can often be distinguished: those nutrients that are found in small quantities in a large number of foods, such as iron and most of the B vitamins, and those that are found in large quantities in a small number of foods, such as cholesterol and vitamin A. It is very difficult to estimate the intake of the latter type of nutrient by many of the conventional methods because of the large day to day variation. Thus, specific food frequency methods need to be developed (Chapter 6). Although such estimates are not generally very precise, food and nutrient scores may indicate whether average daily intake is adequate.[39]

These scores are calculated as follows:

$$\text{Food score} = \text{Frequency} \times \text{Portion size}$$

$$= \frac{\text{Weight of food consumed}}{\text{Time interval}}$$

$$= \frac{\text{Number of portions consumed}}{\text{Time interval}} \times \frac{\text{Estimated average weight}}{\text{Number of portions}}$$

$$\text{Nutrient score} = \text{Food score} \times \text{Nutrient composition}$$

$$= \frac{\text{Weight of nutrient consumed}}{\text{Time interval}}$$

$$= \frac{\text{Weight of food consumed}}{\text{Time interval}} \times \frac{\text{Nutrient content of food}}{\text{Unit weight of food}}$$

Generally, the time interval chosen is 1 day, 1 week or 1 month.

4.6 CONCLUDING REMARKS

The disadvantage of using food composition tables and nutrient databases is that each value in the table/database is the average of a value for a limited number of samples of each food. As explained in section 4.3.5, sampling errors are large, especially for mixed dishes and meals. These errors contribute to the total error and variation in results from dietary intake studies, but as long as no measure of spread is given for values in food composition tables, it will not be possible to calculate what proportion of random error is attributable to variation in food composition. This

Food consumption tables

Table 4.2 Differences between the composition of a one-day experimental diet determined by analysis of a duplicate portion and by the use of food composition tables[*]

	Analysed a	Calculated c	Difference c−a	Difference c−a in %	Difference c−a in energy %
Energy (kJ)	8895	9050	155	1.7	
Protein (g)	60	64.9	4.9	8.1	0.5
Fat (g)	103	110.7	7.7	7.5	2.6
Carbohydrate (g)	233	220.0	−13.0	−5.6	−3.2
Mono- and disaccharides (g)	108	103.1	−4.9	−4.5	−1.2

[*] Unpublished data cited in Van Staveren and Burema.[41]

variation differs from food to food and from nutrient to nutrient. It is well known that differences in water content are the main cause of variation in the content of other nutrients. Thus, data on the nutrient composition of foods containing large amounts of water are always subject to large variation. The least variable nutrient is probably protein and the other proximate constitutents. Table 4.2 presents data in which analysed and calculated values for energy and proximate constituents of an experimental diet are compared. The data indicates that the differences are all within 10 per cent, which is not sufficient for a metabolic ward study but, as the differences are generally consistent, data derived from using food composition tables are probably adequate for epidemiological studies aimed at classifying individuals or groups of individuals on the basis of their nutrient intake.

Variation in the vitamin content of foods is generally much greater than that for macronutrients. Therefore, an assessment of the vitamin content of a diet based on data in food composition tables/nutrient databases is, for most vitamins, not very reliable. At best, classification of intake into high and low is all that can be done.

For minerals, tables/databases are also of limited value, although calcium may be an exception because the main source of calcium in many cultures is milk and milk products, and the calcium content of milk products is relatively constant.

The situation for minerals is complicated by the large variation in the mineral content of foods and also by the wide variation in the biological availabilty of minerals in different diets and in different people. The whole subject of bioavailability is one that, as yet, has hardly been addressed.

Thus it can be concluded that food composition tables/nutrient databases can be of great value in epidemiological research, but knowledge of how they are constructed and their limitations is necessary to make intelligent use of them. In general, it is better to use food composition tables compiled for local use. However, for international studies, data on food composition should be comparable and the efforts of organizations such as INFOODS and EUROFOODS are directed towards this goal.

REFERENCES

1. Thomas, R. U., Rutlege, M. M., Beach, E. F., Moyer, E. Z., Drummond, M. C., Miller, S., Robinson, A. R., Miller, O. N., Coryell, M. N., and Macy, I. G. (1950). Nutritional status of children. XII. Accuracy of calculated intakes of food components with respect to analytical values. *J. Am. Diet. Ass*, **26**: 889–96.
2. Leitch, I. and Aitken, F. C. (1950). Technique and interpretation of dietary surveys. *Nutr. Abstr. Rev.*, **19**: 507–25.
3. Southgate, D. A. T. (1974). *Guidelines for the preparation of tables of food composition*, p. 57ff. Karger, Basel.
4. Greenfield, H. and Southgate, D. A. T. (1991). *Guidelines for the production, management and use of food composition data*, in press. (Prepublication draft available from INFOODS Secretariat.)
5. Arab, L., Wittler, M., and Schettler, G. (1987). *European food composition tables in translation*, pp. viii and 155. Springer-Verlag. Heidelberg.
6. Southgate, D. A. T. and Durnin, J. V. G. A. (1970). Caloric conversion factors: an experimental evaluation of the factors used in the calculation of the energy value of human diets. *Br. J. Nutr.*, **24**: 517–35.
7. Southgate, D. A. T. (1985). Criteria to be used for acceptance of data in nutrient data bases. *Ann. Nut. Metab.*, **29**: Suppl. 1: 47–53.
8. Truswell, A. S., Bateson, D., Madafiglio, K., Pennington, J. A. T., Rand, W. M., and Klensin, J. C. (1991). INFOODS guidelines for describing foods: a systematic approach to describing foods to facilitate international exchange of food composition data. *J. Food Comp. Anal.*, in press.
9. Hollman, P. C. H. and Katan, M. B. (1988). Bias and error in the determination of common macronutrients in foods: an interlaboratory trial. *J. Am. Diet. Assoc.*, **88**: 556–63.
10. Greenfield, H. and Southgate, D. A. T. (1985). A pragmatic approach to production of good quality food composition data. *ASEAN Food J.*, **1**: 47–54.
11. Meyer, B., Van Oosten-Van der Goes, H. J. C., Van Staveren, W. A., and West, C. E. (1988). Missing values in European food composition tables and nutrient data bases: preliminary results of a survey. *Food Sci. Nutr.*, **42F**: 29–34.
12. Paul, A. A. and Southgate, D. A. T. (1978). *McCance and Widdowson's the composition of foods*, fourth edn. Her Majesty's Stationery Office, London.
13. USDA. (1976). *Composition of foods, Agricultural Handbook No. 8*. United States Department of Agriculture, Washington.
14. NEVO. (1989). NEVO tabel: Nederlands voedingsstoffenbestand. NEVO (Stichting Nederlands Voedingsstoffenbestand), CIVO-instituten, Zeist and Voorlichtingsbureau voor de Voedings, Gravenhage.

15. Bergström, L. (1985). NLG project (Nutrient losses and gains in the preparation of foods) report. *Food Sci. Nutr.*, **42F**: 8–12.
16. Southgate, D. A. T. (1989). Bioavailability: conceptual issues and significance for the nutritional sciences. In Kim Wha Young (ed.) *Proceedings of the 14th International Congress of Nutrition*, pp. 777–80. The 14th ICN organizing committee, Seoul.
17. FAO. (1975). *Food composition tables: updated annotated bibliography*. FAO, Rome.
18. EUROFOODS. (1985). Review of food composition tables and nutrient data banks in Europe. *Ann. Nut. Metab.*, **29**, Suppl. 1: 11–45.
19. West, C. E. (1990). Inventory of European food composition tables and nutrient database systems. National Food Administration, Uppsala.
20. Heintze, D., Klensin, J. C. and Rand, W. M. (1988). *International directory of food composition tables*, second edn. INFOODS Secretariat, Massachusetts Institute of Technology, Cambridge, MA.
21. Wu Leung, W. T., Busson F. and Jardin C. (1968). *Food composition table for use in Africa*. US Dept. of Health, Education and Welfare, Bethesda, MD and FAO, Rome.
22. Wu Leung, W. T., Butrum R.. R. and Chang F. H. (1972). *Food composition table for use in East Asia*. U. S. Dept of Health, Education and Welfare Bethesda, MD, and FAO, Rome.
23. Pollachi, W. McHargue J. S. and Perloff B. P. (1982). *Food composition tables for the Near East*. FAO Food and Nutrition Paper No. 26. FAO, Rome and USDA, Washington.
24. Pollachi, W., McHargue J. S. and Perloff B. P. (1972). *Amino acid content of foods and biological data of proteins*, second edn. FAO, Rome.
25. Platt, B. S. (1962). *Tables of representative values of foods commonly eaten in tropical countries*. Medical Research Council Special Report Series No. 302. Her Majesty's Stationery Office. London.
26. Caribbean Food and Nutrition Institute. (1974). *Food composition tables for use in the English-speaking Caribbean*. Caribbean Food and Nutrition Institute, Kingston, Jamaica.
27. Wu Leung, W. T. and Flores, M. (1961). *INCAP-ICNND* food composition table for use in Latin America. INCAP, Guatemala and Bethesda, MD: National Institutes of Health.
28. West, C. E., Pepping, F. and Temalilwa, C. R. (1988). *The composition of foods commonly eaten in East Africa*. Wageningen Agricultural University, Wageningen.
29. Rand, W. M. and Young, V. R. (1984). Report of a planning conference concerning an international network of food data systems (INFOODS). *Am. J. Clin. Nutr.*, **30**: 144–51.
30. Rand. W. M., Pennington, J. A. T., Murphy, S. P., and Klensin, J. C. (1988) *Compiling data for food composition databases*. INFOODS Working Paper. INFOODS, Cambridge MA.
31. Klensin, J. C., Feskanich, D., Lin, V., Truswell, A. S. and Southgate, D. A. T. (1988). *Identification of food components for INFOODS data interchange*. INFOODS Working Paper INFOODS/IS N40, Cambridge, MA.
32. Klensin, J. C. (1988). International interchange language for food composition

data. Working Papers INFOODS/IS N6 and N16. INFOODS, Cambridge MA.

33. Rand, W. M., Windham, C. T., Wyse, B. W., and Young, V. R. (1988). *Food composition data: a user's perspective*. United Nations University, Tokyo.
34. West, C. E. (ed.) (1985). Eurofoods: towards compatibility of nutrient data banks in Europe. *Ann. Nut. Metab.*, **29**, Suppl. 1: 1–72.
35. Fox, K. and Stockley, L. (1988). EUROFOODS: Proceedings of the Second Workshop. *Food Sciences and Nutrition*, **42F**: 1–82.
36. Becker, W. and Danfors, S. (1990). *4th Eurofoods Meeting May 31–June 3. 1989. Uppsala. Sweden: Proceedings*. Swedish National Food Administration, Uppsala.
37. University of Washington Computer Services. (1989). *Computer Programs and Databases in the Field of Nutrition*. University of Washington Computer Services. Seattle WA.
38. Arab, L. (1988). Analyses, presentation, and interpretation of results. In M. E. Cameron and W. A. van Staveren (eds). *Manual on Methodology for Food Consumption Studies*. Oxford University Press, Oxford.
39. Bazzarre, T. and Myers, M. (1979). The collection of food intake data in cancer epidemiology studies. *Nutr. Cancer*, **5**: 201–14.
40. Van der Haar, F. and Kromhout, D. (1985). Food intake, nutritional anthropometry and blood chemical parameters in three selected Dutch school children populations. *Meded. Landbouwhogeshool Wageningen*, (1985), **5**: 78–9.
41. Van Staveren, W. A. and Burema, J. (1985). Food consumption surveys: frustrations and expectations. *Näringsforskning*, **29**: 38–42.

5. Use of existing nutritional data and household-based surveys

Measures of exposure relevant to nutritional epidemiology are often collected in the course of monitoring food consumption or health for non-epidemiological purposes. As a consequence, there are large bodies of data that are sufficient, in their own right, for epidemiological analysis or that provide the basis for investigations for which only a portion of the data need then be collected. For example, the National Food Survey provides detailed information on food acquisition at the household level, and this has been used in conjunction with existing health statistics to examine the aetiology of appendicitis.[1] To have collected this data *de novo* would have been a long and costly exercise.

Data available at national level are discussed in Chapter 10; this chapter focuses on data available in Britain collected at both household and individual level by the Department of Health (DoH) and the Ministry of Agriculture, Fisheries and Food (MAFF). It also discusses the collection of food consumption data at the household level, as this can be more economical than individual surveys (See Chapter 6) for obtaining information for ecological studies. It also opens possibilities for assessing diet–disease relationships in a number of different subgroups within the population if the distribution of food and nutrients within households can be properly assessed.

The use of existing health data is discussed elsewhere.[2]

Household data and the National Food Survey

M. Nelson

5.1 INTRODUCTION

Aggregate data based on surveys of groups of people rather than individuals can be used in ecological, geographical, and community trial studies to assess diet–disease relationships. The unit in which this data is collected is usually the household, although information can be usefully collected at the institutional level.[3] These studies often shed light on the diversity of food consumption patterns between communities at far less cost than individual surveys. They can also provide opportunities to aggregate data along regional or socio-economic lines. Such studies are often carried out by government or other bodies for non-epidemiological purposes, but can provide a ready-made database with epidemiological applications. Their principal drawback is that the relationships between diet and disease cannot be assessed at the level of the individual. They are therefore more appropriate for hypothesis-generating studies rather than for testing specific hypotheses concerning the causation of disease in particular individuals (see Chapter 10 for more detailed discussion of ecological studies).

Many household food consumption studies focus on economic rather than nutritional aspects of diet.[4-6] This is clearly not adequate for most epidemiological studies, in which the minimum requirement is an estimate of the quantity of food available for consumption. To be of use in nutritional epidemiology, therefore, studies of this nature must have as their basis the quantitative measurement of food acquired for consumption over a given time period, and the number of people sharing the food must be known, so that standardized estimates of food availability can be calculated for purposes of comparison between groups. Questions about the distribution of food within the group, and the importance of the age structure in comparing groups are discussed later in the chapter.

5.2 TECHNIQUES, USES, AND LIMITATIONS

Four principal methods of assessment have been used: food accounts, inventories, household recall, and list-recall.[3] They vary in respondent and interviewer burden, and each has its advantages according to the degree of accuracy required at the household level, the degree of literacy and numeracy within the population, and the extent to which food is consumed outside the household or institution food supply. The bulk of this section of the chapter is devoted to a discussion of the National Food Survey, a food account survey conducted annually in Great Britain, but other techniques are described.

5.2.1 Food account method

This method is based upon the household. The main respondent (housewife, or person responsible for food purchasing and/or preparation), or the interviewer, keeps a detailed record of the quantities of food entering the household, including purchases, food from allotments or gardens, gifts, payments in kind and other sources.

In its most widely used form, no attempt is made to assess changes in stocks (see section 5.2.2). The method assumes that, within a given category of household composition, over a sufficient number of households, there is no change in the *average* levels of food stocks, although it is recognized that some households will acquire more food than they consume over the survey period, while others will acquire less and use existing stocks to make up for any shortfalls in acquisition. Efforts are made to estimate the proportion of the diet consumed from outside the household food supply, but usually no attempt is made to measure the food consumption directly. It is generally assumed that the quality of the diet obtained away from home is similar in nature to that consumed within the home. The nutrient content of the home diet can be estimated by using appropriate nutrient conversion tables and allowing for preparation losses and waste, and again, that proportion of the diet obtained from outside the home is assumed to have a composition similar to the home food supply.

The National Food Survey   The Household Food Consumption and Expenditure Survey (The National Food Survey (NFS)) has been conducted annually in Great Britain for half a century.[7-10] The Survey was begun in 1940 to monitor the nutritional quality of the diets of urban working class households[8] in order to assess the value of the wartime food policy, but by 1950 it had been extended to cover virtually all sectors of the population. In its original form it included a larder inventory (see section 5.2.2), but this was dropped in 1952, and the survey has continued essentially unchanged since then. Reports are published annually and provide an excellent unbroken record of British food habits since 1950. The published results afford opportunities to conduct time trend, [11,12] social class,[13] and regional[14] analyses in relation to epidemiological questions, and some methodological issues in its use have been discussed by Derry and Buss.[15]

The respondents are selected by the Office of Population Censuses and Surveys in a three-stage cluster sampling scheme, and the survey itself is carried out by a private market research company. In the first stage, 52 local authority districts are selected in proportion to their population to provide a representative sample of areas covering Wales, Scotland, Greater London, and eight further regions, balanced according to the distribution of the population density (rural, semirural, and urban). At the second stage, 16 postal sectors within each of the districts are selected, to provide clusters that facilitate the visiting of households by the interviewer. At the final stage, 18 individual addresses are selected within each sector. Response rates average about 55 per cent (65 per cent of households actually contacted), and there is no replacement of non-responders. The effect of non-response was examined in a study[16] in which it was shown that, when the results were reweighted to the characteristics of the entire sample (based on census data describing the non-responding households), the national averages for food and nutrient consumption remained essentially unchanged. The effect of differential non-response by income group was not assessed.

Method of recording

Households are recruited 'on the doorstep' by specially trained interviewers who are provided with a list of addresses (no preliminary letter is sent). The respondent is asked to complete a questionnaire, and to keep a record for seven days of the description, quantity, and cost (if any) of all food items entering the home for human consumption. Sweets, chocolates, and alcohol are excluded from the record as they are often purchased by individual household members, outside the respondent's knowledge, and soft drinks, although recorded, are not included in the final analyses of cost or nutrients. Data on the national consumption of these items are available.[7] Free food from employers, gardens, and allotments is included, although only that portion of garden produce actually consumed (not harvested) is recorded. Menus are recorded at each of four meals (breakfast, lunch, tea, and supper), together with the number of household members and visitors consuming the meal. This provides information with which to cross-check the food acquisition record, as well as data on the age and sex of people consuming the food that is used subsequently in estimating the dietary adequacy of the home food supply. Over 200 separate food categories are coded.

Nutritional estimates

MAFF has determined the approximate nutritional content for each food or food group coded, based primarily on McCance and Widdowson's *The Composition of Foods*[17] but also from additional unpublished food composition data, information from manufacturers, and, for composite groups (e.g. 'frozen cereal convenience foods'), an estimate of the contribution of the different foods to the nutrient content of the food group. These data are updated annually to take advantage of new analytical data and to keep up with the changing profile of food purchases. The nutrient conversion factors allow for inedible material such as bones and potato skins, but not for household wastage.

The nutritional results are calculated in two ways. In the first, the total nutrient available within a given household type is divided by the total number of household members in the survey within that category, ignoring the presence of visitors. This is expressed as nutrient available per head per day. No account is taken of waste or food eaten away from home. In the second method, the nutrient available is compared with the Recommended Daily Amounts (RDA).[18] This takes into account, within each household composition category, the age and sex of those actually consuming meals from the household food supply (including visitors), and also the proportion of food eaten away from home. A 10 per cent allowance is made for waste.

Presentation of results

Results are presented as average consumption of food (ounces per person per week, or pint equivalents of milk, milk products and cream, or number of eggs); as average nutrient availability (nutrient per person per day); and as a percentage of the RDA. Additional tables show nutrient density of the diets (Nutrients per 1000 kcals) and the percentage of food energy derived from protein, fat, and carbohydrate. Nutrients reported include dietary fibre and saturated, mono- and polyunsaturated fatty acids.

Because the survey collects data on the socio-economic background of each household, it is possible to aggregate the data in a wide variety of ways. Within the annual report, therefore, results are presented not only for national averages but also according to region, household income group, population density, age of housewife, etc. Moreover, since 1979, the basic data of food acquisitions plus socio-economic and demographic information—but not nutrient intakes—has been stored on magnetic tape at the University of Essex Data Archive. These are available for research purposes for a modest handling fee and royalty. Full documentation on the survey methods, coding, etc., is provided.

Strengths and limitations

The principal strengths of the NFS are its availability and continuity. It is unique in providing an up-to-date record of consumption patterns of representative samples of the British population stretching back in an unbroken record for 40 years. It is accessible and cheap for analysing food and nutrient consumption trends in epidemiological studies. With the availability of the data on magnetic tape, detailed geographical[19] or income group[20] comparisons can be undertaken.

The limitations of the NFS deserve close attention, so that misinterpretation of results based on its analysis can be avoided.

1. Validity of the method

Two surveys that have compared the average level of purchases with average consumption, one in elderly single women[21] and one in families with two adults and two or three children,[22] suggest that the survey tends to stimulate overpurchasing, i.e. foods are purchased in excess of requirements during the survey week. For many groups of households, it is likely that the degree of over-purchasing is roughly equal to the amount consumed outside the home, so that when average food or nutrient availability is calculated, it approximates the actual level of consumption (less any waste). However, the over-purchasing appears to be greater in households on low incomes[23] and amongst the elderly,[21] so comparisons between income or age groups are likely to be less reliable than those between regions (assuming no major demographic differences), or over time within given groups of households of a consistent socio-economic mix.

2. The data provide information on households, not individuals.

In the calculation of dietary adequacy, the NFS tacitly assumes that nutrient is distributed to individuals within households according to the RDAs, but this is likely to overstate the dietary adequacy of some groups (such as women and young girls) and understate it in others (men and boys).[24] Alternatives to the RDAs can be used for estimating nutrient distribution within groups of families in epidemiological studies,[24,25] but the reliability of these methods needs further assessment.

3. The data must be aggregated over groups of households.

Because no measure is made of changes in larder stocks, the results for a single household over one week are unlikely to represent the usual consumption levels in that household. This means that households cannot be selected for analysis of disease risk to individuals within the household on the basis of high or low consumption of a particular food or nutrient. The NFS queries the reliability of results for groups of fewer than 20 households, and any analysis of small groups should ensure that the grouping of the households does not depend in any way on the apparent level of purchases (or expenditure).[20]

4. The data are confined to food brought into the home.

Although the analyses of nutrient adequacy take into account the amount of food consumed outside the home, this amount is probably an underestimate, because foods eaten between meals are not taken into account.[23] Time trend analysis and comparisons between large regions are likely to be less subject to differential misclassification. However, when comparing smaller groups of households or assessing differences between household types, it is sensible to ensure that any differences observed are not due to differences in the proportion of the diet consumed away from home.

5. The NFS results do not include sweets, chocolates, alcohol, soft drinks, and vitamin and mineral supplements.

Apart from the supplements, these foods can be regarded primarily as sources of energy and, if food energy deficiency was a problem, it would be likely to become apparent from medical evidence long before it was reflected in the results of the NFS. If comparisons between groups include an analysis of energy, fat, or carbohydrate, attempts must be made to ensure that these missing items are unlikely to provide a significantly different proportion of energy or nutrient in the different groups. The survey is, therefore, arguably better for monitoring trends in protein, dietary fibre, mineral, and vitamin consumption, taking into account the limitations of the food tables (see Chapter 4).

Conclusions regarding the National Food Survey

The NFS is a valuable epidemiological resource unique in Britain. It warrants careful use to avoid falling into potential traps of misinterpretation. Several aspects of the NFS results need further investigation, such as the contribution of sweets, soft drinks, alcohol, and foods eaten away from home to total consumption; and the likely distribution of foods and nutrients within households so that more extensive use of the data can be made in descriptive epidemiological studies.

The survey is carried out continually throughout the year and, in previous years, special studies have been undertaken in relation to health issues when these were warranted (e.g. milk consumption in children and mothers, etc.)[7] The possibility of collecting additional data utilizing the NFS in this way can be explored with MAFF in relation to specific hypotheses that are testable using data collected at the household level.

5.2.2 Inventory method

The inventory method is similar in nature to the food account method in that respondents are asked to keep records of all foods coming into the house. In addition, a larder inventory is carried out at the beginning and end of the survey period. This was the method used by the NFS prior to 1952, including the first study on urban working class households.[8]

5.2.3 Comparison of food account and food inventory methods

Both methods are appropriate to communities in which a high proportion of food is purchased rather than home-produced, and where the level of literacy is high. Where the interviewer has regular access to the respondent, it may be possible to obtain information (by recall) concerning the amounts of foods removed from stores.

The principal advantage of the food inventory over the food account method is that it provides a direct measure of the amount of food and nutrient available for consumption within a single household. In contrast to the food account method, this allows single households to be identified on the basis of the nutrient available to the household members, and so to correlate food or nutrient availability (making appropriate assumptions concerning distribution within the household) with disease occurrence within the household.

Most household surveys cover a period of one week. This is likely to be associated in the food account method with an initial reaction to 'stock up' on items.[21,22,26] This can be taken into account in the food inventory method by subtracting those foods that have been acquired but not consumed from the total available. However, the food inventory draws to respondents' attention items in the larder that would otherwise have remained unused, and therefore distorts the purchasing pattern.[3,27]

5.2.4 Household record

In the household record method, the foods available for consumption (whether raw or processed) are weighed, or estimated in household measures, allowing for preparation waste (discarded outer leaves, peel, trimmed fat, etc.). Any food consumed by visitors is estimated and subtracted from the total, and an allowance should also be made for food waste (food prepared but not consumed), either by collecting the waste directly (which is likely to underestimate the true amount[28]), or by estimating the proportion of the total prepared food believed to be wasted.

The technique is often a combination of recall and record and a recommended approach has been outlined.[3] Briefly, the interviewer calls in the morning, establishes the household composition, and asks the respondent to recall the quantities of food used to prepare breakfast. The foods to be used in the preparation of lunch can then be weighed or recorded in household measures. An afternoon interview allows the waste at lunch to be estimated, and the foods for the evening meal to be measured and recorded.

Uses and limitations　The technique is well suited to populations in which a substantial proportion of the diet is home-produced rather than preprocessed. It lends itself to use in populations where the level of literacy is variable or low, because the number of visits to each household can easily be tailored to obtain the necessary degree of detail. Because the technique provides a direct measure of food available for consumption and makes no assumptions about changes in food stocks, it can be used, like the inventory method, to identify houses with particular consumption characteristics (subject, of course, to a knowledge of the day to day or week to week variability in consumption within households).

As with other household food assessment methods, no information is obtained concerning the distribution of foods to individuals within the household, nor about consumption of foods outside the home. As it is more likely to be used in less developed countries where literacy is low, there may be seasonal variations in consumption that need to be taken into account. This is especially important in epidemiological studies where regional comparisons are undertaken, or where it is proposed to examine diet–disease relationships within households.

5.2.5 List-recall method

This is a structured survey in which the respondent is asked to recall the amount and cost of food obtained for household use over a given period, usually one week. In addition to food purchases and acquisitions, it takes into account the use of food. It can therefore be used to provide an estimate of food costs and, for nutritional epidemiological purposes, net household consumption of both foods and nutrients. The technique has been used in the United States Food Consumption Surveys.[29]

Uses and limitations The technique is well suited to populations in which most food is purchased rather than home-produced. It is relatively quick and cheap, as it requires only a single interview. It is helpful to notify the respondent of the study in advance, so that he or she may keep records of purchases (such as supermarket receipts) to aid the recall, but this may have the effect of distorting food consumption patterns. The information on food use helps to overcome problems about movement of foods into and out of stock, but distortions in recall, which are characteristic of any memory-based survey, will inevitably influence the outcome, although perhaps less so than in individual surveys. Questions about foods eaten away from home, consumption of food by visitors, and distribution of nutrients within families persist.

Studies on the validity and reliability of list-recall surveys have been reviewed by Burk and Pao.[30] These suggest that list-recall methods give values some 20 per cent lower than inventory methods. On the other hand, comparison of the 1965–6 United States household food consumption survey results with food disappearance data suggest that the list-recall gives values some 5–10 per cent higher. This lack of consistency in comparative validity suggests that substantially more work needs to be done to characterize the nature of the error in list-recall surveys.

5.3 USING HOUSEHOLD SURVEYS IN EPIDEMIOLOGICAL STUDIES

Household food consumption surveys provide a powerful, economical tool for obtaining information about the food consumption characteristics of a wide cross-section of the population. Where survey data have already been collected (as in the National Food Survey), the costs are enormously reduced and relate solely to the collection of non-nutritional information and analysis of the data.

Household food surveys fail in two major areas: completeness of data, and knowledge of distribution of food and nutrient within households. In addition, little is known about the within-household repeatability of measurements. It is worth considering ways in which these problems can be addressed.

Lack of completeness in household surveys relates to foods not recorded, foods obtained and eaten away from home, food consumed by visitors, and waste. Where data have already been collected, as in the NFS, the investigator is restricted in interpretation of data by the assumptions inherent in the survey design. However, if there is the opportunity to undertake a household survey *de novo*, then it may be possible to collect data on *all* food consumed, not just those items under the purview of the respondent. This requires a record from every individual within the household, in household measures, of foods obtained and eaten away from home and of foods, such as chocolate, sweets, soft drinks, and alcoholic beverages, not included in the record of household food acquisitions or consumption. For children, the responsibility for the record would have to lie with an adult. Information concerning the consumption of food by visitors should also be obtained, again, if possible, in household measures. This information, particularly in conjunction with an inventory or household record method, will substantially improve the quality of the data for relatively little effort on the part of the respondents. It also enables a more accurate calculation of the proportion of food in the diet obtained from outside the household food supply, which, for epidemiological purposes, would be of value in interpreting other surveys in which this information has been estimated. The data resulting from the introduction of such measurements would need to be compared with the outcomes from other, more established, techniques. The matter of waste remains a thorny one and, until less invasive techniques are established, we will have to rely on existing estimates.[22,28]

The other major problem with household surveys is the inability to determine the exact distribution of consumption within individual households. It is clear that nutrient distribution is not in accordance with the RDAs,[24] and the RDAs provide no clues as to the distribution of foods within households. Nelson *et al.*[31] describe a 'semi-weighed' technique that has addressed this problem by recording the diet of every household member individually. It has been used to establish patterns of distribution of nutrient intake in different age–sex groups in households with two adults and two or three children.[3] While it is too labour intensive to consider using in a large epidemiological study, it could be effectively carried out in a subset of households from a larger survey in which household food acquisition data were being obtained. This would then allow a more accurate estimate of distribution of food consumption and nutrient intakes within the whole survey sample. This could considerably enhance the value of a geographical study, for instance, by allowing diet–disease comparisons to be made in a number of age–sex subgroups, rather than in the population as a whole.

One final point worth mentioning is that virtually no studies have been carried out to assess the ideal period for recording household food data, nor to assess the within-household variability in purchases or food and nutrient distribution. Most studies in industrialized countries obtain data from each household covering a period of one week. The variability of nutrient intake, and especially the variability of food consumption, means that for a given period of recording, the error in the estimate of intake or consumption will differ substantially between nutrients or foods. For a given difference in intake or consumption between groups of households, the ability to demonstrate a significant risk of disease in relation to diet is inversely related to the size of the within-household variability. New nutritritional epidemiological studies based on households should attempt to assess within- as well as between-household variance in consumption or intake. Any analysis that includes estimates of the distribution of foods or nutrients within households should also consider the errors associated with such estimates.

The generation and use of nutritional data by the Department of Health

R. W. Wenlock

5.4 INTRODUCTION

Although Boyd Orr had carried out dietary surveys in Great Britain before the Second World War,[32] the first large scale surveys of the nutritional condition of various age and sex groups in Britain made by the Ministry of Health were carried out between 1948 and 1951[33] when food rationing was still in force. The state of nutrition in populations in subsequent years could, to some extent, be inferred from running indices, such as the National Food Survey, but these indices suffer from a number of limitations as indicated earlier in the chapter; for example, it is not possible to separate age and sex groups. Accordingly, in 1961, the Chief Medical Officer's Committee on Medical and Nutritional Aspects of Food Policy, now the Committee on Medical Aspects of Food Policy (COMA), advised that a programme of nationwide dietary surveys of various population groups should be undertaken. The evolution of this programme over the next 28 years is described below. The data generated by these surveys were used by the Department of Health and Social Security (DHSS) in assessing aspects of social policy. Some of the key findings and aspects of dietary survey methodologies are discussed.

5.5 FOOD AND NUTRITION SURVEILLANCE

The first of these dietary surveys was carried out on preschool children under the auspices of working groups specially convened by COMA for this purpose. However, when the Government announced changes in 1971 to the provision of welfare milk for pregnant women and preschool children, and of school milk and school meals, there was concern that these changes might have a detrimental affect on the nutritional status of children. Accordingly, COMA was asked to consider the best method of assessing the changes and to make recommendations as were deemed necessary. It convened a standing Subcommittee on Nutritional Surveillance. The Subcommittee's terms of reference were:

1. To advise COMA of the steps that should be taken to detect the effects upon the nutritional state of the community of changes that became effective from April 1971, in the arrangements for the provision of welfare milk, school milk and school meals, at a time when any harmful effects of the changes are likely to be mild and reversible.

2. To consider the long term arrangements that would be required for the prediction and assessment of the nutritional effects of changes in relevant Government policy, whether social, economic, or other.

The responsibility for overseeing surveys recommended by COMA was taken on by this subcommittee, which had subsequently presented three reports to COMA.[34–36] By 1971, the interest of COMA was focused on studies of the elderly but in 1973, following the setting up of the COMA Subcommittee on Nutritional Surveillance, COMA's attention was turned towards monitoring the growth of children. In 1982, major changes in Government policy led the Subcommittee to recommend another national survey of diets. Prior to 1980, the meals provided by schools in Britain had to conform to prescribed nutritional standards. The 1980 Education Act released Local Authorities from this requirement and left them free to decide the form, content, and price of school meals. In the debate on this Act, Ministers agreed that the effect of the new school arrangements and the proposals of the Bill would be monitored. The proposals of the Bill were referred to the Subcommittee on Nutritional Surveillance, who recommended that a 7-day weighed measurement of food intake, together with a study of the heights and weights, of a nationally representative sample of school children should be carried out. This was done in 1983.

During the period since 1984 the dietary surveys carried out by Government have been commissioned by the Ministry of Agriculture, Fisheries and Food (MAFF). The National Food Survey, described previously, has been MAFF's main tool for assessing diets in Britain. However, in 1984 a Working Party on Nutrients was convened under the MAFF Steering Group on Food Surveillance. Its terms of reference, given below, were designed to include advising on dietary surveys:

1. To identify areas in which information on the content and availability of nutrients in foods is required to ensure that the nation's food supplies and diets can be adequately monitored; to review programmes for maintaining *McCance and Widdowson's 'The Composition of Foods'* and the Ministry's nutrient databank; to assess priorities, and to propose means of obtaining information.

2. To propose or, when requested, advise on planning of dietary surveys for the Steering Group of Food Surveillance in order to determine normal and extreme intakes of dietary constituents in groups of the population; and to oversee the Total Diet Study.

3. To advise other committees and Departments as appropriate.

The Working Party has been responsible for several studies of population groups since 1984. The details have been published and a summary of the survey programme has been published in the Report of the Working Party.[37]

In 1984, another development in Government food policy was brought about by the publication by COMA of its Report on Diet and Cardiovascular Disease.[38] Along with recommendations to the population to reduce total fat and saturated fatty acid intakes it also contained a recommendation to Government on research into the identification of risk factors. In 1985, in response to this, the expertise of OPCS, MAFF, and DHSS in carrying out surveys was brought together to carry out a dietary and nutritional survey of British adults. The fieldwork was carried out in 1986 and 1987 and covered a nationally representative sample of people aged 16 to 64 years. A full 7-day weighed account of all food and drink consumed was obtained from about 2200 respondents. In addition, anthropometric and blood pressure measurements were made and blood and urine samples were collected and analysed. The dietary aspects of this survey were carried out under the auspices of the MAFF Working Party on Nutrients, while the health aspects were carried out under the auspices of the COMA Subcommittee on Nutritional Surveillance. The survey expertise of OPCS is now available to both in the future. The results of this joint project will be of direct relevance to the policies of both MAFF and the Department of Health. A report was published in 1990.[54]

By 1987, it was clear to COMA that developments since 1971 had made the terms of reference of the Subcommittee on Nutritional Surveillance out of date. The following new terms of reference were given and the responsibility for future dietary surveys and other types of nutritional surveillance for COMA and the Department of Health were subsumed within them:

To advise COMA on the nutritional implications of changes in society and of proposed changes in legislation or Government provisions, having due regard to the responsibilities of other Government Departments and COMA Panels, Subcommittees and Working Groups and to advise and oversee nutritional and anthropometric, biochemical and other studies recommended by COMA, and to collaborate with other Government Departments where appropriate.

5.6 SURVEYS OF PRESCHOOL CHILDREN

The following sections describe in detail two of the dietary surveys carried out by the Ministry of Health and the Department of Health and Social Security (now the Department of Health), on the recommendation of COMA and its Subcommittee on Nutritional Surveillance; and the implications of several other studies are discussed. A number of studies of the growth of children and other anthropometric studies have been carried out under the auspices of the Subcommittee but, as they deal with aspects of nutritional status other than dietary measurements, they are outside the scope of this chapter. Details are given in the Reports of the Subcommittee.[34-36] A list of all the dietary surveys carried out since 1963 by the British Government is given in Table 5.1. None of these studies was designed as an epidemiological tool but all were commissioned to examine aspects of food policy or as part of the Government's Nutritional Surveillance Programme.

5.6.1 A pilot survey of the nutrition of young children in 1963

To implement the original recommendation of COMA in 1961, a pilot survey of 429 children between the ages of 9 months and 5 years was carried out by the then Ministry of Health between May and September 1963. Details of the methodology and the results of this survey were published by the Ministry of Health.[39] Much was learned from the pilot study, both with regard to sampling technique and to the problems of a dietary study in the field.

Experience from the pilot study showed that it was not necessary to stratify the sample by age to obtain approximately equal numbers in each age group. Nevertheless, if it was deemed necessary to study, for example, nutrient intakes and family size, then some means of stratification should be devised if efficiency and economy were to be combined. It was estimated that not less than 200 subjects were likely to be required in any one family size category.

Table 5.1 Dietary surveys carried out by the British Government

Sample description	Date	Commissioning department	Numbers	Reference
Pilot survey of children aged 9 months to 5 years	1963	Ministry of Health	434 children	Ministry of Health, 1968[39]
Survey of pre-schoolchildren, nationally representative	1967/68	Department of Health and Social Security	673 boys 648 girls	DHSS, 1975[40]
Survey of primary schoolchildren Bristol, Croydon, Sheffield	1971	Department of Health and Social Security	163 boys 158 girls	Darke et al., 1980[43]
Survey of secondary schoolchildren Newcastle-upon-Tyne	1970	Department of Health and Social Security	93 boys 85 girls	Darke et al., 1980[43]
Survey of secondary schoolchildren Birmingham	1971	Department of Health and Social Security	390 boys 402 girls	Darke et al., 1980[43]
Survey of pregnant women 39 areas in Great Britain	1967/68	Department of Health and Social Security	435 women 6–7 months pregnant	Darke et al., 1980[43]
Survey of the elderly 4 areas in England, 2 areas in Scotland	1967/68	Department of Health and Social Security	396 men 431 women 65 years and over	DHSS, 1972[42]
Follow up survey of the elderly survivors of 1967/68 survey	1972/73	Department of Health and Social Security	169 men 196 women 69 years and over	DHSS, 1979[45]

Survey	Date	Organisation	Subjects	Reference
Follow-up survey of the elderly survivors of 1967/68 survey	1977/78	Department of Health and Social Security	85 women 69 men 75 years and over	Unpublished
Survey of the elderly, nationally representative	1973/74	Department of Health and Social Security	1000 people 65 and over	Unpublished
Survey of Orkney Islanders	1980	Ministry of Agriculture Fisheries and Food	78 women 40 men	Barber et al., 1986[52]
Teenagers and young adults, nationally representative	1982	Ministry of Agriculture Fisheries and Food	452 men 461 women 15/25 years	Bull, 1985[51]
Dietary survey of British school children, nationally representative	1983	Department of Health and Social Security/Office of Population Censuses and Surveys	902 boys 821 girls 10/11 years 513 boys 461 girls 14/15 years	Wenlock et al., 1986[46] DoH, 1989[47]
Survey of pregnant women, Edinburgh and London	1983/85	Ministry of Agriculture Fisheries and Food	260 women Early and late pregnancy and post partum	Schofield et al., 1987[53]
Dietary and nutritional survey of British adults, nationally representative	1986/87	Department of Health, Ministry of Agriculture Fisheries and Food, Office of Population Censuses and Surveys	1087 men 1110 women 16 to 64 years	Gregory et al., 1990[54]

The pilot study was carried out in early summer, but it was concluded that for a satisfactory picture a survey should run continuously for one year.

Experience from field work revealed that the most pressing and unresolved problem was that of rapid detection of mistakes in the dietary records.

Mothers kept records of what their children ate and the opportunities to describe inadequately recorded meals were limited. Meals eaten away from home presented particular difficulties, which required detailed instruction of mothers by field-workers in the techniques of diet recording.

The scales used were capable of recording to only one-third of an ounce (9 g) but this was shown not to be precise enough and scales weighing to one-sixth of an ounce (5 g) were recommended for future surveys. Cumulative weighing was employed and was particularly successful; it was recommended for future surveys. This technique has recently declined in popularity with the introduction of battery operated digital food weighing scales.

Mothers found the methods used to record uneaten food and leftovers difficult to deal with and it was concluded that, for young children, it would be best to ask only for the total weight of leftovers, with some description of the food that was left.

The dietary data from the survey were analysed to yield nutrient intakes using tables of food composition especially compiled for the study. These were based on the published data of McCance and Widdowson, plus standard recipes for which moisture loss was either determined experimentally or calculated. The food tables were never published, but copies were made available to *bona fide* investigators by the Ministry of Health and, later, the Department of Health and Social Security.

5.6.2 A nutrition survey of preschool children 1967–68

In 1967, COMA called upon the experience gained during the 1963 pilot study to carry out a larger comprehensive survey. The sample of children studied was nationally representative of Great Britain: the 2321 preschool children were selected from 39 areas in England, Wales, and Scotland. Of these, complete and usable 7-day diet records were produced by 1321 mothers or guardians in respect of 673 boys and 648 girls. A further 560 were interviewed but did not produce a diet record. In addition, heights and weights were measured for 1627 and 1622 boys and girls, respectively.

The food composition table used in the 1963 pilot study was revised and updated for this survey. A total of 630 food codes were available, giving values for the following nutrients:

Energy	Iron
Protein	Thiamin
Animal protein	Riboflavin
Fat	Nicotinic acid
Carbohydrate	Vitamin A
'Added sugars'	Vitamin C
Calcium	Vitamin D

In the survey, medical and dental examinations were also carried out on all the children, and full details of the sample, methods, and results are given in the published report.[40] The main nutritional findings are shown in Table 5.2. The average intakes of most nutrients reached or exceeded the Recommended Daily Intakes (RDI) for all the age/sex groups of children.[41] The exceptions were vitamin D and iron. Children from small families, those from social classes I, II, and III non-manual and those with higher income levels derived a greater percentage of their energy from protein. Children from larger families and from social classes IV and V had higher average daily energy intakes but these children did not weigh more than others and it was concluded that this difference in intakes could be due to a difference in energy requirement because children with more siblings and fewer social amenities might be physically more active.[40]

The survey was particularly designed to study the role, if any, of milk in the diet but, although a possible relationship between milk intake and height had been noted in the 1963 pilot study,[39] this was not established by this survey. There was a tendency for height to increase with milk intake, but this did not achieve statistical significance.[40]

5.7 SURVEYS BETWEEN 1968 AND 1971

A further five surveys were carried out between 1968 and 1971 on groups of people who could have been at risk of malnutrition (Table 5.1). The methodology developed after the pilot study and fully tested in the main survey on preschool children was used throughout this period. All the studies were cross-sectional in design. Trained dietary investigators visited each respondent in their own home to explain the purpose of the survey and to make periodic checks on the keeping of the dietary records. Full participation in a study yielded socio-economic information and a weighed record of all food (solid and liquid) ingested for a period of seven days. The same, specially compiled food composition table was used in all the surveys.

Except for some preschool children, all subjects were assessed for clinical signs of malnutrition and height, weight, and skinfold measurements were made. In addition, in the surveys of elderly people, a blood sample

Table 5.2 Mean daily intake, for total food energy and selected nutrients from 7-day

	Preschool children 1967/68							
	12–23 months				24–35 months			
	Boys		Girls		Boys		Girls	
	Mean	SD	Mean	SD	Mean	SD	Mean	SD
Energy: MJ	5.05	1.22	4.74	1.16	5.73	1.49	5.37	1.
kcal	1207	291	1133	277	1370	357	1284	310
Total protein (g)	37.8	10.4	35.3	9.4	39.7	10.9	38.5	10.
Animal protein (g)	27.4	8.6	26.0	8.7	27.4	9.0	27.1	8.
Fat (g)	51.2	15.2	48.7	13.6	57.9	17.8	55.5	16.
Carbohydrate (g)	157	42	146	42	182	51	167	42
Calcium (mg)	744	233	704	272	678	216	660	210
Iron (mg)	7.0	3.4	6.5	3.1	6.8	2.4	6.4	2.
Retinol (μg)	821	570	798	623	656	430	704	635
Thiamin (mg)	0.63	0.32	0.57	0.20	0.65	0.25	0.68	0.
Riboflavin (mg)	1.21	0.66	1.10	0.46	1.06	0.33	1.04	0.
Nicotinic acid (mg)	6.56	5.54	5.78	3.01	7.08	3.15	6.80	3.
Pyridoxine (mg)	0.65	0.34	0.60	0.21	0.70	0.20	0.66	0.
Ascorbic acid (mg)	42.6	34.9	41.0	31.3	36.3	31.0	38.8	37.
Cholecalciferol (μg)	3.14	3.85	3.84	4.96	2.29	3.02	2.63	4.

Nutrient	Children aged 14–15 years, 1970				Children aged 14–15 years, 1970/71			
	Boys		Girls		Boys		Girls	
	Mean	SD	Mean	SD	Mean	SD	Mean	SD
Energy: MJ	11.19	2.30	8.64	1.83	10.25	2.47	8.00	1.
kcal	2674	549	2063	437	2451	589	1911	454
Total protein (g)	75.1	15.2	60.4	14.8	71.2	17.4	57.2	13.
Animal protein (g)	45.8	12.5	37.1	12.0	42.0	13.3	35.1	11.
Fat (g)	114.6	29.2	91.8	22.2	101.8	28.2	84.7	23.
Carbohydrate (g)	356	82	264	61	330	87	243	64
Calcium (mg)	950	306	705	218	870	299	667	238
Iron (mg)	13.4	3.4	10.9	2.7	12.4	3.5	10.1	2.
Retinol (μg)	832	539	737	414	860	610	780	574
Thiamin (mg)	1.16	0.27	0.90	0.24	1.17	0.35	0.92	0.
Riboflavin (mg)	1.61	0.56	1.18	0.44	1.48	0.57	1.13	0.
Nicotinic acid (mg)	13.64	3.08	10.61	2.86	13.31	4.22	10.53	5.
Pyridoxine (mg)	1.41	0.31	1.15	0.29	1.40	0.35	1.17	0.
Ascorbic acid (mg)	58.3	37.2	47.2	26.0	53.3	29.2	48.8	27.
Cholecalciferol (μg)	2.10	1.66	2.18	1.70	2.11	1.67	1.81	1.

eighed studies obtained from dietary surveys carried out by the British Government

				Pregnant women 1967/68		Children aged 10–11 years, 1971			
	36–47 months						Boys		Girls
Boys		Girls				Boys		Girls	
Mean	SD	Mean	SD	Mean	SD	Mean	SD	Mean	SD
6.40	1.58	5.80	1.49	9.01	2.10	9.08	1.63	8.02	1.56
529	378	1387	355	2152	503	2169	390	1916	372
43.9	12.1	39.2	10.5	70.5	16.7	62.4	12.5	55.4	11.2
29.4	9.6	26.7	11.3	47.8	14.3	39.1	9.9	35.6	9.2
64.0	20.2	58.6	18.6	97.9	26.4	90.7	19.6	82.8	19.9
204	49	186	48	260	69	292	58	252	52
704	225	618	202	959	320	899	231	787	224
7.4	2.6	6.7	2.1	11.7	3.1	10.8	2.6	9.7	2.3
764	630	636	458	1269	975	893	548	812	453
0.75	0.27	0.64	0.24	1.04	0.28	1.03	0.28	0.88	0.21
1.16	0.39	1.00	0.36	1.60	0.67	1.43	0.40	1.24	0.36
8.26	3.35	7.29	3.04	14.30	5.30	11.19	3.13	9.57	2.46
0.77	0.23	0.69	0.20	1.27	0.32	1.16	0.24	1.05	0.23
40.0	34.4	35.8	30.9	54.9	24.7	48.5	24.4	46.2	23.4
1.94	2.62	1.94	2.59	2.28	2.01	1.66	1.02	1.44	0.74

| Elderly aged 65–74 years, 1967/68 | | | | Elderly aged over 75 years, 1967/68 | | | |
| Men | | Women | | Men | | Women | |
Mean	SD	Mean	SD	Mean	SD	Mean	SD
9.82	2.44	7.48	1.91	8.80	2.31	6.81	1.72
2347	528	1788	456	2103	551	1627	410
74.8	17.8	59.2	14.4	67.6	18.4	53.6	13.0
50.9	13.9	41.1	11.6	45.9	14.1	37.4	10.4
110.0	32.8	87.4	26.3	97.9	29.2	77.6	22.0
267	75	200	61	244	73	187	59.0
911	282	796	244	883	302	726	253
12.2	3.3	9.4	2.6	10.9	3.2	8.5	2.5
1142	686	1027	676	1094	741	888	588
1.05	0.35	0.82	0.23	0.93	0.29	0.74	0.23
1.55	0.48	1.27	0.42	1.40	0.51	1.13	0.39
16.91	7.42	11.49	4.56	13.55	5.04	10.18	3.80
1.37	0.41	1.01	0.28	1.18	0.36	0.93	0.27
42.8	26.0	40.5	27.8	37.7	23.1	33.7	20.0
3.34	3.62	2.32	2.18	2.28	2.13	2.09	1.79

was taken for biochemical and haematological analysis and radiology of the metacarpal was done.[42]

The main nutritional results for these surveys are given in Table 5.2 but the data were also reanalysed by Darke *et al.* to show centile distributions.[43] As early as 12–23 months of age there was a statistically significant difference in the mean energy intake between the sexes, the mean energy intake of the boys being, as for older males, greater than that of the girls of the same age. The differences were more pronounced in the older age groups. In general, except for preschool boys and elderly men, more than half the groups had daily energy intakes that were less than the recommended intake (RDI).[41]

There were a number of important implications from these studies. First, in an environment where the motor car, television, and domestic and industrial work-saving appliances were common, individual energy requirements seemed less than they had been a decade before. Second, from the age of 12 months, mean energy intakes of males were shown to be greater than those of females of the same age. Third, the distributions of nutrient intakes showed that many individuals in the different groups surveyed were eating less than the RDI without any signs of malnutrition.[43] The 1969 RDI was defined as the amount sufficient, or more than sufficient, for the nutritional needs of practically all healthy persons in a population. The survey findings suggested that a more practical definition of the recommended intake of a nutrient would be the average amount of the nutrient that should be provided per head in a group of healthy people if the needs of practically all members of the group are to be met. This definition as agreed by the Committee on Medical Aspects of Food Policy and, in 1979, using the data from these surveys, a new report on Recommended Daily Amounts (RDA) was published in which energy recommendations were reduced, those for males being made larger than for females from infancy onwards, and revised RDA for a number of nutrients were also estimated.[44]

5.8 STUDIES OF THE ELDERLY

When the elderly who had been studied in 1967 and 1968 were resurveyed in 1972, all but three of the original responding sample of 879 people were traced and, although one-third had died, over half of the survivors (365 subjects) were willing and able to take part in a follow-up study, which included detailed dietary, social, medical, biochemical, and haematological assessment.[45] The results confirmed that the nutrient intakes of these elderly people were not very different from those of the general population. The mean daily energy and nutrient intakes are given in Table 5.3. Those under 80 years old showed few differences from the data for

Table 5.3 Mean daily intakes of energy and nutrients, and the percentage of energy derived from protein, fat, and added sugars, for all men and all women in the 1972 survey of the elderly in two age groups

Daily intake	Sex and age group							
	Under 80 years (111 men)		80 years and over (58 men)		Under 80 years (125 women)		80 years and over (71 women)	
	Mean	SD	Mean	SD	Mean	SD	Mean	SD
Energy (MJ)	9.3	2.20	8.5	2.10	7.0	1.70	6.5	1.50
(kcal)	2217	522	2024	498	1679	416	1559	358
Total protein (g)	71.2	15.6	68.9	17.5	57.5	13.7	52.6	12.1
Animal protein (g)	47.5	12.9	47.8	14.3	39.3	10.7	36.4	9.5
Fat (g)	100.0	27.4	93.0	27.9	81.0	23.8	72.0	19.1
Carbohydrate (g)	255	67.5	235	63.1	189	56.8	182	52.8
Calcium (mg)	890	285	870	311	780	251	690	184
Iron (mg)	11.6	3.01	11.0	3.06	9.3	3.09	8.6	2.74
Vitamin A (μg)	1120	728	1050	689	1050	1161	980	776
Thiamin (mg)	1.0	0.27	0.9	0.26	0.8	0.27	0.7	0.20
Riboflavin (mg)	1.5	0.62	1.4	0.47	1.3	0.53	1.1	0.40
Nicotinic acid (mg)	14.4	5.97	12.3	4.02	10.3	3.45	9.8	2.86
Pyridoxine (mg)	1.3	0.41	1.2	0.37	0.9	0.26	0.9	0.29
Ascorbic acid (mg)	46.0	28.2	38.0	31.1	40.0	29.3	37.0	25.1
Cholecalciferol (μg)	2.4	1.64	2.7	2.01	2.1	1.79	2.3	2.61
Added sugars (g)	71.6	35.7	66.0	33.0	48.8	27.0	48.5	28.3
% energy from protein	13.1	2.29	13.7	2.59	13.9	2.52	13.7	2.30
% energy from fat	40.6	5.98	41.0	5.50	43.2	5.63	41.8	5.51
% energy from added sugars	12.7	5.34	13.2	6.76	11.5	5.47	12.2	6.04

From DHSS (1979)[45]

75-year-olds given in Table 5.2, those over 80 years had smaller total food energy intakes and lower intakes of several nutrients. COMA concluded that this reflected a decline in physical activity with increasing age but was also due in part to impaired health, because the incidence of diagnosed diseases was much higher in this older age group.

5.9 THE DIETARY SURVEY OF BRITISH SCHOOL CHILDREN IN 1983

Ten years after this survey of the elderly, the plan for the Dietary Survey of British Schoolchildren, devised in 1982, called for a nationally representative sample. The COMA Subcommittee on Nutritional Surveillance recommended that, in keeping with the DHSS dietary surveys described previously, a full 7-day weighed record of all food consumed should be made because this method would provide data on dietary intakes of greater precision than any other available method of measurement (such as 24-hour recall, a food frequency questionnaire, or shorter periods of weighed intakes). Because of the intensive field-work required for a 7-day weighed dietary survey of this size, it was impossible to cover all ages within the school population, so two age groups were selected comprising, children aged 10 to 14 years at the start of the school year. These were chosen in the hope that most of the younger girls would be sampled prior to the onset of menarche, and older boys would be sampled after most of them had entered their adolescent growth spurt. The two age groups were thereby also comparable with those selected in the previous DHSS dietary studies of school children carried out in 1970 and 1973.[43]

A full account of sampling and of methodologies was published in 1986, together with the results of a nutritional analysis[46] and the complete Report covering the dietary findings was published in 1989.[47] The survey covered a nationally representative sample of 4597 children. Of these, 3285 (including an enhanced sample of 884 10 and 11 year olds from Scotland), provided a full 7-day weighed record of all the food they consumed. This made it the largest 7-day dietary survey ever and the enormous quantity of information collected provided much experience in coding and computing very large volumes of dietary data.

The sample of 64 Local Authority Districts in England and Wales was drawn and a multistage procedure selected areas, then schools, and finally children in the two age groups. Some clustering of schools within districts was necessary and, to ensure a representative sex balance, single sex secondary schools were linked with nearby schools with children of the other sex to make a single 'secondary school unit'. These were then clustered with nearby primary schools so that the primary schools' population was in proportion to the size of the secondary school unit with which they were clustered. One cluster was then randomly selected within each district with a probability proportional to the size of the school population aged 11 to 15 years in each cluster. The result of this process was that children in the sample were not selected with equal probability, so the sample was reweighted by calculating factors based on the number of children on the school roll in each selected cluster. The numbers of children forming the final sample are given in Table 5.4. The overall response rate in England and Wales was 75.2 per cent.

In Scotland the area north of the Caledonian Canal was excluded because operational costs in this sparsely populated area were too high. An enhanced sample of Scottish primary schoolchildren was required by the Scottish Home and Health Department (SHHD), to provide more representative data; this meant that all primary schools in the rest of Scotland were grouped in clusters to provide reasonably sized geographical areas and 52 of these schools were selected with probability proportional to cluster size. A sample of 40 children was then selected at random from these schools. No enhanced sample of secondary schools was required by SHHD, so the sample reflected only the relative population sizes of Scotland and the rest of Great Britain. A sample of eight Local Education Authorities was selected, with probability proportional to the number of children aged 12 to 15 years, rather than 11 to 14 years as in England and Wales, as this is the age range on which central Scottish records are kept. The numbers of children forming the final sample are given in Table 5.5. The overall response rate in Scotland was 75.4 per cent.

The field-work was undertaken between January and June 1983. By this time the Medical Research Council and the Ministry of Agriculture, Fisheries and Food (MAFF) had completed the revision of the British tables of food composition and the fourth edition had been published.[17] This superseded the DHSS tables of food composition, which had been used for all the surveys previously described. The Nutrition Branch of the Ministry of Agriculture, Fisheries and Food collaborated in producing a specially designed nutrient data base for analysing food intakes. This was based on the fourth edition of *McCance and Widdowson's 'The Composition of Foods'*[17] and was used to recalculate recipe data and the nutrient content of composite dishes contained in the nutrient data bank used by the DHSS in all its preceding surveys.

The field-work was carried out by the Office of Population Censuses and Surveys (OPCS) whose field-workers were specially trained in the techniques of 7-day weighed record dietary surveys. With all children, the first step was to explain the nature of the survey to one or both parents following up an introductory letter. The questionnaire interview then followed, at which a field sift was used to exclude ineligible children. This included questions on basic socio-economic matters and about diets and eating patterns. Following this interview, children and their parents were

Table 5.4 The dietary survey of British schoolchildren, 1983

Sample response rates—England and Wales	Number	Percent
Children sampled from school registers	4597	
Children who would have been sampled if their school had not refused to cooperate	+ 187	
Total potential sample	4784	
Subtract ineligibles (ill all survey period or moved out of sampled area)	− 50	
Subtract children found to be in the higher social classes I–III non-manual in the sifted sampled (see sample design)	−1436	
Subtract estimated number of refusals and non-contacts that would have been in the higher social classes I–III non-manual and have been ineligible if they had cooperated	− 174	
Total eligible sample	3124	100.0
Estimated number of children from refusing schools who would have been eligible	129	4.1
Estimated number of non-contacts who would have been eligible if they had been contacted	29	0.9
Estimated number of refusals who would have been eligible if they had cooperated	229	7.3
Number of children who dropped out during the recording period having previously promised to keep 7-day records	179	5.7
Total cooperating sample	2558	81.9
Number of children who did not keep records accurately enough	138	4.4
Number of children whose recording week included less than three schooldays	78	2.3
Number of children for whom satisfactory records were obtained	2348	75.2

shown how to use the weighing scales and how to fill in the three different dietary record books used in the survey. Everything consumed was to be recorded. Children were shown how to zero the scales after each weighing so that a series of items could be put on the same plate and weighed. After 24 hours, the field-worker returned to the child's home for a checking call to assess progress.

Table 5.5 The dietary survey of British schoolchildren, 1983

Sample response rates—Scotland	Number	Percent
Children sampled from school registers	1915	
Children who would have been sampled if their school had not refused to cooperate	+ 155	
Total potential sample	2070	
Subtract ineligibles (ill all survey period or moved out of sampled area)	− 4	
Subtract children found to be in the higher social classes I–III non-manual in the sifted sampled (see sample design)	− 590	
Subtract estimated number of refusals and non-contacts that would have been in the higher social classes I–III non-manual and have been ineligible if they had cooperated	− 83	
Total eligible sample	1393	100.0
Estimated number of children from refusing schools who would have been eligible	108	7.8
Estimated number of non-contacts who would have been eligible if they had been contacted	28	2.0
Estimated number of refusals who would have been eligible if they had cooperated	55	3.9
Number of children who dropped out during the recording period having previously promised to keep 7-day records	78	5.6
Total cooperating sample	1124	80.7
Number of children who did not keep records accurately enough	66	4.7
Number of children whose recording week included less than three schooldays	8	0.6
Number of children for whom satisfactory records were obtained	1050	75.4

The number of checking calls made in the 7-day period varied but after each call the field-worker coded each food item with reference to the food code list prepared for the nutrient data bank. Queries were referred to nutritionist advisers who also checked completed records after the field-worker had sent them in to OPCS. Apart from checking calls, field-workers also monitored record keeping in schools, where children were consuming lunch.

Each food was given a code number from the nutrient data base that enabled the computer to identify the energy and nutrient intake which it represented, and there were a number of codes for prepared dishes. For each of these codes a nutrient content was available from one of five sources:

1. *McCance and Widdowson's 'The Composition of Foods'* (Eds Paul and Southgate), London: HMSO, 1978.[17]

2. The DHSS Food Composition Tables by M. M. Disselduff (unpublished).

3. Wiles S., Nettleton P., Black A. Nutrient composition of some cooked dishes eaten in Britain: A supplementary food composition table.[48]

4. *Immigrant Foods*. Second supplement to *McCance and Widdowson's 'The Composition of Foods'* S. P. Tan, R. W. Wenlock, D. H. Buss. London: HMSO, 1985.[49]

5. *Cereals and Cereal Products*. Third supplement to *McCance and Widdowson's 'The Composition of Foods'* B. Holland, I. D. Unwin, D. H. Buss. London: HMSO, 1988.[50]

Interviewers were issued with a food code list describing foods in sufficient detail to distinguish about 1080 different foods or food dishes. All details of foods eaten were obtained at the time of the field-work, when the precise nature of the items consumed could be recalled. Sometimes the foods had to be 'split' into components that could be coded separately. So, for example, a cheese, ham, and tomato pizza was split into a cheese and tomato pizza, for which there was a code, and an entry, of, say, 'tinned ham', for which there was also a code.

Experience with the earlier surveys had confirmed the importance of measuring leftovers. However, some respondents are apt to forget leftovers no matter how diligent the interviewer may be in reminding them of them. Interviewers always probed for a description of leftovers but there was often little chance of securing the weight. Most commonly, this problem arose when the subject neglected to weigh the natural wastage such as the bones in fish, the skin of a banana or the core of an apple. Food composition tables can cope with this problem by the 'as purchased' codes that contain allowances for the non-edible part in the food composition analysis. Such codes are particularly useful but interviewers had to be trained to be especially careful that these 'as purchased' codes were only used in appropriate circumstances.

The survey showed that the main sources of dietary energy in diets of

British school children were bread, chips, milk, biscuits, meat products, cake and puddings. Almost all children in the survey recorded consumption of chips, crisps, cakes, and biscuits. Boys recorded more chips consumed than girls, along with more milk, breakfast cereals, and baked beans; girls recorded more fruit consumed and more girls drank fruit juice than boys. Yogurt, fizzy drinks, and sweets were more popular among younger children. Older children recorded consumption of more tea and coffee.

Scottish primary schoolchildren appeared to have a distinctive dietary pattern, with higher consumption of beef, soups, milk, cheese, sausage, chocolate, and sweets and lower consumption of cakes, biscuits, puddings, potatoes, and in particular, of vegetables of all kinds than children in the other regions of Great Britain.

Mean energy intakes were about 90 per cent of the 1979 RDA[44] but there was no evidence, from height and weight data, to suggest that these intakes were inadequate. Average intakes of iron were below the RDA in younger and older girls, but in the absence of biological measurements of iron status, the clinical significance of these findings is not clear. Mean intakes of riboflavin in the older girls were also below the RDA. This survey added to evidence that the 1979 RDA for the UK were in need of revision. COMA, recognizing this, convened a panel on RDA in 1987, which is currently reviewing them.

To some extent, dietary patterns were dependent on the composition of school meals. Older children obtained over half the chips that they ate in the survey week from school meals. Younger children obtained over half the buns and pastries they ate from this source. However, the total average daily intakes of energy and nutrients did not vary with the kind of meal eaten at weekday lunchtimes.

Older children, especially girls, who ate out of school at places such as cafes, take-away or 'fast food' outlets chose meals that were low in many nutrients, particularly iron. Their average daily nutrient intake was not made up of the levels of intake of the rest of the population by the meals they consumed at other times during the week. The overall nutritional quality of their diets was the poorest of any group surveyed.

This survey of children highlighted the importance of ensuring that school meals, and indeed all meals and snacks consumed outside the home, are included in any dietary survey. Other lessons arise from the evidence it provided of very similar intakes of nutrients among the children. There were few significant differences in energy and nutrient intakes for any age and sex group according to region, social class, receipt of benefits, employment status or the provision and type of school meal. This again highlighted the need, recognized from the 1963 pilot study of COMA, for a weighed dietary survey methodology to increase the precision of estimates and to allow the demonstration of small differences among a population group with almost identical nutrient intakes and very homogenous dietary patterns. Although a 7-day period of weighing is desirable, it is extremely costly, and a 4-day weighing period would produce results with only marginally less precision, as long as the period included a weekend. Analyses of foods consumed showed that no food was eaten by all the 3000 or so children sampled in the survey week. Most foods were eaten by less than half the sample. Median values of foods consumed are more useful in these circumstances than the mean for groups. However, where less than 50 per cent of a group actually ate the food, the median intake was zero, so the best way to express consumption is as the mean among those in the group who consumed the food. Interpretation of any differences in the diets of groups is therefore extremely complicated. Increasing sample sizes will not provide more precise data where only a very low proportion are consumers.

5.10 STUDIES SINCE 1983

The Ministry of Agriculture, Fisheries and Food commissioned dietary surveys during the period of 1980 to 1985. These covered groups of the population who were considered vulnerable or of particular interest namely teenagers and young adults aged 15 to 25 years;[51] Orkney Islanders[52] and pregnant women.[53] Data from the surveys were made available by the Working Party on Nutrients to COMA for consideration. It was concluded that there was a need for re-evaluation of the energy and nutrient RDA for pregnancy.[53] The Panel convened by COMA in 1987 is carrying out a review of all the RDA including those for pregnancy.

5.11 SUMMARY AND CONCLUSIONS

Since 1963, the Government studies have been designed for surveillance purposes and have all utilized the 7-day weighed dietary survey methodology. They have shown that nutrient intakes among different socio-economic groups of populations of the same age and sex are very similar. They have also provided data that have been used in two revisions of the RDA for energy and nutrients, and for a third review currently underway. Food intakes show more variation than nutrient intakes, and in all samples of people studied there were many who consumed very small amounts, or even none, of otherwise popular foods. Interpretation of dietary information on groups is therefore extremely complex.

Since 1982, the emphasis of Government dietary surveillance has shifted towards the study of people on extremes of dietary intakes, for whom the 7-day method is particularly suited. In particular, information has been sought on those who eat large quantities of foods such as liver, shellfish and semi-skimmed milk, which are relatively unpopular. On the nutrient intake side, the emphasis is on variation in intakes of fat and saturated fatty acids as proportions of energy intakes as indicators of possible risk for cardiovascular disease.

For the future, the results of the joint DH/MAFF/OPCS Dietary and Nutritional Survey of British Adults are awaited. These could point to potentially vulnerable subgroups that may warrant further study. In the meantime, COMA is reconsidering its requirement for nutritional surveillance of all kinds, including dietary assessments. The kind of programme that will develop in the 1990s has yet to emerge from these deliberations.

REFERENCES

1. Barker, D. J. P., Morris, J. A., and Nelson, M. (1986). Vegetable consumption and acute appendicitis in 59 areas in England and Wales. *Br. Med. J.,* **292:** 927–30.
2. Alderson, M. (1983). An introduction to epidemiology, second edn. Macmillan, London.
3. Flores, M. and Nelson, N., (1988). Methods for data collection at household or institutional level. In M. E. Cameron and W. A. van Staveren, (eds). *Manual on methodology for food consumption studies.* Oxford University Press, Oxford.
4. Department of Employment. (1989). Family Expenditure Survey 1988. HMSO, London.
5. Community of Greater New York. (1982). A family budget standard. Budget Standard Service of New York Community Council, New York.
6. Montreal Diet Dispensary. (1982). Budgeting for basic need. Montreal Diet Dispensary, Montreal.
7. Ministry of Agriculture, Fisheries and Food. (1955–1991). Household food consumption and expenditure: 1953–1989. HMSO, London.
8. Ministry of Food. (1951). The urban working-class household diet 1940–1949. HMSO, London.
9. Ministry of Food. (1952–1954). Domestic food consumption and expenditure: 1950–1952. HMSO, London.
10. Ministry of Food. (1956). Studies in urban household diets 1944–49. HMSO, London.
11. Ingram, D. M. (1981). Trends in diet and breast cancer mortality in England and Wales 1928–1977. *Nutr. Cancer,* **3:** 75–80.
12. Key, T. J. A., Darby, S. C., and Pike, M. C. (1987). Trends in breast cancer mortality and diet in England and Wales from 1911 to 1980. *Nutr. Cancer,* **10:** 1–9.
13. Marmot, M. G., Adelstein, A. M., Robinson, N., and Rose, G. A. (1978). Changing social class distribution of heart disease. *Brit. Med. J.,* **2:** 1109–12.
14. Bingham, S., Williams, D. R. R., Cole, T. J., and James, W. P. T. (1979). Dietary fibre and regional large bowel cancer mortality in Britain. *Brit. J. Cancer,* **40:** 456–63.

15. Derry, B. J. and Buss, D. H. (1984). The British National Food Survey as a major epidemiological resource. *Brit. Med. J.*, **288:** 765–7.
16. Kemsley, W. F. F. (1976). *Statistical News No. 35.* HMSO, London.
17. Paul, A. A. and Southgate, D. A. T. (1978). *McCance and Widdowson's the composition of foods*, fourth edn. HMSO, London.
18. Department of Health and Social Security. (1979). Report on Health and Social Subjects No. 15: recommended daily amounts of food energy and nutrients for groups of people in the United Kingdom. HMSO, London.
19. Barker, D. J. P., Morris, J. A., and Margetts, B. M. (1988). Diet and renal stones in 72 areas in England and Wales. *Br. J. Urol.*, **62:** 315–18.
20. Nelson, M. and Peploe, K. A. (1990). Construction of a modest-but-adequate food budget for households with two adults and one preschool child: a preliminary investigation. *J. Hum. Nutr. Diet.*, **3:** 121–40.
21. Platt, B. S., Gray, P. G., Parr, E., Baines, A. H. J., Clayton, S., Hobson, E. A., Hollingsworth, D. F., Berry, W. T. C., and Washington, E. (1964). The food purchases of elderly women living alone: a statistical inconsistency and its investigation. *Brit. J. Nutr.*, **18:** 413–29.
22. Nelson, M., Dyson, P. A. and Paul, A. A. (1985). Family food purchase and home food consumption: comparison of nutrient contents *Brit. J. Nutr.*, **54:** 373–87.
23. Nelson, M. (1983). PhD Thesis. University of London, London.
24. Nelson, M. (1986). The distribution of nutrient intake within families. *Brit. J. Nutr.*, **55:** 267–77.
25. Jensen, O. M., Wahrendorf, J., Rosenquist, A., and Geser, A. (1984). The reliability of questionnaire-derived historic information and temporal stability of food habits in individuals. *Am. J. Epidemiol.* **120:** 281–90.
26. Sudman, S. and Ferber, R. (1971). Experiments on obtaining consumer expenditures by diary methods. *Am. Stat. Assoc.*, **66:** 725–35.
27. Hollingsworth, D. F. and Baines, A. H. J. (1961). A survey of food consumption in Great Britain. Family Living Studies, A Symposium. Studies and Reports No. 63. International Labour Office, Geneva.
28. Wenlock, R. W., Buss, D. H., Derry, B. J., and Dixon, E. J. (1980). Household food wastage in Britain. *Brit. J. Nutr.*, **43:** 53–70.
29. United States Department of Agriculture. (1983). Food consumption: households in the United States, seasons and years 1977–8. Nationwide food consumption survey 1977–8. Report No. 4–6. US Government Printing Office, Washington DC.
30. Burk, M. C. and Pao, M. (1976). Methodology for large-scale surveys of household and individual diets. Home Economics Research Report No. 40. Agricultural Research Service, US Department of Agriculture, US Government Printing Office, Washington.
31. Nelson, M., Nettleton, P. A. (1980). Dietary survey methods. I. A semi-weighed technique for measuring dietary intake within families. *J. Hum. Nutr.*, **34:** 325–348.
32. Orr, J. B. (1936). *Food, health and income.* Gollancz, London.
33. Ministry of Health (1957). *Report of the sub-committee on welfare foods.* HMSO, London.

34. Department of Health and Social Security. (1973). *First report by the sub-committee on nutritional surveillance.* Reports on Health and Social Subjects No. 6. HMSO, London.

35. Department of Health and Social Security. (1981). *Sub-committee on nutritional surveillance: second report.* Report on Health and Social Subjects No. 21. HMSO, London.

36. Department of Health, (1988). *Third report the sub-committee on nutritional surveillance.* Report on Health and Social Subjects No. 33. HMSO, London.

37. Ministry of Agriculture, Fisheries and Food. (1988). *The British diet: finding the facts.* Food Surveillance Paper No. 23. HMSO, London.

38. Department of Health and Social Security. (1984). *Diet and cardiovascular disease.* Report on Health and Social Subjects No. 28. HMSO, London.

39. Ministry of Health. (1968). *A pilot survey of the nutrition of young children in 1963.* Reports on Public Health and Medical Subjects No. 118. HMSO, London.

40. Department of Health and Social Security. (1975). *A nutrition survey of pre-school children 1967–68.* Report on Health and Social Subjects No. 10. HMSO, London.

41. Department of Health and Social Security. (1969). *Recommended intakes of nutrients for the United Kingdom.* Report on Public Health and Medical Subjects No. 120. HMSO, London.

42. Department of Health and Social Security. (1972). *A nutrition survey of the elderly.* Reports on Health and Social Subjects No. 3. HMSO, London.

43. Darke, S. J., Disselduff, M. M., and Try, G. P. (1980). Frequency distributions of mean daily intakes of food energy and selected nutrients obtained during nutrition surveys of different groups of people in Great Britain between 1968 and 1971. *Br. J. Nutr.,* **44:** 243–52.

44. Department of Health and Social Security. (1979). *Recommended daily amounts of food energy and nutrients for groups of people in the United Kingdom.* Reports on Health and Social Subjects No. 15. HMSO, London.

45. Department of Health and Social Security. (1979). *Nutrition and health in old age,* Reports on Health and Social Subjects No. 16. HMSO, London.

46. Wenlock, R. W., Disselduff, M. M., Skinner, R. K., and Knight, I. (1986). *The diets of British schoolchildren.* Department of Health and Social Security, London.

47. Department of Health. (1989). *The diets of British schoolchildren.* Reports on Health and Social Subjects No. 36. HMSO, London.

48. Wiles, S. J., Nettleton, P. A., and Black, A. A. (1983). Nutrient composition of some cooked dishes eaten in Britain: a supplementary food composition table. *J. Hum. Nutr.,* **34:** 189–223.

49. Tan, S. P., Wenlock, R. W., and Buss, D. H. (1985). *Immigrant foods.* Second Supplement to *McCance and Widdowson's the composition of foods.* HMSO, London.

50. Holland, B., Unwin, I. D., and Buss, D. H. (1988). *Cereals and cereal products.* Third Supplement to *McCance and Widdowson's the composition of foods.* The Royal Society of Chemistry, Nottingham.

51. Bull, N. L. (1985). Dietary habits of 15 to 25 year olds. *Hum. Nutr: Appl. Nutr.,* **39A,** Suppl. 1: 1–68.

52. Barber, S. A., Bull, N. L., and Cameron, A. M. (1986). A dietary survey of an isolated population in the UK: the islanders of Orkney. *Hum. Nutr: Appl. Nutr.*, **40A,** 462–9.
53. Schofield, C., Wheeler, E. F., and Stewart, J. (1987). The diets of pregnant and post-pregnant women in different social groups in London and Edinburgh: energy, protein, fat and fibre. *Br. J. Nutr.*, **58:** 369–81.
54. Gregory, J., Foster, K., Tyler, H., and Wiseman, M. (1990). *The dietary and nutritional survey of British adults.* HMSO, London.

6. Assessment of food consumption and nutrient intake

INTRODUCTION

A major challenge facing the nutritional epidemiologist is the correct measurement of dietary exposure. [1-3] An apparently straightforward task is fraught with difficulties and plagued by a seemingly endless list of factors that will introduce error into the simplest measurement. If the aim is to measure current diet, the Heisenberg uncertainty principle rears its head: as you stop something to measure it, you change its behaviour. If the aim is to measure past dietary exposure then one is reliant on the memory, conceptual abilities, and ruthless honesty on the part of respondents. It thus would seem that no direct measure of what people eat will provide a true picture of their dietary habits. And this is before one considers the error introduced by the use of food composition tables.

Nevertheless, in the absence of truly objective measures of diet, it is the task of the nutritional epidemiologist to obtain the best measure of diet possible. This chapter is devoted to an exploration of how such measurements can be obtained with the minimum error. Equally important, it addresses the question of how best to measure the error itself, because a knowledge of the size of the error in individual dietary assessments will provide valuable information about the likely attenuation of risk estimates based on imprecise measurements. The first section of the chapter looks at measures of current diet. It questions in a positive way the notion that 'current' is equivalent to 'valid' by examining the relationship between current records and external standards that offer scope for assessing the validity of dietary records. The second section considers the assessment of past diet, using a variety of techniques, and addresses the problems of deciding which measures are appropriate in which circumstances, and how best to measure the validity of measures based on recall.

Current intake

Sheila A. Bingham

6.1 INTRODUCTION

Most individuals who are the subject of an investigation can be trained to make records of everything they eat and drink over a defined period. Records may be written, verbal, or visual but in situations where subjects are unable to keep records themselves, trained field-workers are necessary. Such 'observed' records are particularly required in rural areas of developing countries, or in the study of individuals living in institutions.[4] As with all methods of dietary assessment, some estimate of the weight of food consumed is required and, for the determination of nutrient or other food component intake, either an appropriate description for use with food tables or an aliquot for chemical analysis (see Chapter 4) is necessary.

Records of food consumption are associated with fewer sources of error than estimates of past intake and hence are particularly appropriate for research purposes and for assessing the accuracy of epidemiological methods.[1,5] Precoded food records are currently under investigation for large scale prospective trials and are discussed in section 6.6.

All methods for assessing habitual food intake in free-living individuals rely on information supplied by the subjects themselves, which may not be correct. Recent findings show that results obtained from even the method that has been considered to be the most accurate, the weighed dietary record, is associated with substantial bias in western societies (see section 6.5.1). Furthermore, 'simple' epidemiological methods tend to give results that are as low, or lower, than results obtained from the weighed dietary record. Hence, bias may not be overcome by simplifying methods in order to reduce the burden of work for the individual under observation.

Bias in the overall average may well be due to errors in reports from some individuals in the distribution (differential misclassification), rather than a systematic rendering of biased information from all individuals (non-differential misclassification). Biological markers for determining bias at an individual level are now available and it is worthwhile to incorporate these into future protocols, particularly those that set out to use records to assess the accuracy of methods for large scale epidemiological uses.

6.2. DESCRIPTION: WEIGHED AND ESTIMATED RECORDS

Detailed descriptions of methods for obtaining records of food intake are given elsewhere, together with practical information on equipment, timing, protocols, etc.[5,6] In these methods, subjects are taught to describe and give an estimate of the weight of food immediately before eating, and to record any leftovers. Details of recipes are necessary, and a data bank of average recipes used in a particular locality, together with manufactured foods, greatly simplifies the procedure. Records, either weighed or described, are very different from the so-called 'precise weighing' that is necessary if food composition tables with values for cooked foods are not available. Raw ingredients, the cooked food, meal, or snack, plus the individual portions must all be weighed,[7] and aliquots for chemical analysis may also be necessary. It is usual for skilled field-workers to carry out this survey, rather than the subjects themselves.

Records are generally written, although portable tape recorders have been used.[8] Novel approaches have included food photography. In one procedure, photographs of meals consumed by the survey subject are projected alongside standard slides showing a variety of portion sizes of the same foods.[9] The other procedure uses a computer to convert photographs of foods into volumetric and weight equivalents.[10] Food photography avoids the use of scales or other measures and might reduce the disruption resulting from weighed and measured surveys, although these methods are not yet in common use. The PETRA (Portable Electronic Tape Recorded Automatic) scales combine both a tape recorder and an electronic scale, which automatically records both a verbal description and the weight of food on a dual track cassette (Cherlyn Electronics, Cambridge). The weight of food consumed is not available to the subject, in contrast to the usual procedure where the subject is given a set of spring balances or dietary electronic scales and records the weight of food him- or herself in a notebook. Where scales are not used, portions of food are described in terms of household measures, volume models, photographs, average portions, units, or pack sizes.[1,11] This involves the investigator in a considerable amount of work to convert the various descriptions used into weights of food eaten.[11] Larger scale surveys generally incorporate standard descriptions and weight equivalents into computer databases of the chemical composition of foods.

Detailed manual coding of food records is rapidly becoming superseded by 'menu' computer programs based on food groups, usually characterized by their source and nutritional composition (cereal, meat, etc.). These should remove much of the time, tedium, and considerable error associated with manual coding of food records. Systems that use aggregated food codes for major categories of foods are also available. The FRED (Food Recording Electronic Device) is an electronic scale linked to a personal computer modified with designated keys for major items of foods ('potatoes', etc.). The subject places the food on the scale and presses the appropriate key. Nutrient intakes are then calculated directly by the computer using the weight of food and the aggregated data base.[12] The NESSy (Nutritional Evaluation Scale System) is a similar system, except that foods are identified and entered into the computer via a bar code reader.[13] Bar code readers have also been used with a record book, weights of food being estimated as small, medium, or large portions.[14]

6.3 ACCURACY

Records require a high degree of cooperation from subjects, partly because their low day-to-day repeatability, (see below) may require many days of record from each subject. Nevertheless, cooperation rates in excess of 80 per cent from randomly selected samples have been achieved both from records with weights of food and records with estimated weights of food, over 4–7-day periods.[1,11] If a precise measure of an individual's average intake is required, studies of longer duration are necessary, and compliance is likely to be substantially reduced.

The weighed dietary record has generally been regarded as the 'gold standard' of dietary assessments and, for this reason, the accuracy (repeatability and validity) of other methods has usually been measured by comparison with it. Hence, there have been no assessments of the validity of records using estimated weights of food with independent markers of food intake, such as the doubly labelled water or 24-hour urine nitrogen. On balance, there appears to be little or no systematic bias in group averages of nutrients obtained by records with estimates of food, compared with group averages obtained by weighed dietary records.[1,11] Nevertheless, despite the absence of overall bias in a population, the estimation of portion size rather than direct weighing is associated with imprecision at the individual level. In general, this is in the order of 50 per cent (co-efficient of variation) for foods, but less, about 20 per cent, for nutrients, probably due to cancellation of error from the use of food tables. Table 6.1 shows a summary of comparisons between estimated and direct weights of food. Models and photographs may incur less error in the estimation of portion weights, at least when compared with estimations from household measures and dimensions. For example, Rutishauser showed that when nutrition students were asked to estimate portion size, the coefficients of variation of differences between actual and estimated weights were from 16 to 53 per cent with household measures and 10 to 27 per cent with models and photographs.[15] However, using a book of photographs alone, Brock and Ellery found that the variance on any one food item was high, from 30 to 50 per cent (Table 6.1).[16] Bollard *et al.* trained students to estimate food portions using either food models or household measures.[17] There was no difference in the accuracy of either method in assessing predetermined weights of food and coefficients of variation ranging from about 20 per cent for cornbread to 70 per cent for sugar (Table 6.1). However, these trained

Table 6.1 Coefficients of variation of differences in estimated versus measured weights of food eaten

Foods		Nutrients
Household measures	Photographs	
1–96[a]	9–44[f]	7–11[h]
13–32[b]	30–50[g]	11–16[i]
16–53[c]	10–27[c]	19–28[j]
21–70[d]		
21–91[e]		

(a) Minimum value cookies, maximum casseroles;[21] (b) Minimum value heaped tablespoons, maximum level teaspoons;[45] (c) [15] (d) Minimum value corn bread, maximum sugar;[17] (e) Minimum value drinks, maximum cake;[18] (f) [46] (g) [16] (h) Minimum value energy, maximum iron;[19] (i) Energy 11%, protein 16%;[8] (j) Minimum value protein, maximum vitamin C.[20]

students performed significantly better than untrained students in estimating portion size.[17]

Blake et al. asked 94 women, 46 of whom were overweight, to estimate the weight of foods eaten in a cafeteria, and foods on display.[18] No difference in the ability of the overweight subjects to estimate portion size could be discerned when compared with normal weight subjects. Coefficients of variation were the same as found elsewhere, from 20 to 90 per cent (Table 6.1).

From Table 6.1 it can be seen that the coefficients of variation for nutrients assessed ranged from 7 to 16 per cent in two studies,[8,19] where averages of 3 and 15 days were compared, much less than those for foods. The errors incurred in Bransby et al.'s study[19] were likely to be conservative, because all the estimations were done by trained field-workers. When untrained subjects, such as the housewives in the study by Eppright et al.,[20] make the estimations, and when only a single day was considered, coefficients of variation were from 20 to 30 per cent, and there was a systematic overestimation of nutrient intake (Table 6.1). In the study by Young et al.,[21] of the subjects who were unaware that their food intake was being observed, less than half were able to estimate their portions of food with sufficient accuracy to enable nutrient intake to be calculated to within 10 per cent of the correct value. In more than two-thirds of subjects, erroneous estimates of portion weights gave results greater than 20 per cent of the correct value.

The use of food photographs may improve precision. For example, Edington et al. incorporated a series of photographs of small, medium and large portions of many commonly used foods that are not readily estimated

Table 6.2 Percentage of subjects whose nutrient intakes estimated from household measures is within ± 10 per cent of the value based on weighed records of consumption[11]

Nutrient	Study		
	Bransby et al.[19]	Eppright et al.[20]	Nettleton et al.[24]
Energy	71	33	92
Protein	49	41	87
Fat	41	37	71
Carbohydrate	82	37	89
Calcium	69	35	100
Iron	35	–	84
Thiamin	–	32	87
Ascorbic acid	–	29	79
No.	49	25	38

– indicates value not published

in household measures into a food record book.[22] Twenty-two subjects kept weighed records of their food intake for 7 days, 3 to 7 months after completing the 7-day food record book. Correlation coefficients for nutrients calculated by the two methods were in the order of 0.7, with little evidence of misclassification into thirds of the distribution.

The 'semiweighed' technique, in which information from prepacked foods is used, is associated with smaller errors, 2 to 5 per cent.[11,23,24] Table 6.2 shows that the percentage of subjects within ± 10 per cent of the value based on weighed records of consumption is greatly increased compared with the studies of Bransby and Eppright mentioned above.[19,20] Furthermore, the remaining error associated with the semiweighed technique is small compared with that from daily variation (see below). This indicates that the variance and therefore ranking of individuals within a distribution of nutrient intake, seems little affected whether or not weighed or semiweighed records are used.[11]

6.4 REPEATABILITY

The error associated with the estimation of weight of food is generally assumed to be random. If this is the case, error will be reduced by increasing the number of observations on each individual. In addition, as has been detailed elsewhere,[1,25] individuals vary substantially from day to day in

Table 6.3 Detectable difference*† in means for sample size of 500, $\alpha = 0.05$, $\beta = 0.20$

	% detectable difference in averages from different numbers of observations on each subject		
	One day	Three days	Seven days
Energy	6	5	4
Protein	6	5	5
Fat	7	5	5
Dietary fibre	7	5	5
Riboflavin	8	5	4

* Variances[47]; † Formulae[48,49]
(see also eqns 2.1, 2.4)

their intake of foods and nutrients. Daily variation is one of the main factors in reducing precision of record methods of assessing diet. The variability from day to day is closely related to the nutrient under study. The early descriptions of record techniques specified that subjects should be observed for seven days and this practice has been followed for nearly 50 years.[26,27] Nevertheless, when only the average intake of a group of individuals is required for cross-sectional studies, it is difficult to justify gathering this amount of data, even for the more variable nutrients such as cholesterol, or polyunsaturated fatty acids. A 3- to 4-day record, randomized to cover seasonal and weekday variations, seems to be the optimum, there being little decrease in the difference between averages that can be detected from a given sample size if the number of observations on each subject is increased to 7 days (Table 6.3).

In some circumstances, a 1-day record collected from a large number of subjects, may suffice for the assessment of group means, although it is generally more useful to obtain at least two days of record to be able to estimate the within-subject component of error.

Longer periods of observation on each individual are necessary for cohort and dietary validation studies. Table 6.4 shows the number of recording days necessary to classify 80 per cent of subjects correctly into the extreme thirds of the distribution, based on data from three population groups. The actual number of records in any specific population will depend on the specific ratio between the average within-person daily variation and the between-person variation. Nevertheless, it is clear from Table 6.4 that, whereas a 7-day record is probably sufficient to classify into

Table 6.4 Number of daily food records necessary to correctly classify 80 per cent of men into the extreme thirds of the distribution $P < 0.05$

	British Civil Servants (Marr, 1981[50])	Random selection of British men (Bingham et al., 1981[47])	Random selection of Swedish men*
Energy	7	5	7
Protein	6	5	7
Fat	9	9	7
Carbohydrate	4	3	3
Sugar	2	2	–
Dietary fibre	6	10	–
P:S ratio	11	–	–
Cholesterol	18	–	–
Alcohol	4	–	14
Vitamin C	–	6	14
Thiamin	–	6	15
Riboflavin	–	10	–
Calcium	–	4	5
Iron	–	12	9

*Callmer, Personal communication. 58×7-day weighed records from middle-aged men randomly selected in Stockholm, Sweden.

thirds of the distribution for energy and energy-yielding nutrients, longer periods are necessary for items such as alcohol, some vitamins and minerals, and cholesterol. Only if a less precise estimate of individual mean intakes is acceptable, and correct classification into extreme fifths of the distribution is adequate, would a 7-day record be sufficient for these more variable food constituents.[28]

6.5 VALIDITY

6.5.1 Weighed records

Since the weighed dietary record has in the past been regarded as the 'gold standard' of dietary methodology, there has been little questioning of its accuracy. The error in estimating individual nutrient intakes from 7-day measurements has been well documented but, in addition, the validity of this method used to assess the habitual diet of free-living individuals has come increasingly to be questioned, following the introduction of two biological markers of food intake that are sufficiently accurate in themselves to compare with detailed weighed food records.

The doubly-labelled water method is an important advance in the measurement of energy expenditure and it can be used on free-living individuals with virtually no interference with everyday life, in contrast to previous procedures. Subjects are given a carefully weighed oral dose of $^2H_2^{18}O$ and are then required only to donate timed urine samples over the next 15 days. Carbon dioxide production is measured as the difference in the water pool (measured by $^2H_2$) and the bicarbonate plus water pool (measured as ^{18}O). Changes in body weight and the water pool can be used to correct measured energy intake in relation to energy expenditure from the doubly-labelled water method. When this is done, energy expenditure should equal energy intake.

In early reports, energy expenditure assessed from this method was unexpectedly low, 1.4 times the basal metabolic rate (BMR) on average in a small group of sedentary women.[29] In women of normal weight, energy intake from weighed dietary records agreed with energy expenditure data but in obese women, energy intake assessed from 7-day weighed records was about 2 MJ (465 kcal) lower than expenditure, suggesting that over-weight women do not report their habitual food intake.[30]

In a more recent study, energy expenditure also exceeded energy intake measured from 7-day records in 31 normal individuals, on average by 20 per cent.[31] As a ratio to BMR, energy intake was 1.46 ± 0.31, and energy expenditure was 1.82 ± 0.24, greater than previously found in sedentary women.[29] Reported energy intakes agreed with energy expenditure in about one-third of these subjects, predominantly those who were at the higher end of the distribution of energy intake.[31]

The doubly-labelled water method is too expensive for routine use for validation of dietary intake measurements but the usefulness of the 24-hour urine nitrogen method is currently being assessed. Isaksson first proposed that 24-hour urine nitrogen (N) should be used as an independent validity check on dietary survey methods.[32] This depends on the assumption that subjects are in nitrogen balance, with no loss due to starvation or injury and with no gain, and it has been used to validate dietary survey methods used to estimate average dietary intakes of groups in a number of population studies in Gothenburg.[32] Further studies from this group have confirmed the difficulties of dietary assessments of patients in clinical work. For example, reported protein intake in obese subjects (from a diet history) was only 46 g but on the basis of 24-hour urine collections it was 87 g.[33] In another study, subjects who were overweight or diabetic seemed to report their prescribed diet rather than what they were actually eating as judged by their urine N excretion.[34]

In an ongoing study of the validity of various methods of dietary assessment in individuals in Cambridge, subjects are asked to weigh their food using PETRA scales for 4 days and to collect 24-hour urine samples, once when weighing their food (Urine I) and once when not weighing their food (Urine II). The completeness of the urine samples is assessed by the

Table 6.5 Analytes in complete versus incomplete 24-hour urine collections

Specimens from:		Mean	Standard deviation	Significance of difference
Hospital outpatients				
Volume (ml)	1[a]	1788	663	ns
	2	1692	971	
PABA (%)	1	94	6	0.001
	2	70	12	
Potassium (mmol)	1	63	19	ns
	2	56	13	
Sodium (mmol)	1	134	51	0.03
	2	103	51	
Creatinine (mmol)	1	10.8	3.0	0.06
	2	9.3	2.7	
Urea (mmol)	1	301	78	0.001
	2	223	63	
Nitrogen (g)	1	10.1	2.7	0.01
	2	8.3	2.4	
Randomly selected healthy men				
PABA (%)	1[b]	95	6	0.001
	2	69	9	
Potassium (mmol)	1	74	23	ns
	2	66	15	
Sodium (mmol)	1	172	52	0.001
	2	131	31	
Urea (mmol)	1	380	104	0.001
	2	281	64	

[a] 1 'Complete' group: 30 female and 15 male patients; total 45 collections; duration 23.6 ± 0.6 h; 2 'Incomplete' group: 9 female and 9 male patients; total 18 collections; duration 23.5 ± 1.0 h.
[b] 1 'Complete' group: 71 men, duration 23.5 ± 2.2 h; 2 'Incomplete' group: 12 men, duration 21.7 ± 5.0 h.
ns, not significant.

PABAcheck method.[35] Subjects are asked to repeat this four times per year, and so far 80 subjects have been studied. Body weight is also obtained, together with a fasting blood and breath sample, at each dietary season.

The importance of including a measure of the completeness of the urine collections themselves is shown in Tables 6.5 and 6.6, where data from another epidemiological study[36] and some clinical work[37–38] has been collated in Table 6.5 with that from the present study in Table 6.6. In urines that have been classified as incomplete, there are systematically

Table 6.6 Specimens collected by dietary validation volunteers

		Mean	Standard deviation	Significance of difference
Season One				
PABA (%)	1[a]	92.2	6.0	0.001
	2	70.1	11.4	
Nitrogen (g)	1	10.4	2.4	0.001
	2	8.9	2.1	
Season Two				
PABA (%)	1[b]	92.7	7.2	0.001
	2	74.4	10.7	
Nitrogen (g)	1	10.6	2.2	0.001
	2	9.2	2.1	

[a] 1 'Complete' group, 94 females; 2 'Incomplete' group, 64 females.
[b] 1 'Complete' group, 88 females; 2 'Incomplete' group, 67 females.

lower contents of nearly all analytes compared with those that are complete. The consistently lower values for nitrogen are particularly important from the point of dietary validation, because it shows that omission of an objective check on 24-hour urine collections in a dietary validation study will under-estimate the extent of bias in a dietary assessment method.

On completion of the study, the average N intake from the 16 days of records is then compared with the average N excretion in the complete 24-hour urine collections, with the expected ratio of urine N to dietary N being 81 ± 5 per cent.[39] So far, 31 of the 80 individuals have excreted more than two standard deviations in excess of the expected ratio of 81 per cent (91 per cent) of their reported dietary N intake in urine, and have been classified as 'under-reporters'. Of these, eight lost from 2 to 4 kg body weight over the year, but seven gained 2–4 kg. No changes occurred in the other 16 subjects.

Table 6.7 compares daily dietary intake data and body weight (mean and standard deviation) for the 31 'under-reporters' and 49 other subjects. The under-reporters were significantly heavier than the other subjects and differences were evident between average reported intakes of energy, protein, fat, and sugars from records obtained from under-reporters and those subjects whose records appeared to be valid from the 24-hour urine nitrogen. There were no differences in alcohol, non-starch polysaccharide (NSP), and starch consumption.

Hence, bias in reports of food intake obtained from weighed dietary

Table 6.7 Nutrient intakes from weighed records and body weights of 31 individuals classified as under-reporters from 24-hour urine N, compared with 49 individuals with satisfactory records

	Energy (MJ)	Protein (g)	Fat (g)	Alcohol (g)	Sugars (g)	Starch (g)	NSP (g)	Weight (kg)
Under-reporters (n = 31)								
Mean	6.89	62	65	9	88	103	14	74
SD	1.46	12	18	14	35	30	6	13
Others (n = 49)								
Mean	8.68	73	86	9	124	112	15	62
SD	1.68	15	22	16	37	30	5	8
P	<0.001	<0.001	<0.001	ns	<0.001	ns	ns	<0.001

records can be detected by the use of 24-hour urine nitrogen. Simultaneous use of both the 24-hour urine N and doubly-labelled water has shown that both methods identify the same subjects who under-report their food intake when asked to keep weighed records.[40] Only some, not all, nutrients may be under-reported and the range of individual values within the distribution will be artefactually extended. For example, Figure 6.1

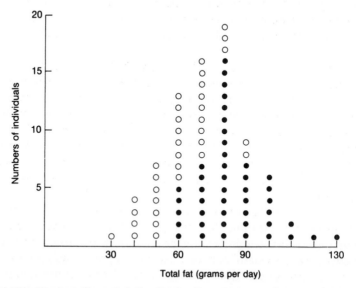

Fig. 6.1 Distribution of total daily dietary fat (g) in 86 volunteer women aged 50–65 measured over 16 days by weighed food records using the PETRA system. Open symbols are under-reporters, as judged by 24-hour urine nitrogen excretion.

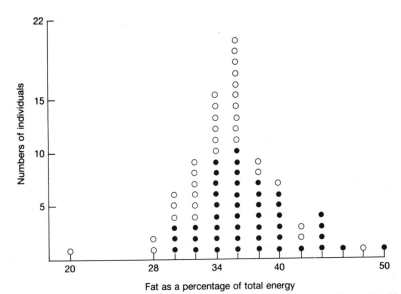

Fig. 6.2. As Figure 6.1, except values are for fat as a percentage of total energy.

shows the distribution of reported intakes of fat where it can be seen that under-recording has a particular effect on the distribution of the absolute intake of fat, although there is less truncation of the distribution when expressed as a proportion of total energy (Fig. 6.2).

In this survey, under-reporting was more likely to occur in overweight individuals, and could have arisen either from failure to report all food eaten during the 16-day period, or because the subjects decided to diet whilst weighing their food, causing a negative nitrogen balance. Long term slimming can also cause negative nitrogen balance, although only three subjects lost from 2 to 4 kg during the survey year. Adiposity may not be a universal predictor of the tendency to under-report; Livingstone *et al.* found no association between body mass index and the extent of under-reporting from the 7-day weighed record assessed by the doubly-labelled water method.[31]

Validated 24-hour urine collections are feasible and, increasingly, a prerequisite for validation studies of dietary methods in nutritional epidemiology. Body weight can also be measured, and an approximate (± 12 per cent) estimate of basal metabolic rate calculated from the equations in Table 6.8. Energy intakes of less than 1.2 × the BMR calculated in this way can be excluded from analyses with certainty as erroneous estimates of habitual food intake. However, greater accuracy in predicting cut-off values is not possible in the absence of accurate measures of BMR.

Table 6.8 Equations for estimated basal metabolic rate from weight

Ages of subjects	n	R	SE
Under 3 years			
m BMR = 0.249 wt − 0.127	162	0.95	0.2925
f BMR = 0.244 wt − 0.130	137	0.96	0.2456
3 − 10 years			
m BMR = 0.095 wt + 2.110	338	0.83	0.2803
f BMR = 0.085 wt + 2.033	413	0.81	0.2924
10−18 years			
m BMR = 0.074 wt + 2.754	734	0.93	0.4404
f BMR = 0.056 wt + 2.898	575	0.80	0.4661
18−30 years			
m BMR = 0.063 wt + 2.896	2878	0.65	0.6407
f BMR = 0.062 wt + 2.036	829	0.73	0.4967
30−60 years			
m BMR = 0.048 wt + 3.653	646	0.60	0.6997
f BMR = 0.034 wt + 3.538	372	0.68	0.4653
Over 60 years			
m BMR = 0.049 wt + 2.459	50	0.71	0.6865
f BMR = 0.038 wt + 2.755	38	0.68	0.4511

From Schofield et al.[51] m, male; f, female; n, sample size; R, correlation coefficient; SE, standard error. BMR is expressed in MJ/24 h; weight (wt) is expressed in kg.

6.5.2 Estimated records

The validity of other types of records of food intake using estimated weights of food has rarely been assessed. However, these and other methods, with the possible exception of the diet history, tend to give the same or lower values as weighed diet records on an average basis.[5,11] For example, Hallfrisch et al. found that a record with estimated weights of food kept by 24 men and women underestimated true intake (as assessed by the amount of energy required to maintain weight in a controlled study) by 3.8 MJ (900 kcals) in women and by 2.1 MJ (500 kcals) in men.[41]

6.6 RECORDING TECHNIQUES FOR COHORT STUDIES

To obtain the required accuracy of dietary exposure in individuals, 5–10 days of diet record would be required for energy and macronutrients, and considerably more days for some micronutrients (see Table 6.4). Often, because of the size of cohort studies required to obtain sufficient numbers of outcome units, it is not feasible to assess diet using record techniques.

One solution is to conserve resources by using a nested case control design (see Chapter 11) and only code and analyse data for cases and matched controls several years after the dietary data has been obtained. Another solution may be to use a record system, precoded according to the most frequently consumed foods or food groups. For example, Johnson *et al.* developed such a technique for use with women, each of whom is provided with a precoded daily record form which is filled out as food is eaten.[42] Up to 72 records per person have been obtained.[43] Unpublished work of Elmer is quoted as showing very high correlation coefficients, 0.8 to 0.9, between nutrient intakes calculated from weighed records, and the record form in institutionalized women.[42] Agreement between average nutrient intakes calculated from weighed records and the precoded record form in 162 free-living women was also almost complete, although the extent of agreement on an individual basis does not seem to have been reported in these free-living individuals.[42,44] Ongoing studies comparing similar types of precoded recording systems suggest rather better agreement on an individual basis between these and 16 days of PETRA records (see section 6.5) than other simplified methods, such as the 24-hour recall and food frequency questionnaire.

Past intake

Michael Nelson

6.7 INTRODUCTION

The majority of nutritional epidemiological studies require detailed information on diet and nutrient intake from large numbers of subjects. Furthermore, the aim is frequently to characterize the diet at a time in the past that coincides with the induction of disease (although recent dietary factors that may influence the progress of disease may also be of interest). The methods for collecting records of current diet outlined in the first part of this chapter are often expensive in terms of staff and time, and address questions of current diet only; and, if past diet is the relevant exposure, forcing the investigator to assume that current and past diet are closely correlated, or to make an assessment of the ways in which current and past diet are related. For these reasons, relatively inexpensive methods that characterize past diet are needed, and the aim of this section of the chapter is to describe those methods and to highlight their strengths and weaknesses in nutritional epidemiological studies. Most of the discussion that follows concerns dietary assessment in the relatively recent past, and only a few studies have addressed the question of methodology and validity of recall of diet in the distant past.

The methods available for assessing past diet all have at their core the need to ask individuals to recall accurately the frequency and/or quantities of food that were consumed on previous occasions. The simplest of these is the 24-hour recall, in which subjects are asked in a systematic way to recall their food consumption from the previous day. The most complex is the diet history, in which subjects are asked, during the course of a long and detailed interview, to describe as fully as possible their usual pattern of consumption, including day to day and seasonal variations. In between, there are methods such as the food frequency questionnaire (FQ) and the food frequency and amount questionnaire (FAQ), which assess diet using a fixed number of questions, and which usually aim to characterize subjects according to their position in the distribution of intake for purposes of grouping or ranking. These methods commonly have a highly structured format and are often completed by the respondent without the need for an interviewer.

Because these methods depend entirely on the ability of the subject to provide accurate information, none of which is easily corroborated, it is necessary to establish the relative validity of the responses obtained. This can be done in two ways. The first is to include markers of internal validity in the assessment process. This involves asking the subject for the same information in different ways (without being too obvious!) to see if the evidence from one question is consistent with another. The second is to use an external marker of validity, usually a so-called 'objective' measure (such as the weighed record), against which the retrospective method can be checked. The purpose of the validation process is to assess the extent to which subjects may be misclassified using the chosen measuring instrument. Some studies that assess measurement error are limited to measures of repeatability, an important part of the validation process, but not in itself sufficient to show whether differential misclassification is likely to affect the interpretation of results in an epidemiological study. A full discussion of the validation process is given in Chapter 8.

6.8 ADVANTAGES AND DISADVANTAGES OF RETROSPECTIVE METHODS

Table 6.9 summarizes the advantages and disadvantages of retrospective methods. To the epidemiologist, the methods are attractive because they are cheap in comparison with most of the methods for assessing current diet; they are usually quick to administer, whether in an interview or by post; the respondent burden is characteristically low, which usually en-

Table 6.9 Advantages and disadvantages of retrospective
methods of dietary assessment

Advantages	Disadvantages
Quick	Reliant on memory
Cheap	Conceptualization skills needed
Low subject motivation	Observer bias possible
Low literacy and	Reported diet may be a distortion
numeracy skills	No measure of day to day
Good cooperation	variation in diet
	Requires regular eating habits
	Dependent on food composition
	tables

hances the rate of cooperation, thereby increasing the representativeness
of the sample; and, if conducted by interview, they overcome problems
related to limited literacy and numeracy skills in the population.

However, there are many disadvantages, necessitating validation in most
circumstances. First, responses are dependent upon subjects' ability to
remember food consumption accurately, which varies in an unsystematic
way from person to person, although it can be said generally that children
under the age of about 12 and elderly people are less likely to recall diet
well. Children under 12 should not be asked to recall their diets without the
help of an adult, and subjects over the age of 60 should be given a simple
mental ability test (such as the Hodkinson Abbreviated Mental Test
Score[52]) to ensure that basic memory skills are intact. The problem of
memory relates primarily to the omission of foods, particularly sauces and
condiments that may contribute significantly to micronutrient intakes in
some diets. The number of foods recalled is often correlated with the total
intake of energy and nutrients,[53] and important differential misclassification will occur between those with good memories and those with poor
memories. It could nevertheless be argued that, in a case-control study, the
distribution of people with good and bad memories is likely to be similar
amongst both cases and controls, and that the only effect will be attenuation of relative risk estimates. However, if the disease process or drugs
used in treatment affect memory only in the cases, then it is possible that
the calculation of disease risk in relation to diet could be severely distorted,
and over- or under-estimated. Validation of retrospective measure of diet
in hospitalized patients is particularly problematic.

Like memory, conceptualization skills, or the ability to relate actual
consumption to descriptions of portion sizes and estimates of frequency,
will vary substantially between individuals. Children under 12 are again
likely to be poor at conceptualization, even when visual aids in the form of

photographs, portion models, or actual food models are used. Some aid to describe portion sizes is usually necessary. Particularly when regional differences in diet are being assessed, what may be regarded as a small portion in one area may be medium in another; an 'average' portion for a woman is typically smaller than an 'average' portion for a man.

Observer bias can take two forms. In the first, one observer may ask a different set of questions from another. This is again a problem of special importance in regional studies, when it is likely that different interviewers will be used in different regions to save on time and travel costs. In the second form, the interviewer in case-control studies may change the emphasis of questions if he or she is aware of the hypothesis being tested. The first problem can be overcome principally by adequate training, making the likely contribution of observer bias small.[54] The second problem can be overcome by blinding the observer to the status of the patient (if that is possible), i.e. the cases are not all being interviewed in hospital and the controls at home. Where this is not possible, a more structured interview can reduce the problem, or, if observer bias is likely to be a severe problem, it may even be an advantage to substitute a self-completing questionnaire with a follow-up interview.

Subjects may distort their reported diet for several reasons. First, they may not wish to confess to the consumption of certain types of foods, particularly sweets and alcohol, which are notoriously under-reported, often by 50 per cent or more. Second, subjects may more generally wish to report a diet that they believe will be acceptable in the eyes of the interviewer (for example, reporting less consumption of fried foods and more of fruit and vegetables). These distortions may be greater in a face to face interview than when filling in a self-completing questionnaire or using a computer terminal interactively. Third, people often idealize their consumption by reporting a diet that they believe reflects what they usually do, or would like to achieve, but which in fact represents their activity only a small proportion of the time. This is of particular concern in subjects who are overweight, where the level of consumption reported has been shown to be inversely proportional to their weight.[55] Distortions of this type can only be brought to light by careful validation, using methods that are not liable to reporting or recording errors (see 6.5.1 and Chapter 7).

Most retrospective methods do not provide a measure of day to day variation in diet. The exception is repeat 24-hour recalls,[54,56] but these are in essence the application of a retrospective method to the assessment of current diet. Given that a diet history or questionnaire will, to some extent, misclassify individuals according to their true intake, it is important to have a measurement of error associated with each individual's estimate of mean intake. Repeat interview or application of questionnaire will provide an estimate of error associated with the measuring tool but not with the variability of each individual's intake. Thus, retrospective techniques are generally less effective than prospective techniques in identifying within-subject sources of measurement error, and it is therefore more difficult to adjust for attenuation of risk in epidemiological analyses. Approaches to this problem are discussed in Chapter 8.

All of these methods, apart from the 24-hour recall, require that subjects have sufficiently regular habits for the concept of 'usual' intake to have meaning, to allow successful completion of an interview or questionnaire in which regular frequency of consumption is the key to accuracy. Subjects whose diets consist primarily of a small number of foods eaten very regularly are more likely to have their dietary intakes assessed accurately than subjects who eat a wide variety of foods relatively infrequently.[57] Interview or questionnaire responses give no immediate clues as to the true characteristics of the subject's diet, and differential misclassification is likely to occur in regional comparisons of diet if meal patterns and the availability of foods differ substantially between regions.

Finally, it is important to remember that all estimates of nutrient intakes based on retrospective methods are dependent upon food composition tables. The problems inherent in their use are discussed in detail in Chapter 4.

6.9 METHODS, APPLICATIONS, AND VALIDITY

In addition to the general features of retrospective methods described above, each technique has particular attributes that make it more or less appropriate to different investigations. These attributes are discussed below.

6.9.1 24-hour recall

Originally attributed to Wiehl,[58] the technique for administering a 24-hour recall is deceptively simple. Each subject is asked, through a systematic series of questions, to recall and describe all food and drink consumed in the 24 hours prior to the interview. Typically, the respondent is asked to recall diet from waking up to the time of the interview, and then to recall diet from exactly 24 hours previously until going to bed. The detail of description must be consistent with the food tables upon which nutrient calculations are to be based, and the interviewer must be thoroughly familiar with the food habits of the population from which the sample has been drawn. Photographs or food portion models portraying likely portion sizes (and based on previous surveys of food consumption within the population) are likely to improve estimation of portion size, and respondents should be given as wide a latitude as possible to describe portions in their own terms, rather than the interviewer suggesting measures with which the respondent may be unfamiliar. Interviews should be conducted in the subject's native language where this will facilitate more complete and accurate responses. It is essential that interviewers receive adequate training in the technique, as it is easy to bias subjects' responses through ill-judged or leading questions, or by failing to probe adequately for items not initially mentioned.

The Nordic Cooperation Group of Dietary Researchers suggests a recommended procedure that is intended to minimize differential misclassification and facilitate the collection of representative results:[6]

1. Subjects should be given no prior warning that they will be interviewed because they may choose to alter their habits.
2. The recall should be conducted as an interview (either in person or by telephone).
3. The interview should take place in a quiet, relaxed atmosphere and, in so far as possible, should follow the same format for every subject.
4. In the sample as a whole (and within any strata on which data will be analysed), interviews should be evenly distributed over the days of the week.
5. The order of recall should commence with the first food or drink taken in the day (or, for night workers, from midnight to midnight).
6. The interviewer should ask neutral questions and should be aware of combinations of foods likely to be eaten together so as to be able to probe effectively for items not mentioned.
7. Aids to description of portion sizes should be provided.
8. An open-ended form with precoded foods listed may aid speed of recording and subsequent coding.

The principal advantages of the 24-hour recall are its speed and ease of administration. This allows large numbers of subjects to be interviewed with the minimum of resources. Compliance is usually excellent because of the small amount of information required from each respondent. This has made its use particularly attractive in very large-scale studies such as the Ten-State Survey, NHANES I and II, and Nutrition Canada.[59–61]

The principal limitation of the 24-hour recall is that it does not provide a reliable estimate of an individual's intake because of day to day variation. 24-hour recall data cannot, therefore, be used to rank subjects reliably.[62] If used for this purpose in epidemiological studies, the ability to describe significant relationships between diet and disease risk will be severely reduced (although not entirely lost). This holds true even if subjects are grouped according to their intake (high, medium, and low) based on their 24-hour recalls, as the degree of misclassification will persist. The problem is compounded by the fact that 24-hour recall results exhibit the 'flat-slope' syndrome:[63] subjects with true low intakes tend to report higher than usual intakes, and those with true high intakes tend to report lower than usual intakes. While this may not significantly influence the mean, the variation in intakes between subjects is further underestimated. The problem can in part be overcome by obtaining repeat 24-hour recalls,[56] but the advantages in terms of cost and inconvenience quickly begin to evaporate and make other techniques more attractive.

The validity of group mean nutrient intakes based on 24-hour recalls has been assessed by comparing results with weighed records[64,65] and diet histories.[62,66,67] The results are not always consistent, but across a wide variety of samples, including children, adults, and elderly people, suggest that 24-hour recalls tend to underestimate group intakes, the extent of the underestimation varying with different nutrients.[68] What is striking in the Acheson study[64] is that the men, all scientists, underestimated their energy intakes by an average of 21 per cent on the day after they had actually weighed their food and drink. The repeatability of 24-hour results on a group basis is generally good.[62,67,69]

Twenty-four-hour recalls are thus appropriate for measuring current diet in groups of subjects, and are therefore particularly well suited to studies where differences between group means are to be assessed, either in cross-section or longitudinally. The number of subjects needed in a study is a function of the likely size of the difference between means, and the within- and between-subject variance (which will vary with the nutrient in question). The methods of calculating n are given in Chapter 2 and in Nelson *et al.*[70] If information on variation in diet within or between subjects is needed, as few as two repeat measures may help to elucidate the likely extent of misclassification of individuals, although the more repeats, the better the classification is likely to be. Estimates of intake are generally lower than with other methods, particularly diet histories, and if information on intake in relation to dietary cut-off or threshold values is needed, this must be taken into account.

6.9.2 Diet history

The research diet history, attributed to Burke,[71] consists of a three-part assessment: (i) a detailed interview to assess usual consumption of a wide variety of foods; (ii) a cross-check food frequency list; (iii) a 3-day record. Most allusions to the 'diet history' in the literature refer to the interview alone, and the food frequency list and 3-day record, used by Burke as markers of internal validity, tend to be forgotten.

The diet history is typically a detailed interview to establish 'usual' food consumption patterns. Often starting with a 24-hour recall, the interviewer probes carefully for food consumption meal by meal, seeking day to day and seasonal variations to build up the 'usual' pattern. As with the 24-hour recall, aids to memory and conceptualization, in the form of food lists and photographs or models, contribute significantly to the accuracy of the assessment. Interviews often last for 1 to 2 hours, and are best recorded on prepared forms that allow for the meals, foods, and variations to be noted clearly and systematically. Interviewer training is vital, both to ensure that diet histories are complete and that differences between interviewers are minimized. It is not acceptable for untrained interviewers to undertake diet histories, however straightforward they may at first appear.

The diet history has numerous theoretical and practical advantages over prospective methods and over 24-hour recalls and questionnaires. A single, extended interview can provide detailed information about meal patterns, food consumption, and nutrient intake for an individual. Depending upon the quality of the food composition tables used to calculate nutrient intake, diet histories can provide data on the usual intakes of a wide variety of nutrients. Subject involvement is kept to a minimum and no literacy or numeracy skills are needed. The information is representative of diet over specified periods, regarding both the interval and point in time, which can be varied to suit the needs of the study. Particular attention can be paid to foods or nutrients that may be of special interest (for example, sources of dietary selenium), or that are notoriously under-reported (such as sweets and alcohol). An individual's consumption of foods relatively infrequently eaten but that may be important sources of nutrient (liver and offals, for example), or highly seasonal foods, is better assessed by diet history than by other methods.

The disadvantages of the diet history are common to those relating to other recall methods as regards memory, conceptualization, regular habits, etc. Moreover, the complexity of the procedure makes it particularly prone to interviewer bias, and subjects are likely to recall diet that relates to the immediate past and not necessarily to the period of interest. Diet histories may also exaggerate the regularity of dietary habits,[6] and do not provide information about day to day variations in diet. Assessment of the likely error of misclassification is more difficult than in prospective methods, requiring both repeat measures within individuals using the diet history, and comparison with a more 'objective' external standard.

The repeatability of diet histories is generally good for assessing group means of energy and macronutrients for periods up to two years before the interview,[72–74] although the repeatability of ranking is less consistent, correlations for repeat interviews ranging from 0.57 to 0.9 in the study by Reshef and Epstein[73] and up to 0.92 in the study by Morgan[74], to as low as 0.13 for protein in a study of elderly subjects.[75] The results for micronutrients are generally poorer than those for macronutrients,[75,76] Beyond two years, it becomes difficult to separate sources of error relating strictly to repeatability from factors which relate to real changes in diet over time.[77]

Relative validity has been measured in relation to weighed records. Mean intakes by diet history are usually higher than by weighed intake,[76,78,79] although not always.[6,80] Thus, it seems probable that diet histories will overestimate true intakes, but the average error is likely to be consistent between groups, allowing valid comparisons of group means.

Correlations between individuals' estimates of intake based on histories and weighed records sometimes show poor agreement, in part because of the variation between individuals in the factors that determine the success with which they are likely to complete the two types of assessment, and in part because diet histories are designed to assess 'usual' diet while weighed records assess diet for a limited period only. Morgan et al.[74] showed only modest correlations for energy, fat, and fat fractions between diet histories and 4-day records (0.27–0.42). In a study comparing 30-day records kept by spouses with the diet histories of 16 men,[76] correlations ranged from 0.24 for fibre to 0.63 for vitamin C.

While the results in the first part of this chapter suggest that weighed records may not be as reliable as once believed, they have provided the only widely accepted standard of comparison. It is now clear that part of the error in correlations between diet histories and weighed records is due to error in the determination of the standard, raising the possibility that diet histories may actually perform better as a tool for ranking subjects than has been believed previously. More thorough validation studies are needed to discover the truth of this possibility.

The repeatability and relative validity of diet histories suggest that the method is robust enough to be of value in epidemiological studies, either to compare group means or to rank subjects according to levels of current or recent food consumption or nutrient intake. The probable error in ranking is more difficult to judge than when using methods that provide information on within-subject day to day variations in diet, because the sources of error are less readily amenable to measurement. A particular advantage of the diet history method in epidemiological studies is that the comprehensive assessment of diet allows for nutrient interactions or confounding to be taken into account at the level of the individual; this is not always possible with 24-hour recall or questionnaire techniques.

6.9.3 Questionnaires

The most widely used technique for assessing diet in epidemiological studies has been the questionnaire. These have ranged from very short questionnaires with only nine food items to assess a single nutrient (calcium)[81] in a study of osteoporosis,[82] to comprehensive food lists numbering 190 items or more for assessing a wide variety of nutrients[83–85] in studies on vascular disease and cancer. The main reason for choosing a questionnaire approach to dietary assessment has been the limitation of resources in relation to the number of subjects. But it is equally important to recognize that a weighed record or full diet history is not always necessary for measuring a limited range of nutrients, while the ability to rank subjects demands more than a simple 24-hour recall.

Questionnaires have generally been of the frequency and amount type (FAQ), in which subjects are asked to say how often they usually consume an item of food or drink, and how much they typically have on the days they consume it. A few attempts have been made at classifying subjects according to nutrient intake on the basis of frequency of consumption alone,[86-90] but these have generally been regarded as too insensitive to differences in diet between subjects to have been of value.

The basic principles of questionnaire design have been outlined in Chapter 1, Appendix 2, and it is worth restating the major points in relation to FAQs.

1. The purpose of the questionnaire should be clearly defined: to assess food consumption or nutrient intake, frequency or amounts, group means or individual intakes, one nutrient or a range of nutrients, etc.

2. The foods included in the questionnaire should be the minimum number that includes the major sources of nutrient for the majority of subjects. Extraneous questions take up valuable time and provide little information.

3. Questions on frequency and portion size should be closed rather than open. This reduces coding time, transcription errors, and the number of questionnaires that have to be rejected because the responses are incomplete or cannot be adequately interpreted.

4. Frequency categories should always be continuous, e.g. 'Never', 'Less than once per month', 'One or two times per month', 'Three to four times per month', followed by categories indicating the number of days per week on which the item was consumed. Other groupings of frequency may be appropriate according to the items being measured, but there should never be gaps, e.g. 'Once or twice per month', 'Once or twice per week', 'Every day', as the sensitivity of the questionnaire will be reduced and respondents will be frustrated if they cannot find a response that corresponds to their own habits.

5. Portion sizes should reflect known consumption patterns in the population and the questionnaire should allow for a sufficient range of expression of portion size to enable subjects with the same frequency of consumption but different portion sizes to be adequately distinguished.

6. Aids to the assessment of portion size are essential in the form of photographs, line drawings, or models of portions (neutral shapes) or foods.

7. Questionnaires may be either interviewer- or self-administered, according to the needs of the study. Self-administered questionnaires require more careful preparation and pretesting.

A useful way of overcoming limited interviewer resources is to design a questionnaire that is self-administered but to include in the study protocol an opportunity for the responses to be reviewed and any queries clarified in a face to face or telephone interview.

Every questionnaire should be rigorously pretested to ensure that the meanings of the food names and the portion size descriptors are clear to the subjects and that the method for recording responses is unambiguous. Questionnaires must also be validated against a standard of known accuracy. The matter of questionnaire validation, a vital stage in the design of many nutritional epidemiological studies, is covered in depth in Chapter 8.

The main advantages of questionnaires are their ease and uniformity of administration (which can overcome problems of interviewer bias), their low cost (especially if self-administered), and their use with geographically widespread samples (through the use of postal questionnaires). The primary disadvantage is the amount of work that it is necessary to devote to their development and validation.

Substantial effort has gone into assessing the repeatability and validity of questionnaires. Repeatability measures help to assess the contribution of within-subject error to misclassification of subjects based on questionnaire responses in studies where rank order is important (e.g. case-control and cohort studies). In the absence of repeatability measures, the degree of attenuation of risk estimates will be under-stated, and therefore the true relative risk under-estimated. Most repeatability studies show correlations between repeat nutrient intake assessments consistently above 0.5,[73,84,85,91] although this is not always so.[92] These errors in repeatability are substantial, and in the process of validation, when questionnaire results are compared with those from a standard (more 'objective') measurement, the contribution of within-subject variation should be distinguished from the estimate of error of questionnaire results with 'true' intake (see Chapters 3 and 8).

A number of recent questionnaire validation studies are summarized in Table 6.10. Willet et al.[91] have compared the performance of a general purpose 61-item dietary questionnaire with 28-day (4 × 7-day) diet records collected over the course of one year, and more recently Pietinen has compared a comprehensive 276 item 'food use' questionnaire[84] and an abbreviated 44-item 'food frequency' (and amount) questionnaire[85] with 24-day (12 × 2-day) weighed records. Numerous studies published have also looked at questionnaires designed to assess a more limited range of nutrients. It can be seen from the ranges of values for the correlation coefficients shown in Table 6.10 that a large number of items in a question-

Table 6.10 Summary of food frequency and amount questionnaire (FAQ) validation studies

Reference	Sample	FAQ	Standard	Nutrients (r_{min}, r_{max})*
Balogh et al., 1968[102]	Israeli men aged 40–59	'short' DH interview	DH ($n = 48$) 7-day WI ($n = 14$)	Energy, animal protein, fat, SFA, PUFA (0.69 PUFA, 0.94 fat)
Morgan et al., 1978[74]	Canadian women $n = 400$	DHQ	4-day HM	Energy, fat, SFA, 18:1, 18:2, cholesterol (0.34 energy, 0.42 cholesterol)
Jain et al., 1980[76]	US men $n = 16$	DHQ	30-day record kept by spouse	Energy, protein (total, animal, vegetable), fat (total, animal, vegetable), 18:1, 18:2, cholesterol, fibre, vitamin C (0.24 fibre, 0.61 cholesterol)
Jain et al., 1982[103]	US women aged 40–59 $n = 50$	69-item SA	DH	Energy, protein (total, animal, vegetable), fat (total, animal, vegetable), 18:1, 18:2, cholesterol, fibre, vitamin C (0.50 cholesterol, 0.64 energy)
Barasi et al., 1983[104]	Welsh women aged 18–75 $n = 102$	27-item SA	4-day WI	Dietary fibre (total, cereal, fruit/vegetable) (0.34 fruit/veg, 0.69 cereal)
Stuff et al., 1983[105]	US pregnant women $n = 40$	105-item	7-day HM	Energy, protein, fat, carbohydrate, calcium, phosphorus, iron (r_I, 0.42 protein, 0.66 phosphorus)
Yarnell et al, 1983[106]	Welsh men $n = 119$	54-item SA	7-day WI	Energy, protein, fat, SFA, carbohydrate, sucrose, dietary fibre, cereal fibre, vitamin C, alcohol (0.27 carbohydrate, 0.75 alcohol)
Gray et al., 1984[107]	California aged 58–95 men $n = 19$ women $n = 31$	56-item SA	DH	Vitamins A and C (0.43 A, 0.38 C)
Shepherd et al., 1985[108]	UK men and women $n = 33$	15-item SA	7-day urine sodium	Salt (0.66)

Table 6.10 (continued)

Reference	Sample	FAQ	Standard	Nutrients (r_{min}, r_{max})
Willett et al., 1985[91]	US female nurses aged 34–59 n = 173	61-item SA	28-day WI (4 × 7-day) over 1 year	Energy, protein, fat, SFA, PUFA, cholesterol, carbohydrate, sucrose, crude fibre, vitamins A, B_6, C (0.18 protein, 0.53 vitamin C)
Cummings et al., 1987[109]	California women aged 65+ n = 37	34-item	7-day HM	Calcium (0.76)
Nelson et al., 1987[110]	UK women aged 25–64 n = 56	22-item SA	24-hour urine iodine	Iodine (0.24, 0.50)
Willett et al., 1987[111]	US men n = 12 women n = 15	61-item SA	1-year HM record	As per ref. 91 plus 18:1, vitamins B1, B2, niacin, Ca, P, K, Fe (0.38 vitamin C, 0.76 fat)
Nelson et al., 1988[81]	UK women aged 65–74 n = 30; aged 72–90 men n = 13 women n = 15	9-item	7-day WI 5-day DD	Calcium (0.69) Calcium (0.76)
Pietinen et al., 1988[84]	Finnish men aged 55–69 n = 190	276-item SA	24-day WI (12 × 2-day)	Energy, protein, fat, SFA, MUFA, PUFA, cholesterol, carbohydrate, starch, sucrose, dietary fibre, alcohol, vitamins A, C, D, E, Na, K, Ca, Mg, Cu, Zn, Se, Pb, % energy from protein, fat, carbohydrate, alcohol, P/S ratio (0.38 fat % energy, 0.80 alcohol)
Pietinen et al., 1988[85]	Finnish men aged 55–69 n = 190	44-item SA	24-day WI (12 × 2-day)	Energy, fat, SFA, PUFA, vitamins A, C, E, Se, dietary fibre, % energy from fat, carbohydrate, P/S ratio (0.33 Se, 0.81 P/S ratio)
Boutron et al., 1989[83]	French men and women aged 30–79 n = 40	190-item by meal (n = 20) by food (n = 20)	14-day HM	Energy, protein (total, animal, vegetable), fat SFA, MUFA, PUFA, carbohydrate saccharose, sugar, starch, dietary fibre, alcohol (0.08 fat, 0.90 alcohol)

Table 6.10 (continued)

Reference	Sample	FAQ	Standard	Nutrients (r_{min}, r_{max})
Stigglebout et al., 1988[112]	Dutch women aged 30–49 $n = 82$	30-item	DH	Retinol, beta-carotene (0.54 retinol, 0.59 beta-carotene)
O'Donnell et al., 1991[114]	UK aged 25–64 men $n = 24$ women $n = 28$	196-item SA	16-day WI (4 × 4-day)	Energy, protein, fat, SFA, PUFA, carbohydrate, sucrose, dietary fibre, vitamins A, B1, B2, C, D, E, niacin, folate, carotene, % energy from fat P/S ratio (0.26 vitamin D, 0.73 alcohol)
O'Brien and Nelson, 1991[113]	UK aged 60–75 men $n = 14$ women $n = 15$	133-item SA	7-day WI	Energy, fat, SFA, retinol, carotene, vitamins A, C, E (0.45 vitamin E, 0.59 fat)

DD, duplicate diet; DH, diet history (after Burke); DHQ, diet history questionnaire; HM, household measures food record; WI, weighed food record; SA, self-administered (otherwise interview administered); SFA, saturated fatty acids; MUFA, monounsaturated fatty acids; PUFA, polyunsaturated fatty acids; 18:1, oleic acid; 18:2, linoleic acid; P/S ratio, polyunsaturated to saturated fatty acid ratio.
* r = Pearson correlation coefficient; r_I = Intraclass correlation coefficient.

naire is no guarantee of success, and that macronutrients are not consistently better correlated with the standards than micronutrients. Most of the values shown are Pearson correlations (not always appropriate for some of the higher values shown for non-normally distributed variables such as alcohol intake or P/S ratio, even after log transformation). Further discussion of techniques for evaluating agreement between questionnaire responses and standards is presented in Chapter 8.

What is important here is that the validity of questionnaire estimates of nutrient intake (or food consumption) varies between items between communities. There are no clear-cut reasons why questionnaires perform as differently as they do with the groups to be assessed (apart from the more obvious limitations concerning inadequate assessment of frequency of consumption or portion size). The variability in the findings emphasizes the need to assess the performance of a questionnaire in *every* study in a new population, and not to assume that its performance will mimic that in a previous investigation.

6.9.4 Assessment of intake in the distant past

The aim in many case-control studies is to assess dietary exposure at the time relevant to the induction of disease. While it is in practice possible to simply ask questions concerning the time in question, (and Moore et al.[93] have devised a scheme to assist subjects in remembering the characteristics of a particular period in the past) it is difficult to know (i) how well the responses correspond with the true intake in the past; and (ii) the extent to which recent diet may have biased responses. A number of studies have addressed these questions, the results of which are summarized in Table 6.11. The ages shown for the samples are those when the original dietary assessment was made.

The results show that the level of agreement between recall and original diet varies considerably between studies, being of the order of 0.5–0.8 in those by Van Leeuwen et al.,[94] Byers et al.,[95] and Bakkum et al.[96] but generally lower in the studies by Rohan and Potter,[97] Jensen et al.,[98] and Wu et al.[99] The low values in the latter studies suggest that some attempts to assess past diet may lead to such extensive misclassification of subjects as to substantially understate risks associated with diet in case-control studies. Assessment of variance in both the recalled and original estimates of intake[99] can be used to adjust both the correlations (see Chapters 3 and 8) and risk estimates[100] upwards.

It is also striking from the studies[96–99] in which current as well as past diet was assessed, that the recalled diet agrees more closely with the current than with the past diet. This suggests that the current diet is having a strong influence on the recalled diet. Moreover, the original diet correlates as well with the current diet as it does with the recalled diet, suggesting that the extent of misclassification (and attenuation of risk estimates) would be as great using the recalled diet as it would be using the current diet, although the individuals who were misclassified would be different in the two analyses and there are no reports of the differences in risk calculated using the three measures of diet (original, recalled, and current). Indeed, for three out of four nutrients in the first Bakkum study,[96] any estimate of risk associated with past diet would have been more likely to be detected using an assessment of current diet rather than recall of the distant past. The only potential advantage of using recall from the distant past in a case-control study, therefore, would be the probable identification of individuals whose diets had changed radically over the intervening period, but Linsted and Kuzma (in an analysis of foods rather than nutrients) found that the extent of misclassification was likely to remain the same in cases and controls,[101] and that change in diet was *negatively* associated with an ability to recall accurately. Thus, while the recall of diets in the distant past is theoretically an attractive measurement to make, it

Table 6.11. Summary of questionnaire validation studies of diet in the distant past

Reference	Sample	Assessment methods and dates		Nutrients and correlations			
		Original	Recall	Nutrient	Recall vs Original	Recall vs Current	Current vs Original
Van Leeuwen et al., 1983[94]	Dutch men (n = 44) and women (n = 56) aged 25–65	7-day WI 1977	DH 1981	Energy	0.68	–	–
				Protein	0.47	–	–
				Fat	0.68	–	–
				Cholesterol	0.51	–	–
				Carbohydrate	0.64	–	–
				Dietary fibre	0.54	–	–
				Alcohol	0.82	–	–
Rohan and Potter, 1984[97]	Australian men (n = 37) and women (n = 33) aged 30–74	141-item FAQ	141-item FAQ	Energy	0.62	0.87	0.58
				Protein	0.25	0.82	0.48
				Fat	0.52	0.84	0.53
				Cholesterol	0.32	0.78	0.35
				PUFA	0.34	0.61	0.48
				Starch	0.66	0.77	0.45
				Sugar	0.61	0.91	0.53
				Dietary fibre	0.52	0.74	0.52
				Alcohol	0.87	0.89	0.91
				Retinol	0.48	0.67	0.48
				Iron	0.38	0.74	0.41

Reference	Subjects	Method 1	Method 2	Nutrient			
Jensen et al., 1984[98]	Danish (n = 79) aged 18–50	28-day FPR 1954–57 1964–66	DH 1982	Energy	0.42	0.63	0.41
				Protein	0.31	0.55	0.38
				Fat	0.40	0.66	0.45
				Carbohydrate	0.33	0.64	0.35
Byers et al., 1987[95]	US men (n = 232) and women (n = 91)	129-item FAQ 1975–79	47-item FAQ 1984–85	Fat	0.50	—	0.50
				Vitamin A	0.61	—	0.49
				Dietary fibre	0.61	—	0.53
Wu et al., 1988[99]	US men (n = 378) and women (n = 495)	47-item FAQ 1972	47-item FAQ 1983	Energy*	0.33	0.54	0.32
				Fat*	0.33	0.53	0.30
				PUFA*	0.25	0.58	0.19
				Cholesterol*	0.37	0.55	0.32
Bakkum et al., 1988[96]	Dutch men (n = 37) aged 58–65	DH 1971–72	DH 1984–85	Energy	0.54	0.70	0.75
				Protein	0.65	0.66	0.77
				Fat	0.59	0.74	0.50
				Carbohydrate	0.52	0.75	0.78
	men (n = 22) and women (n = 24) aged 67–82			Energy	0.69	0.69	0.63
				Protein	0.50	0.47	0.31
				Fat	0.64	0.67	0.55
				Carbohydrate	0.63	0.79	0.52

* results for men only; women's results very similar. DH, Diet history; FAQ, food frequency and amount questionnaire; FPR, food purchasing record; PUFA, polyunsaturated fatty acids; WI, weighed inventory.

has yet to be demonstrated that it has advantages over risk analyses based on current diet. Substantially more work needs to be carried out to identify the most useful way in which a meaningful recall of diet in the distant past can be achieved.

6.10 CONCLUSIONS

There are powerful arguments for using retrospective methods of dietary assessment in nutritional epidemiological studies of individuals. They offer a cheap and efficient way of rapidly obtaining data from large numbers of subjects. Their chief drawback is that the error associated with each individual's estimate of diet is less readily assessed than in studies using prospective measures of diet, and care needs to be taken to ensure that this error is properly described. There are three main components to the error: (i) that associated with the method of assessment itself (its repeatability); (ii) that associated with variation in diet over time; (iii) that associated with the ability of the respondent to provide the information required (the main source of differential misclassification). These three components should be identified in every analysis of disease risk, in order to appreciate the extent of attentuation that may be occurring. It is the measurement of this error that adds substantially to the cost of using retrospective methods in epidemiological studies. But failure to assess the components of error, and to undertake proper validation of questionnaire methods, significantly reduces the ability to interpret the results from nutritional epidemiological studies.

REFERENCES

1. Bingham, S. A. (1987). The dietary assessment of individuals: methods, accuracy, new techniques and recommendations. *Nutr. Abs. Rev.*, **57**: 705–42.
2. Black, A. E. (1982). The logistics of dietary surveys. *Hum. Nutr: Appl. Nutr.*, **36A**: 85–94.
3. Black, A. E. (1981). Pitfalls in dietary assessment. In A. N. Howard and I. McLean Baird (eds), *Recent advances in clinical nutrition.* John Libbey, London.
4. Paul, A. A. (1988). Observed weighed records. In M. E. Cameron and W. A. van Staveren, (eds), *Manual for methodology for food consumption studies.* pp. 75–9. Oxford Medical Publications, New York.
5. Gregory, J., Foster, K., Tyler, M., and Wiseman, M. (1990). *The dietary and nutritional survey of British adults.* HMSO, London.
6. Cameron, M. E. and van Staveren, W. A. (eds) (1988). *Manual on methodology for food consumption studies.* Oxford Medical Publications, New York.
7. Pekkarinen, M. (1970). Methodology in the collection of food consumption data. *World Rev. Nutr. Dietet.*, **12**: 145–71.
8. Todd, K. S., Hudes, M., and Calloway, D. H. (1983). Food intake measurement: problems and approaches. *Am. J. Clin. Nutr.*, **37**: 139–46.

9. Elwood, P. C. and Bird, G. (1983). A photographic method of diet evaluation. *Hum. Nutr: Appl. Nutr., 37A*: 474–7.

10. Sevenhuysen, G. P. (1985). Image processing to measure individual food consumption (Abstract), p. 121. Original Communications XIII International Congress of Nutrition, Brighton.

11. Nelson, M. (1988). Estimated records. In M. E. Cameron and W. A. van Staveren, (eds). *Manual for methodology for food consumption studies.* pp. 64–75. Oxford Medical Publications, New York.

12. Stockley, L., Hurren, C., Chapman, R., Broadhurst, A., and Jones F. (1986). Energy protein and fat intake estimated using FRED compared with a weighed diary. *Human Nutr: Appl. Nutr., 40A*: 19–23.

13. Kretsch, M. J. and Fong, A. K. H. (1990). Validation of a new computerized technique for quantitating individual dietary intake. *Am. J. Clin. Nutr., 51*: 477–84.

14. Rivellese, A., Vespasiani, G., Ventura, M. M., Bruni, M., Pacioni, D., Genovese, S., Brunetti, P., and Riccardi, G. (1989). Evaluation of a new computerized method for the seven day food record in insulin dependent diabetic patients. (Abstract) VII Int. Symp. Diabetes Nutn. The Netherlands.

15. Rutishauser, I. H. E. (1982). Food models, photographs or household measures? *Proc. Nutr. Soc. Aust., 7*: 144.

16. Brock, K. and Ellery, C. (1982). Quantitative dietary assessment in human populations: the development and assessment of food photographs to aid in the use of a food frequency questionnaire. *Proc. Nutr. Soc. Aust., 7*: 169.

17. Bollard, J. E., Yuhas, J. A., and Bollard, T. W. (1988). Estimation of food portion sizes: effectiveness of training. *J. Am. Diet. Ass., 88*: 817–20.

18. Blake, A. J., Guthrie, H., and Smicklas-Wright, H. (1989). Accuracy of food portion estimates by overweight and normal weight subjects. *J. Am. Diet. Ass., 89*: 962–4.

19. Bransby, E. R., Daubney, C. G., and King, J. (1948). Comparison of results obtained by different methods of individual dietary survey. *Br. J. Nutr. 2*: 89–110.

20. Eppright, E. S., Patton, M. B., Marlatt, A. L., and Hathaway, M. L. (1952). Dietary study methods. V. Some problems in collecting dietary information about groups of children. *J. Am. Diet. Ass., 28*: 43–8.

21. Young, C. M., Hagan, G. C., Tucker, R. E., and Foster, W. D. (1952). A comparison of dietary study methods. II Dietary history vs. seven-day record vs. 24hr recall. *J. Am. Diet. Ass., 28*: 218–21.

22. Edington, J., Thorogood, M., Geekie, M., Ball, M., and Mann, J. (1989). Assessment of nutritional intake using dietary records with estimated weights. *J. Hum. Nutr. Diet., 2*: 407–14.

23. Nelson, M. and Nettleton, P. A. (1980). Dietary survey methods. 1., A semi-weighed technique for measuring dietary intake within families. *J. Hum. Nutr., 34*: 325–48.

24. Nettleton, P. A., Day, K. C., and Nelson, M. (1980). Dietary survey methods. 2. A comparison of nutrient intakes within families assessed by household measures and the semi-weighed method. *J. Hum. Nutr., 34*: 349–54.

25. Beaton, G. H., Milner, J., Corey, P., McGuire, V., Cousins, M., Stewart, E., de Ramos, M., Hewitt, D., Grambsch, P. V., Kassim, N., and Little, J. A.

(1979). Sources of variance in 24 hour dietary recall data: implications for nutritional study design and interpretation. *Am. J. Clin. Nutr.,* **32:** 2546–59.

26. Widdowson, E. M. (1936). A study of English diets by the individual method. Part I. Men. *J. Hygiene,* **36:** 269–92.

27. Widdowson, E. M. and McCance, R. A. (1936). A study of English diets by the individual method. Part II. Women. *J. Hygiene,* **36:** 293–309.

28. Liu, K., Stamler, J., Dyer, A., McKeever, J., and McKeever, P. (1978). Statistical methods to assess and minimize the role of intra-individual variability in obscuring the relationship between dietary lipids and serum cholesterol. *J. Chron. Dis.,* **31:** 399–418.

29. Prentice, A. M., Coward, W. A., Davies, H. L., Murgatroyd, P. R., Black, A. E., Goldberg, G. R., Ashford, J., Sawyer, M., and Whitehead, R. G. (1985). Unexpectedly low levels of energy expenditure in healthy women. *Lancet,* **ii:** 1419–22.

30. Prentice, A. M., Black, A. E., Coward, W. A., Davies, H. L., Goldberg, G. R., Murgatroyd, P. R., Ashford, J., Sawyer, M., and Whitehead, R. G. (1986). High levels of energy expenditure in obese women. *Br. Med. J.,* **292:** 983–7.

31. Livingstone, M. B. E., Prentice, A. M., Strain, J. J., Coward, W. A., Black, A. E., Barker, M. E., McKenna, P. G., and Whitehead, R. G. (1990). Accuracy of weighed dietary records in studies of diet and health. *Br. Med. J.,* **300:** 708–12.

32. Isaksson, B. (1980). Urinary nitrogen output as a validity test in dietary surveys. *Am. J. Clin. Nutr.,* **33:** 4–6.

33. Steen, B., Isaksson, B., and Svanborg, A. (1977). Intake of energy and nutrients and meal habits in 70 year old males and females in Gothenburg, Sweden: a population study. *Acta Med. Scand.,* Suppl. **611:** 39–86.

34. Warnold, I., Carlgren, G., and Krotkiewski, M. (1978). Energy expenditure and body composition during weight reduction in hyperplastic obese women. *Am. J. Clin. Nutr.,* **31:** 750–63.

35. Bingham, S. and Cummings, J. H. (1983). The use of 4-amino benzoic acid as a marker to validate the completeness of 24 h urine collections in man. *Clin. Sci.,* **64:** 629–35.

36. Williams, D. R. R. and Bingham, S. (1986). Sodium and potassium intakes in a representative population sample: estimates from 24h urine collections known to be complete. *Br. J. Nutr.* **55:** 13–22.

37. Bingham, S., Murphy, J., Waller, L., Runswick, S., Neale, G., Evans, D., and Cummings, J. (1992). Incomplete 24 h urine collections from hospital outpatients. *Eur. J. Clin. Nutr.,* in press.

38. Bingham, S., Welch, A., Cassidy, A., Runswick, S., Gill, C., and Khaw, K. T. (1991). The use of 24h urine nitrogen to detect bias in the reported habitual food intake of individuals assessed from weighed dietary records (Abstract). *Proc. Nutr. Soc.,* **50:** 32A.

39. Bingham, S. and Cummings, J. H. (1985). Urine nitrogen as an independent validatory measure of dietary intake. *Am. J. Clin. Nutr.,* **42:** 1276–89.

40. Black, A., Jebb, S. A., and Bingham, S. (1991). Validation of energy and protein intakes assessed by diet history and by weighed records against total energy expenditure and 24h urinary nitrogen (Abstract). *Proc. Nutr. Soc.,* **50:** 108A.

41. Hallfrisch, J., Steele, P., and Cohen, L. (1982). Comparison of 7-day diet record with measured food intake of 24 subjects. *Nut. Res.,* **2:** 263–73.

42. Johnson, N. E., Sempos, C. T., Elmer, P. J., Allington, J. K., and Matthews, M. E. (1982). Development of a dietary intake monitoring system for nursing homes. *J. Am. Diet Ass.,* **80:** 549–57.

43. Freudenheim, J. L., Johnson, M. E., and Wardrop. R. L. (1987). Misclassification of nutrient intake of individuals and groups using 1, 2, 3 and 7 day food records. *Am. J. Epid.,* **126:** 703–13.

44. Sempos, C. T., Johnson, N. E., Smith, E. L., and Gilligan, C. (1985). Effects of intra-individual and inter-individual variation in repeated dietary records. *Am. J. Epid.,* **121:** 120–30.

45. Lockwood, M. J., Riding, K. H., and Keen, H. (1968). The spoonful as a dietary measure. *Nutrition,* **22:** 7–14.

46. Morgan, S., Flint, D. M., Prinsley, D. M., Wahlqvist, M. L., and Ponsh, A. E. (1982). Measurement of food intake in the elderly by food photography. *Proc. Nutr. Soc. Aust.,* **7:** 172.

47. Bingham, S., McNeil, N. I., and Cummings, J. H. (1981). The diet of individuals: a study of a randomly chosen cross-section of British adults in a Cambridgeshire village. *Br. J. Nutr.,* **45:** 23–35.

48. Ducimetière, P. (1983). Data analysis problems. In *Surveillance of the dietary habits in the population with regard to cardiovascular disease.* Euronut 2 Report, pp. 81–92. Wageningen, The Netherlands.

49. Cole, T. and Black, A. (1984). *Statistical aspects in the design of dietary surveys.* In MRC Report No. 4, Environmental Epidemiology Unit, Southampton.

50. Marr, J. W. (1981). Individual variation in dietary intake. In M. Turner (ed.), *Preventive nutrition and society.* Academic Press, London.

51. Schofield, W. N., Schofield, C., and James, W. P. T. (1985). Basal metabolic rate. *Human Nutr: Clin. Nutr.* **39C,** Suppl. 1: 1–96.

52. Hodkinson, H. M. (1975). An outline of geriatrics. Oxford University Press.

53. Epstein, L. M., Reshef, A., Abrahamson, J. H., and Bialik, O. (1970). Validity of a short dietary questionnaire. *Israel J. Med. Sci.,* **6:** 589–97.

54. Beaton, G. H., Milner, J., Corey, P., McGuire, S., Cousins, M., Stewart, E., de Ramos, M., Hewitt, D., Grambsch, P. V., Kassium, N., and Little, J. A. (1979). Sources of variance in 24-hour dietary recall data: implications for nutrition study design and interpretation. *Am. J. Clin. Nutr.,* **32:** 2546–59.

55. Keen, H., Thomas, B. J., Jarrett, R. J., and Fuller, J. H. (1979). Nutrient intake, adiposity and diabetes. *Br. Med. J.,* **1:** 655–8.

56. Balogh, M., Kahn, H. A., and Medalie, J. H. (1971). Random repeat 24-hour dietary recalls. *Am. J. Clin. Nutr.,* **24:** 304–10.

57. Nomura, A., Hankin, J. H., and Rhoads, G. G. (1976). The reproducibility of dietary intake data in a prospective study of gastrointestinal cancer. *Am. J. Clin. Nutr.,* **29:** 1432–6.

58. Wiehl, D. G. (1942). Diets of a group of aircraft workers in Southern California. Millbank Memorial Fund Quarterly, **20:** 329–66.

59. United States Department of Health, Education and Welfare (1975). National Health and Nutrition Examination Survey (NHANES) I and II. DHEW, Washington.

60. United States Department of Health, Education and Welfare. (1972). Ten-state nutrition survey 1968–1970. DHEW, Washington.

61. Nutrition Canada. (1973). Information Canada, Ottawa.

62. Rasanen, L. (1979). Nutrition survey of Finnish rural children. VI. Methodological study comparing the 24-hour recall and the dietary history interview. *Am. J. Clin. Nutr.*, **32:** 2560–7.

63. Rasanen, L. (1982). Validity and reliability of recall methods. In *Report to the EEC Workshop on Methods of Evaluating Nutritional Status with Emphasis on Food Consumption studies.* Wageningen.

64. Acheson, K. J., Campbell, I. T., Edholm, O. G., Miller, D. S., and Stock, M. J. (1980). The measurement of food and energy intake in man – an evaluation of some techniques. *Am. J. Clin. Nutr.*, **33:** 1147–54.

65. Linusson, E. E. I., Sanjur, D., and Erickson, E. C. (1974). Validating the 24-hour recall method as a dietary survey tool. *Arch. Latinoamer. Nutr.*, **24:** 277.

66. Emmons, L. and Hayes, M. (1973). Accuracy of 24-hour recall of young children. *J. Am. Diet. Assoc.*, **62:** 402–15.

67. Karvetti, R. L. and Knuts, L. R. (1981). Agreement between dietary interviews. *J. Am. Diet. Assoc.*, **79:** 654–60.

68. Bazzarre, T. L. and Myers, M. P. (1979). The collection of food intake data in cancer epidemiology studies. *Nutr. Cancer*, **1:** 22–45.

69. Posner, B. M., Borman, C. L., Morgan, J. L., Borden, W. S., and Ohls, J. C. (1982). The validity of a telephone administered 24-hour dietary recall methodology. *Am. J. Clin. Nutr.*, **36;** 546–53.

70. Nelson, M., Black, A. E., Morris, J. A., and Cole, T. J. (1989). Between- and within-subject variation in nutrient intake from infancy to old age: estimating the number of days required to rank dietary intakes with desired precision. *Am. J. Clin. Nutr.*, **50:** 155–67.

71. Burke, B. S. (1947). The diet history as a tool in research. *J. Am. Diet. Assoc.*, **23:** 1041–6.

72. Trulson, M. F., McCann, M. B. (1959). Comparison of dietary survey methods. *J. Am. Diet. Assoc.*, **35:** 672–81.

73. Reshef, A. and Epstein, L. M. (1972). Reliability of a dietary questionnaire. *Am. J. Clin. Nutr.*, **25:** 91–5.

74. Morgan, R. W., Jain, M., Miller, A. B., Choi, N., W., Matthews, V., Munan, L., Durin, J. D., Feather, J., Howe, G. R., and Kelly, A. (1978). A comparison of dietary methods in epidemiologic studies. *Am. J. Epid.*, **107:** 488–98.

75. Bazzarre, T. L. and Yuhas, J. A. (1983). Comparative evaluation of methods of collecting food intake data for cancer epidemiology studies. *Nutr. Cancer*, **5:** 201–14.

76. Jain, M., Howe, G. R., Johnson, K. C., and Miller, A. B. (1980). Evaluation of a diet history questionnaire for epidemiologic studies. *Am. J. Epid.*, **111:** 212–19.

77. Dawber, T. R., Pearson, G., Anderson, P., Mann, G. V., Kannel, W. B., Shurtleff, D., and McNamara, P. (1962). Dietary assessment in the epidemiologic study of coronary heart disease: the Framingham study. 2. Reliability of measurement. *Am. J. Clin. Nutr.*, **11;** 226–34.

78. Young, C. M., Chalmers, F. W., Church, H. N., Clayton,M. M., Tucker, R. E., Werts, A. W., and Foster, W. D. (1952). A comparison of dietary study methods.

I. Dietary history vs seven-day record. *J. Am. Diet. Assoc.*, **28**; 124–8.

79. Huenemann, R. L., and Turner, D. (1942). Methods of dietary investigation. *J. Am. Diet. Assoc.*, **18**: 562–8.

80. Burk, M. C. and Pao, E. M. (1976). *Methodology for large scale surveys of households and individual diets.* Home Economics research report No. 40. US Department of Agriculture. US Government Printing Office, Washington.

81. Nelson, M., Hague, G. F., Cooper, C., and Bunker, V. W. (1988). Calcium intake in the elderly: validation of a dietary questionnaire. *J. Hum. Nutr. Diet.*, **1**; 115–27.

82. Cooper, C., Barker, D. J. P., and Wickham, C. (1988). Physical activity, muscle strength and calcium intake in fracture of the proximal femur in Britain. *Br. Med. J.*, **297**: 1443–6.

83. Boutron, M. C., Faivre, J., Milan, C., Gorcerie, B., and Esteve, J. (1989). A comparison of two diet history questionnaires that measure usual food intake. *Nutr. Cancer*, **12**; 83–91.

84. Pietinen, P., Hartman, A. M., Haapa, E., Rasanen, L., Haapakoski, J., Palmgren, J., Albanes, D., Virtamo, J., and Huttunen, J. K. (1988). Reproducibility and validity of dietary assessment instruments. I. A self-administered food use questionnaire with a portion size picture booklet. *Am. J. Epid.*, **128**; 655–66.

85. Pietinen, P., Hartman, A. M., Haapa, E., Rasanen, L., Haapakoski, J., Palmgren, J., Albanes, D., Virtamo, J., and Huttunen, J. K. (1988). Reproducibility and validity of dietary assessment instruments. II. A quantitative food frequency questionnaire. *Am. J. Epid.*, **128**: 667–76.

86. Wiehl, D. G. and Reed, R. (1960). Development of new or improved dietary methods for epidemiological investigations. *Am. J. Publ. Hlth.*, **50**: 824–8.

87. Marr, J. W., Heady, J. A., and Morris, J. N. (1961). Towards a method for large-scale individual diet surveys. In *Proceedings of the 3rd International Congress of Dietetics*, pp. 85–91. London, 10–14th July 1961, Newman Books.

88. Hankin, J. H., Rhoads, G. G., and Glober, G. A. (1975). A dietary method for an epidemiologic study of gastrointestinal cancer. *Am. J. Clin. Nutr.*, **28**: 1055–61.

89. Abrahamson, J. H., Slome, C., and Kosovsky, C. (1963). Food frequency interview as an epidemiological tool. *Am. J. Publ. Hlth.*, **53**: 1093–1101.

90. Chu, S. Y., Kolonel, L. N., Hankin, J. H., and Lee, J. (1984). A comparison of frequency and quantitative dietary methods for epidemiologic studies of diet and disease. *Am. J. Epid.*, **119**; 323–34.

91. Willett, W. C., Sampson, L., Stampfer, M.J., Rosner, B., Bain, C., Witschi, J., Hennekens, C. H., and Speizer, F. E. (1985). Reproducibility and validity of a semi-quantitative food frequency questionnaire. *Am. J. Epid.*, **122**: 51–65.

92. Hankin, J. H., Kolonel, L. N., and Hinds, M. W. (1984). Dietary history methods for epidemiologic studies: application in a case-control study of vitamin A and lung cancer. *J. Nat. Cancer Inst.*, **73**: 1417–21.

93. Moore, J. V., Prestridge, L. L., and Newell, G. R. (1982). Research technique for epidemiologic investigation of nutrition and cancer. *Nutr. Cancer*, **3**: 249–56.

94. Van Leeuwen, F. E., de Vet, H. C. W., Hayes, R. B., Van Staveren, W. A., West, C. A., and Hautvast, J. G. A. J. (1983). An assessment of the relative

validity of retrospective interviewing for measuring dietary intake. *Am. J. Epid.*, **118**: 752–8.

95. Byers, T., Marshall, J., Anthony, E., Fielder, R., and Zielezny, M. (1987). The reliability of dietary history from the distant past. *Am. J. Epid.*, **125**: 999–1011.

96. Bakkum, A., Bloemberg, B., van Staveren, W. A., Verschuren, M., and West, C. E. (1988). The relative validity of a retrospective estimate of food consumption based on a current dietary history and a food frequency list. *Nutr. Cancer*, **11**: 41–53.

97. Rohan, T. E. and Potter, J. D. (1984). Retrospective assessment of dietary intake. *Am. J. Epid.*, **120**: 876–87.

98. Jensen, O. M., Wahrendorf, J., Rosenquist, A., and Geser, A. (1984). The reliability of questionnaire-derived historic information and temporal stability of food habits in individuals. *Am. J. Epidemiol.*, **120**: 281–90.

99. Wu, M. L., Whittemore, A. S., and Jung, D. L. (1988). Errors in reported dietary intakes. II. Long-term recall. *Am. J. Epid.*, **128**: 1137–45.

100. Freudenheim, J. L. and Marshall, J. R. (1988). The problem of profound mismeasurement and the power of epidemiological studies of diet and cancer. *Nutr. Cancer.*, **11**: 243–50.

101. Lindsted, K. D. and Kuzma, J. W. (1989). Long-term (24 years) recall reliability in cancer cases and controls using a 21-item food frequency questionnaire. *Nutr. Cancer*, **12**: 135–49.

102. Balogh, M., Medalie, J. N., Smith, H., and Groen, J. J. (1968). The development of a dietary questionnaire for an ischaemic heart disease survey. *Israel J. Med. Sci.*, **4**: 195–203.

103. Jain, M. G., Harrison, L., Howe, G. R., and Miller, A. B. (1982). Evaluation of a self-administered dietary questionnaire for use in a cohort study. *Am. J. Clin. Nutr.*, **36**: 931–5.

104. Barasi, M. E., Burr, M. L., and Sweetnam, P. M. (1983). A comparison of dietary fibre intake in South Wales estimated from a questionnaire and weighed dietary records. *Nutr. Res.*, **3**: 249–55.

105. Stuff, J. E., Garza, C., O'Brian Smith, E., Nichols, B. L., and Montandon, C. M. (1983). A comparison of dietary methods in nutritional studies. *Am. J. Clin. Nutr.*, **37**: 300–306.

106. Yarnell, J. W. G., Fehily, A. M., Milbank, J. E., Sweetnam, P. M., and Walker, C. L. (1983). A short questionnaire for use in epidemiological surveys: comparison with weighed dietary records. *Hum. Nutr.: Appl. Nutr.*, **37A**: 103–12.

107. Gray, G. E., Paganini-Hill, A., Ross, R. K., and Henderson, B. E. (1984). Assessment of three brief methods of estimation of vitamin A and C intakes for a prospective study of cancer: comparison with dietary history. *Am. J. Epid.*, **119**: 581–90.

108. Shepherd, R., Farleigh, C. A., and Land, D. G. (1985). Estimation of salt intake by questionnaire. *Appetite*, **6**: 219–33.

109. Cummings, S. R., Block, G., McHenry, K., and Baron, R. B. (1987). Evaluation of two food frequency methods of measuring dietary calcium intake. *Am. J. Epid.*, **126**: 796–802.

110. Nelson, M., Quayle, A., and Phillips, D. I. W. (1987). Iodine intake and

excretion in two British towns: aspects of questionnaire validation. *Hum. Nutr.: Appl. Nutr.,* **41A:** 187–92.

111. Willett, W. C., Reynolds, R. D., Cottrell-Hoehner, S., Sampson, L., and Browne, M. L. (1987). Validation of a semi-quantitative food frequency questionnaire: comparison with a 1-year diet record, *J. Am. Diet. Assoc.,* **87:** 43–7.

112. Stiggelbout, A. M., van der Giezen, A. M., Blauw, Y. H., Blok, E., van Staveren, W. A., and West, C. E. (1989). Development and relative validity of a food frequency questionnaire for the estimation of retinol and beta-carotene. *Nutr. Cancer,* **12:** 289–99.

113. O'Brien, C and Nelson, M. (1991). Validity of a dietary questionnaire for assessing anti-oxidant vitamin intake, in preparation.

114. O'Donnel, M. G., Nelson, M., and Wise, P. H. (1991). A computerised diet questionnaire for use in health education. I. Development and validation. *Br. J. Nutr.,* in press.

7. Biochemical markers of nutrient intake

Chris J. Bates and David I. Thurnham, with
Sheila A. Bingham, Barrie M. Margetts, and Michael Nelson

7.1 PREDICTION OF NUTRIENT INTAKES FROM THE VALUES OF BIOCHEMICAL MARKERS OF NUTRIENT STATUS

It is a reasonable assumption that any valid biochemical, functional, or clinical index of status of an essential nutrient, (i.e. any essential component of the diet) is likely to be related over at least part of the entire range of observed values, to the amount that is present in the diet. Such an index is, therefore, at least potentially a marker of nutrient intake. However, it clearly cannot be assumed that there will be a close or simple relationship between the amount in the diet and the values that can be obtained by laboratory or other quantitative measurements of status indices. Indeed, the primary intention in developing these indices has been not to predict or estimate the amount in the diet, but rather to estimate the amount present in, or available to, the essential and vulnerable tissues of the body, in order to define different states, namely deficiency, adequacy, or possibly overload, at the tissue level. Thus, independent measurements of intake, of biochemical status, and of functional or clinical status indices when added together, give three different windows on the level of 'nutrient adequacy' of the individual (or group of individuals) being studied. Epidemiological studies might independently investigate the three questions: (i) whether diet affects risk; (ii) whether biochemical status affects risk; and (iii) whether functional status affects risk. The answers could well be different in each case.

Although there are links between them, in the sense that each window can be partly observed from the other two, the view from each is different and the overlap of views is only partial. In addition, the degree of overlap differs for different nutrients, and for different types of indices (e.g. urinary nutrients versus plasma levels, versus blood cell levels, versus tests to probe metabolic pathways, etc.), so that it is difficult to generalize about the extent to which intakes can be predicted from status values. In the following section, a brief discussion of some of the factors and, in particular, the potential errors and confounders that blur the relationship between status values and nutrient intakes, is attempted. It should be recognized at the outset that the quantitative and statistical aspects of these relationships have hitherto received very little attention in published studies, so that although we can, in some instances, give an approximate value for the mean intake of a nutrient by a defined human group, as predicted from the mean biochemical index value, we have virtually no data describing the precision of such estimates, especially for micro-nutrients. In many instances, the best that can be attempted at present is a very approximate subdivision into 'deficient' and 'acceptable' intakes, or perhaps into 'low', 'medium', and 'high' intakes, in terms of their relation-ships to the (also poorly-defined) limits of long term nutrient requirements. In the following discussion it should also be recognized that comparisons between mean values for groups or populations of subjects should, by the law of averages, yield closer correlations (e.g. of intakes versus status values) than can be obtained by similar comparisons between individuals.

7.1.1 Validity and reproducibility*

The factors that determine the quality of laboratory data are central to any discussion of quality control in clinical chemistry. The assay procedures used must be sufficiently sensitive, sufficiently robust, sufficiently free from short term fluctuations and long term drift, and sufficiently free from interference by other sample components (especially the variable ones) to yield a reliable data set. Many vitamins are unstable to heat, light, oxygen, etc. and therefore decay during storage (to different extents in different solutions and matrices, and it is difficult to predict the extent of decay from any known values of storage time and temperature). It is therefore especially important to define an optimum storage schedule, e.g. acidification with a metal-chelating acid for vitamin C, addition of vitamin C as preservative for folate, elimination of light-exposure for riboflavin, elimination of haemolysis for vitamin A, etc.

Validity implies that the data are true, unbiased measures of the vari-able. As nutrition is an international discipline, it is important that results in one laboratory are comparable with another, and attention to this aspect of concurrent validity should not be neglected.

Reproducibility (or precision) implies reliability and expresses the varia-bility of results obtained when a single sample is measured many times. In practice, a mean and standard deviation are calculated from several measurements on a sample (commonly 20) and used to obtain the coeffi-cient of variation ($CV = SD/\bar{X} \times 100$). It is ideally calculated for samples at the bottom, middle, and top of the reference range. The CV represents

---

*For consistent use of language throughout the book, we have used the term 'validity' when a clinical chemist would use the word 'accuracy', and 'reproducibility' when the clinical chemist would use 'precision'.

the sum of all the laboratory factors that can influence a result, and ideally should not be greater than 5 per cent. The simplest methods will have the lowest CVs, while those with many steps and requiring a high level of technical skill will be higher. Automation should be used wherever possible because this will lower the CV and, generally speaking, results obtained where the CV is greater than 10 per cent should be examined very carefully. Low CVs may not be obtained when a new method is first used because factors influencing the variance in the technique may not be known, but measuring a CV makes one aware of potential problems and, with time and experience, sources of error will be identified and removed and the CV will improve. The more experienced a laboratory or worker with a particular method, the lower the CV is likely to be. Reproducibility, therefore, is a measure of good laboratory practice.

Validity and reproducibility are both important in any biochemical measurement. Validity may appear to be more difficult to achieve because most biochemical measurements involve many stages when bias may enter the procedure and consistently raise or lower the end result. When national quality control schemes were introduced, measurements of the same material by different methods produced different results, indicating differences in the accuracy of different methods. However, as time passed reproducibility in the participating laboratories improved and, as it did so, differences between the means obtained by different methods fell; that is, as the quality of work in laboratories improved (as measured by CV), so relative validity between methods also improved. This discussion does not include the variability or bias that may be attributable to within-subject variance, or differential misclassification between subjects. For a fuller discussion on laboratory quality control the reader is referred to Whitehead.[1]

Provided that exactly the same method is used to calibrate the relationship between dietary intake and the status index values (as subsequently used to predict the intake of new individuals or groups from the original calibration), then the absolute accuracy of the index values may be of minor importance, provided the calibration is stable and precise. However, it is very important to realize that apparently minor differences in laboratory protocol, which may not be at all apparent from the published descriptions or worksheets, may have a profound effect on the quantitative relationships between nutrient intakes (or tissue levels) and the index values that are obtained by a particular laboratory. A very clear example of this problem is manifested in the differences in values obtained between the Glatzle et al.[2] and Beutler[3] techniques for the assay of riboflavin status by the activation coefficient of glutathione reductase (both of these are widely used variants). At least part of the explanation for this particular difference became apparent from the subsequent studies of Garry and Owen[4] and of Thurnham and Rathakette.[5] However, the problem in more general terms is one of the major pitfalls that can be encountered if a 'calibration' curve obtained in one laboratory is then used uncritically in another, even if the assay protocols appear to be identical on paper.

Reference materials

For most of the substances measured by the clinical chemist there are reference materials available. These are commercially available serum/plasma samples in which the concentrations of the component materials are known having been analysed by one or more reference laboratories. Unfortunately, the nutritional biochemist does not usually have these available because the methods are used by too few people to be commercially justifiable. This situation is changing for some analytes such as retinol, carotene, vitamin E and some trace elements (The National Institute of Standards and Technology, Gaithersburg, MD, USA) but there is nothing to suggest that reference materials for the other vitamins will appear in the near future.

In the absence of standard reference material, attempts should be made to prepare the laboratory's own reference material. This should be as close as possible in its physical form to the substance that is routinely analysed. Compromises have to be made for unstable substances, hence, for vitamin C the authors' reference materials are plasma and standard extracts in metaphosphoric acid, although lyophilized plasma was found to be satisfactory over 12 months at 4°C (unpublished data). For retinol and carotene, portions of normal plasma stored at −20°C proved satisfactory over 6 months[6] but −70°C, or the use of lyophilized plasma,[7,8] is necessary for storage over longer periods. For the riboflavin assay, haemolysates (1 part erythrocytes: 19 parts water) containing the glutathione reductase enzyme are stable when stored at −50°C or lyophilized at 4°C (unpublished). By routinely including such materials in every batch of samples analysed, the routine performance of assays can be monitored and early indications of more subtle drifts in the data can be picked up.[5] Such procedures help to maintain precision and prevent or reduce drift to a minimum, but of course the longer the study, the more difficult this becomes, particularly if the quality control standards are themselves unstable.

7.1.2 Temporal variations in the biochemical, functional and clinical status indices and factors affecting choices

It is clearly important to know whether a particular index will respond rapidly to fluctuations in nutrient intake (or indeed to other factors that may change in the short term, e.g. diurnal cycles or metabolic adjustments by hormonal mechanisms), or whether it will respond more slowly, over weeks or months, so that a single measurement will portray an integrated response of dietary intake (or tissue status) over a period of time, but be less affected by particular meals, or ingestion of supplements at a particular time (Table 7.1).

Table 7.1. Choice of biochemical markers (indices) for nutrients subdivided by their temporal relationships with dietary intake

Compartment	Nutrients[b]	Comments
Short term indices[1]		
Faeces	Inorganic ions Lipids	Balance studies only; for lipids need to consider endogenous production and contributions of colonic bacteria
Urine[a]	B-vitamins (not folate or B_{12}); Vitamin C	Greatest variation and therefore predictive power at moderate-to-high intakes
	Na^+, K^+, (Ca^{2+}) (Mg^{2+})	
	Halides, sulphate, selenium	
	Nitrogen, urea, creatinine, 3-methyl histidine, sulphur amino acids	All require complete collections, adequate days for desired precision
Bile Salts	Cholesterol	Metabolic ward study only
Breath	Fibre (hydrogen, methane)	Validity uncertain
Serum/plasma[c]	All vitamins, but mainly used for vitamin B_6 (pyridoxal phosphate), vitamin C and the fat-soluble vitamins	Intake range for predictive power varies between nutrients, e.g. wide for water-soluble vitamins, narrow for vitamin A
	Most inorganic nutrients except Ca^{2+}, PO_4^{3-}	Variable predictive power between nutrients
	Cholesterol, cholesteryl esters, phospholipids, triglycerides, free fatty acids	May be affected by recent diet (TG FFA). Total FA can be measured, better analysed in subfractions separately
Medium/long term indices[2]		
Red cells[d]	Vitamins B_1, B_2, B_6	Enzyme activation indices
	B_1, B_6, niacin, folate	Total cofactor concentration

Table 7.1. (continued)

Compartment	Nutrients	Comments
	Se	Glutathione peroxidase
	Cu^{2+}	Superoxide dismutase
	$?Zn^{2+}$ etc	?Metallothionein
	Fatty Acids	
White cells[d]	Vitamin C	Entire 'buffy coat' generally
	Zn	used; separated cell types
		probably better
	Fatty Acids	Monocytes; may be only
		short term indicator
Hair, toe-nails finger-nails	(Zn, Cu and other 'trace' elements)	Controversial interpretation
Cheek cells	Phospholipid fatty acids	Validity uncertain
Adipose tissue	Fatty acids	Becoming more widely used in epidemiological studies

[1] Responding within hours or days to changes in intake, especially in the upward direction. Note that serum/plasma indices generally have both short and medium term components.

[2] Responding within weeks or perhaps months to changes in intakes; unresponsive to short term fluctuations. Red cell indices may respond more slowly than white cell indices, but this depends whether individual nutrients can enter or leave during the lifetime of the cell. Hair and finger- or toe-nail indices are medium or long term, depending whether or not specific zones are analysed separately. All of these medium/long term indices are most responsive at the lower end of the intake-range. Adipose tissue levels will reflect intake over the last 2–3 years.

[a] Urine usually requires acidification and refrigeration to prevent bacterial growth and preserve labile nutrients, such as vitamin C.

[b] Indices in parentheses are not strongly recommended, because of difficulties of adequate sample collection or interpretation.

[c] The choice between serum and plasma often depends on arbitrary historical factors, for instance, many clinical chemistry measurements have been validated with serum, but not yet with plasma.

[d] Certain haematological indices; polymorphonuclear cell lobe counts etc. are sensitive to certain nutrient deficiencies, e.g., Fe, folate, B_{12}.

Limitations both of space and of accurate data preclude any detailed or comprehensive discussion of this complex subject, but the following generalizations may be useful:

Faecal analysis Clearly this would not be considered as an option for vitamin status assays, because most vitamins are extensively metabolized, or otherwise destroyed, especially in the large bowel. Some, namely the B vitamins and vitamin K, can be produced there in considerable amounts, but the proportion that is then available for absorption by the host may be small.

For balance studies involving inorganic anions or cations, faecal analysis may be essential, and in such cases the measurement of transit time (for example by faecal markers) will be needed to relate the amount recovered in the faeces to that in the ingested food. Present understanding of the origins of faecal lipid and nitrogen and their relationship with dietary intake is limited. Faecal lipid levels are derived from maldigested and malabsorbed dietary intake, endogenous secretions, and from colonic bacteria, and levels of output may be quite different in different subjects despite similar intakes (Murphy, unpublished data). Faecal analyses are difficult, laborious, and demanding in terms of subject cooperation; their usefulness in most types of epidemiological studies is limited.

Urine analysis   For water-soluble substances that are readily transported into the renal glomerular filtrates, e.g. the water-soluble vitamins and a range of inorganic ions, the analysis of a well defined urine collection may be informative, particularly about recent dietary intake. Clearly, at equilibrium the difference between the net amount of a nutrient that is absorbed and the amount retained in the tissues must equal the amount excreted in the urine plus other, usually minor, excretory routes. For those nutrients (like iron) which cannot be removed by this route, there has to be a strict control of net absorption, but for those that can be removed (like the water-soluble vitamins and alkali metals), the renal excretion route is continually adjusting the balance, and ensures an appropriate level of retention, provided that the kidneys are functioning correctly. A new bolus of intake in an already nearly saturated subject will produce a bolus of urinary excretion, generally beginning in less than an hour, so that a 6-hour urine collection may then reflect quite accurately the dietary intake over the same period. However, this generalization presupposes that only a small proportion of the nutrient intake is either stored in the tissues or is metabolized.

For instance, in the case of water-soluble vitamins the amount recovered in the urine exhibits a much closer relationship with intake and a more sensitive response to changes in intake when the previous long term intakes (and body stores) are above the 'saturation threshold' for the nutrient in that individual or group. Therefore, the urinary excretion of vitamins like thiamin, riboflavin, and vitamin C tend to reflect intake fairly well when the intakes are moderate to high when compared with requirements, but the variation in excretion is much less informative when the intake is habitually low. Indeed, one approach to the definition of requirements is the measurement of a break-point between the small slope of increase of urinary excretion with increasing intake when the tissues are unsaturated, and the much larger slope when saturation is surpassed.[9,10]

Use of urine analyses in an epidemiological study presupposes that the subjects are able and willing to provide a satisfactory sample, and that the nutrients of interest are stable, or can be satisfactorily preserved. A complete 24-hour urine sample is usually more informative than, say, a random or 'overnight' sample, but is much more difficult to collect. Young infants or demented elderly and certain other human groups are obviously unable to cooperate. Bacterial growth will destroy organic nutrients and unstable substances like vitamin C may require a combination of acidification and cold storage after collection. These constraints frequently tip the balance of choice in favour of blood-sampling. Severe tissue-depletion can be detected by the percentage recovery of an oral test dose of the nutrient in the urine for some nutrients, but this older method has now been largely superseded by blood analysis.

Blood analysis   Blood has the advantages of rapid sampling, with a minimum amount of active participation by the subject. It can provide several fractions representing different compartments and hence presents a wide choice both of analytical possibilities and timescale viewpoints. Although some nutrient assays can, with advantage, be performed on whole blood (e.g. 'red cell' folate), the vast majority employ an initial separation procedure to look at a single compartment within the blood sample.

The most common choice of sampling compartment is plasma or serum, and this is also the most responsive to recent dietary intake, or at least to intestinal lumen contents assuming that absorption is normal. Serum can have certain advantages over plasma, namely of avoiding anticoagulant additives (which may interfere with certain assays) and of 'clean' storage in the frozen state (without the formation of insoluble protein precipitate). However, it has the disadvantages of contamination with platelet contents, of a possibly greater risk of haemolysis, which can seriously affect certain assays, and it entails losing both the red and white cells in the clotted fraction. With respect to temporal variations, serum or plasma often exhibit major fluctuations following meals because nutrients are usually transported from the site of absorption to the tissues via the acellular compartment of the bloodstream, but there will also be an equilibrium set up with tissue nutrient levels, and this will exhibit longer term fluctuations, if tissue status fluctuates. Thus, plasma or serum nutrients usually exhibit rather complex kinetics, with two or more input compartments, representing (i) the gut lumen and (ii) the tissue pool, in even the simplest case.

It is thus an oversimplification to say that plasma levels only reflect recent intake, whereas other compartments only represent long term status, although it would be true to say that plasma levels can often respond rapidly (and transiently) to the intake of nutrient-rich foods or supplements, just as urinary excretion does. Of course, for certain nutrients (e.g. calcium) the homeostatic control mechanisms are so tight that variations in intake over a huge range have a negligible effect on plasma levels, and in the case of vitamin A, for instance, plasma levels depend primarily on the steady-state level of retinol-binding protein. Thus, plasma retinol levels reflect tissue vitamin A status only when tissue stores are very low (i.e. moderate-to-severe deficiency in functional terms), whereas plasma retinyl ester levels normally reflect only very recent intake, although only for as long as the chylomicrons are in the process of transporting them from the site of intestinal absorption to the liver, for storage, or for release as the retinol–RBP complex.

The second possible choice of compartments within an anticoagulated blood sample is the red cell compartment, whose advantages, especially in the water-soluble vitamin field, have become increasingly evident during the past couple of decades. Erythrocytes contain a variety of enzyme systems that depend on B vitamin-derived cofactors, and these have proved very sensitive to variations in tissue and body status of individual vitamins, in a manner that has made them eminently suitable for status-index development. Thus, the total red cell concentrations of vitamin-derived cofactors, or the extent of stimulation of specific enzymes by their vitamin-containing coenzymes (e.g. glutathione reductase by flavin adenine dinucleotide) have yielded status assays that are robust, very sensitive at the borderline of deficiency, and an accurate reflection of body stores. Another approach is the use of red cell enzyme stimulation tests. Here, activity of a red cell enzyme is measured in the presence and absence of its appropriate vitamin coenzyme. In nutritional adequacy, the added coenzyme has little effect on the overall enzyme activity, so the ratio of the two measurements is very close to unity. However, in vitamin deficiency, added coenzyme increases enzyme activity to a variable extent, depending on the degree of deficiency. The test thus measures the extent to which the red cell enzyme has been depleted of coenzyme, and the result is expressed either as the Activation coefficient (AC, or 'α'), where

$$\text{Activation coefficient (AC)} = \frac{\text{Activity of the coenzyme-stimulated enzyme}}{\text{Activity of unstimulated enzyme}}$$

or as Percentage stimulation, where

$$\text{Percentage stimulation} = \frac{\text{Stimulated activity} - \text{Basic activity}}{\text{Basic activity}} \times 100$$

(e.g. TPP effect for thiamin). Table 7.2 gives values for activation coefficients for four vitamins. If the question of risk concerns intakes that can usefully be classified as normal, marginal, or deficient, then functional tests of this type may have value in nutritional epidemiological studies.

For certain vitamins, individual red cells can exhibit gains or losses during their lifetime, although these losses are measured in weeks rather

Table 7.2. Erythrocyte enzyme stimulation tests of nutritional status.

Vitamin	Enzyme/coenzyme	Status measured by activation coefficient	Interpretation	General comments
Thiamin	Transketolase/thiamin pyrophosphate	1.00–1.25 >1.25	Normal or marginal status except when basic transketolase activity is low, then probably chronic deficiency. Biochemical deficiency: high values likely to be acute deficiency	Unstable enzyme. Must be stored at −70°C or measured fresh
Riboflavin	Glutathione reductase/Flavin adenine dinucleotide	1.00–1.30 1.30–1.80 >1.80	Normal status Marginal/deficient status Deficient status associated with intake below 0.5 mg riboflavin/day	Very stable enzyme. Good indicator of tissue status. Possibly unreliable in situations of negative nitrogen balance
Pyridoxine	Aspartate aminotransferase/pyridoxal phosphate	1.00–1.50 1.50–2.00 >2.00	Normal status Marginal status Deficient status	Many modifications of method exist. There is disagreement on thresholds. Uncertain stability at −20°C for more than a few days
Biotin	Pyruvate carboxylase	0.95*(0.85–1.15) 1.25 (1.05–3.8) 2.10 (1.70–2.9)	plasma >60 ng/100ml 45–60 ng/100 ml 30–40 ng/100 ml	From studies on pigs described by Whitehead.[195] Deficiency rare in man

* Values shown are median and ranges corresponding to plasma biotin concentrations. Pigs were fed diets containing varying amounts of biotin (0–900 μg biotin/kg).

than in hours or days (as would be the case with plasma or urine responses). (It is worth noting that dietary supplements of riboflavin, thiamin and pyridoxine may alter the results of red cell enzyme tests within days, as vitamin-deficient red cells may take up vitamins within 24 hours.) For other vitamins, (e.g. red cell folate) the level is determined even before the cell is released from the bone marrow, and it then remains constant until the cell is eventually destroyed. Thus, red cell folate can provide a reasonably good long term reflection of dietary intake and of tissue levels, but it is insensitive to short term fluctuations.

The third possible choice within the bloodstream is the white cell complex. 'Complex' is the operative word, because different white cell types (granulocytes, lymphocytes, platelets, etc.) may not only concentrate many nutrients to different degrees according to the cell type, but they may also exhibit quite different temporal changes in varying situations. For instance, the measurement of 'buffy coat', i.e. total white cell content, of vitamin C can, in certain circumstances, be a good reflection of tissue vitamin C levels, but it may also be severely confounded by a big influx of new granulocytes, e.g. during surgery or acute infection. The exploration of white cells as a biopsy tissue for nutrient status monitoring is at an early stage of development. Provided that new methods of cell-type purification and sensitive assay procedures can overcome the existing problems of contaminated populations and large blood volume requirements, white cell-based status assays may become increasingly useful. Like the red cell compartment, white cells tend to reflect integrated intakes, although their turnover is somewhat more rapid than that of red cells and they may therefore be able to detect medium to long term fluctuations of intake.

Other compartments Breast milk can also provide a useful set of nutrient indices that tend to reflect circulating (plasma) levels and recent nutrient intakes for many nutrients. However, there may also be major effects of the stage of the infant's feeding cycle and stages of lactation that will complicate interpretation and this creates a need for carefully controlled sampling protocols. In some cases (e.g. vitamin A), milk levels can show a wider range of sensitivity than plasma levels, because of the near absence of the retinol binding protein (buffering capacity).

Saliva, semen or term-placental nutrient levels These can give information about some nutrients, but have not been widely used.

Fat biopsies These have been shown to be reasonable markers of long term fatty acid intake, and may be useful for some fat-soluble vitamins, although the latter have not yet been sufficiently well validated.

Hair, finger-nails and toe-nails Levels of trace elements in hair or in finger-nails or toe-nails have been explored, but there is wide disagreement about their usefulness as indices either of status or of intake. More refined technical procedures and a better control of sampling protocols are required in this field.

Table 7.3 has attempted to indicate which biochemical indices are most usefully predictive of intakes for each micronutrient and over what broad range of intakes the relationship is best. To some extent, the choice is necessarily idiosyncratic and personal because the ability to assess the available tests depends on the expertise and equipment available. In addition to considering the 'deficient' and 'normal intake' ranges, Table 7.3 includes some indications of those indices that can recognize the use of dietary supplements, i.e. intakes above the range provided from food alone. Because such supplements might be overlooked during the completion of a diet history or other diet record, it is sometimes important to choose a status index or marker that can recognize 'pharmacological' intakes, and flag the subjects involved. Naturally, the intermittent use of supplements may have only a transient effect on many of the available indices, and could therefore go unrecognized.

Other status indices include 'functional tests' of metabolic pathways, in which a loading dose of a pathway precursor is given, usually by mouth, after which the appearance of metabolic intermediates, usually in the urine, is monitored. This approach can distinguish between long term dietary inadequacy and adequacy, but it is generally insensitive to short term dietary variations. As these tests usually require collection of timed urine samples, they add significantly to the time taken to see subjects, and their use in epidemiological studies needs careful evaluation in terms of both compliance and the restricted nature of the involvement.

Clinical deficiency signs (or physiological abnormalities, e.g. dark adaptation decline) usually represent the extreme lower end of status and intake ranges. Although clinical investigations are very important in defining the status of an individual or population, they frequently have the disadvantage of poor specificity. They are therefore useful only in recognizing prolonged periods of dietary deficiency, and they require biochemical evidence, together with evidence of an improvement during supplementation, to confirm the diagnosis. In some cases, the reversal of clinical deficiency signs (e.g. oedema in beri-beri) may be very rapid, but in others (e.g. mouth signs in riboflavin deficiency) it may be slow and uncertain, because of secondary local infections that require separate treatment.

Finally, no discussion of the temporal aspects of the relationship between dietary nutrients and the status indices that represent the levels in various body compartments would be complete without some discussion of repeat measures. The necessity for time-averaged estimates in dietary measurements is obvious because no nutrient (except in laboratory animal chow perhaps!) is present at exactly the same concentration in all foods, in all meals, on all days of the week, and at all seasons of the year. The extent

Table 7.3. Feasibility of predicting intakes from the biochemical index values of specific nutrients

Nutrient	Range of intakes[1]	Feasibility[2]	Choice of index
Vitamin A	Low	+(L)	Plasma retinol, RDR[3]
	Intermediate	0	
	High (T)	+(S/L)	Plasma vitamin A (mainly esters)
Vitamin D	Low	+[4](L) ⎱	Plasma 25-hydroxy-
	Intermediate	+[4](L) ⎰	cholecalciferol
	High (T)	+(S/L)	plasma vitamin D
Vitamin E	Low	?[5]	
	Intermediate	+(L) ⎱	Plasma vitamin E:cholesterol
	High	+(L) ⎰	ratio
Vitamin K	Low	? +(L) ⎱	Blood clotting (prothrombin)
	Intermediate	+ (S/L) ⎰⎱	time[6]
	High	? +(S/L) ⎰	Plasma vitamin K
B-vitamins (general)	Low	+(L)	Red cell enzyme activation tests; plasma or red cell levels
	Intermediate	+(S/L)	Plasma or red cell levels; urinary levels
	High	++(S/L)	Plasma or urinary levels
B-vitamins (specific)			
Thiamin	Low	+(L)	Red cell transketolase or thiamin level.
Riboflavin	Low	++(L)	Activation of erythrocyte glutathione reductase.
Vitamin B$_6$	Low	+(S/L)	Plasma pyridoxal phosphate or urine pyridoxic acid, or red cell transaminases
Folate	Entire range	+(S/L)	Serum (S/L) or red cell (L) folate.
Vitamin B$_{12}$	Entire range	+(S/L)	Serum vitamin B$_{12}$
Vitamin C	Low	+(L)	Buffy coat vitamin C
	Intermediate	++(S/L)	Plasma or buffy coat vitamin C
	High	+(S/L)	Plasma or urinary vitamin C
Cations:			
Na$^+$ and K$^+$	Entire range	+++(S)	Urinary levels
Ca^{2+} and Mg^{2+}	Low/intermediate	+[7](S)	Urinary levels
Fe^{2+}	Entire range	+/−[8](L)	Serum ferritin, red cell protoporphyrin; transferrin saturation
Zn^{2+}	Entire range	+/−[8](S/L)	Plasma Zn^{2+}
Cu^{2+}	Low	+/−[8](L)	Red cell superoxide dismutase
Ultra trace: (Mn^{2+}, Cr^{2+} etc)	Entire range	+/−[8](S/L)	Plasma levels

Table 7.3. (*continued*)

Nutrient	Range of intakes[1]	Feasibility[2]	Choice of index
Anions:			
F^-, Cl^-, I^-	Entire range	+++(S)	Urinary level
I^-	Low	+(L)	Plasma thyroid hormone levels
$Se^{2-}(SO_3{}^{2-})$	Entire range	++(S)	Urinary level
	Entire range	+(S/L)	Plasma, hair and toe-nail Se
	Low	+(L)	Red cell glutathione peroxidase
$S^{2-}(SO_4{}^{2-})$	Entire range	++(S)	Urinary levels
$PO_4{}^{3-}$	Low/intermediate	+(S)	Urinary levels
Lipids			
Fatty acids[9]	Entire range	++(S/L)	Cholesteryl esters, phospholipid of cell membranes, such as erythrocytes and monocytes. For long term marker adipose tissue.
Cholesterol[10]	Low	+(S/L)	Plasma level, LDL
Protein			
Nitrogen	Entire range[11]	++(S/L)	Urinary level

[1] Uses approximate and arbitrary subdivisions: a) 'low' i.e. intakes that are below the RDA and include the biochemical, functional, and clinical deficiency ranges; b) 'intermediate', i.e. intakes that yield adequate status including the RDA, up to the maximum that could be obtained from a sensible balanced diet; c) 'high' i.e. intakes that can only be obtained by taking supplements, including amounts that are in the pharmacological and in some cases potentially toxic (T) ranges.

[2] Arbitrary subdivisions: 0, not feasible, usually because there is no index that is sensitive over this range; +/− poor predictive power; +, fair predictive power; ++ or +++, good predictive power; ?, insufficient information; S, short term reflection of intake (hours or days); L, long term reflection of intake (weeks or months); S/L, may reflect either short or long term intakes.

[3] Relative dose response, the increase in plasma retinol after a test oral dose.

[4] Assumes that the contribution from sunlight is very small.

[5] Deficiency only encountered in conjunction with a metabolic abnormality; natural human diets do not normally cause overt deficiency.

[6] Or recent variants with improved sensitivity.

[7] Complicated by interference, especially with protein.

[8] Complicated by many other factors, e.g. availability from food matrix, acute phase response for serum ferritin and plasma Zn, etc. Faecal analysis would give better estimates of intake, but this is generally impractical. Hair and finger- or toe-nail analyses may give some long term information.

[9] The best markers of intake are those fatty acids that can not be synthesized endogenously (n6;n3 families). Recent studies have shown good associations between fish oil intake and levels in monocytes.[191] Dietary fatty acids influence levels of serum cholesterol and of cholesterol in lipoprotein fractions.

[10] The relationship between dietary cholesterol and serum cholesterol is complex. Keys et al.[192] and Hegsted et al.[193] have formulae that predict this relationship. Plasma cholesterol rises less steeply as dietary cholesterol intake increases. A recent study[194] has shown that change in cholesterol is strongly influenced by initial levels and that the effect of dietary modification on serum cholesterol was greater in the upper third and lower in the lower third of intake. Other studies have suggested the opposite. Predicting dietary cholesterol intake from serum cholesterol may result in substantial misclassification. As about 65 per cent of cholesterol is carried in LDL, the relationship between dietary cholesterol and LDL cholesterol is similar to that for total cholesterol.

[11] Tissue catabolism when subjects are in negative energy balance will lead to overestimate of intake based on urinary excretion. Extrarenal losses may influence predictive power of urinary measure.

of variability itself varies enormously between nutrients[11] so that the number of days of diet estimation that are needed for a predetermined constant degree of precision for estimation of usual long term intakes also varies greatly between different nutrients. The advantage of repeated dietary measurements on the same individual at intervals during an epidemiological study is that the risk of percentile group misclassification is greatly reduced. It is thus possible to verify the initial classification of individuals in extreme groups of intake by means of a second or subsequent repeat estimate. Likewise, the repetition of biochemical index measurements at intervals during a longitudinal study not only ensures a greater certainty in the classification of individuals by their long term mean status values, but it also permits the estimation of intrasubject variations in status, which can then be compared with the intersubject variation. Clearly, if intersubject variation is large in comparison with the intrasubject variation, the intersubject status classification achieved will be more precise and should have a better predictive power then if the intrasubject variability is large compared with intersubject variation. Thus, studies that attempted to separate intersubject from intrasubject variation for intakes and biochemical indices for riboflavin and vitamin C in elderly people[12,13] demonstrated quite different patterns for these two nutrients, which may have implications for their predictive power in such a population.

7.1.3 Complicating factors in the relationships between dietary nutrient intakes and status indices

A wide variety of complicating factors remain even when the fundamental physiological factors, such as limits on intestinal mucosal transport rates, tissue and renal threshold saturation levels, feedback control of absorption, etc. have all been recognized and defined, and a theoretical relationship has thereby been drawn between the amount of a nutrient in the diet and the amount expected in various tissue or body fluid compartments, with appropriate mathematical treatments of the flux rates through the different body compartments to describe the complex temporal relationships between them. These factors will blur the relationship between intakes and status indices in free-living people (Table 7.4).

The first complication is that of intersubject variations in nutritional physiology and metabolism. This can, of course, occur either at the level of absorption, tissue distribution of uptake, turnover, excretion, or indeed subsidiary elements of these processes. Clearly, it is the combination of individual variations in intake, nutrient deposition, and susceptibility to specific (nutrient-linked) disease, that forms the first and uppermost layer of the science of nutritional epidemiology. Beneath this layer there are important interactions that complicate these relationships:

Table 7.4. Points of measurement at which discrepancies between dietary estimates and biochemical index values may arise.

Point of measurement	Reasons for discrepancy
Diet estimate	Inaccurate recording/recall techniques. Inappropriate time-period for records. Inaccurate or inappropriate food table nutrient values; variations in nutrient content between apparently similar food items; variations in manufacturing techniques, etc. Variations in storage losses, cooking losses, plate wastage, etc.
Absorption	Variation in fundamental bioavailability of the different chemical forms of nutrients. Interactions between nutrients and food components (positive or negative) within the GI tract. Interactions between nutrients and secreted substances in GI tract (digestive enzymes, binding proteins, etc.) Effects of gut flora: contributing to or destroying certain nutrients. Physiological variations in absorptive capacity; feedback control of absorption by size of tissue load for some minerals; effects of transit time, intraluminal concentration and bolus effects, etc.
Disposition, metabolism, and turnover	Variations in distribution between the different tissues (usually via the bloodstream); temporal effects, involving various body pools and rates of transfer between them. Variations in the conversion of nutrients to specific metabolites, to cofactors, or diversion to storage compartments. Variations in degradative pathways. Variations in excretory pathways: renal, biliary, enterohepatic circulation, etc. Effects of xenobiotics. Effects of medical conditions.

1. Nutrients may interact with each other, either in the food or in the intestinal lumen, or they may interact with enzymes or with binding proteins or with other secreted substances. One example of a 'beneficial' interaction is that of food folate polyglutamates with polyglutamylhydrolase (conjugase) enzyme in the intestinal lumen, which liberates the monogluta-

mate and short chain polyglutamates in the form that can then be absorbed. Another is the interaction of vitamin B_{12} with intrinsic factor, which is essential for its absorption. An example of a 'non-beneficial' interaction is that of divalent cations with phytate and other polyvalent anionic substances in food, which thereby diminish nutrient availability. Table 7.5 lists some chemical changes and interactions that may affect the availability of nutrients in food.

The relationships between certain nutrients in the diet and their biochemical index values may also be affected by other nutrients in the diet or in the body. Thus, for instance, vitamin B_6 status indices are greatly affected by dietary protein levels independently of vitamin B_6 intake; other nutrients may compete with each other for absorption, e.g. zinc versus iron. Some nutrients may arise from two or more very different routes, e.g. vitamin D from either the dietary vitamin or ultra-violet light acting on vitamin D precursors in the skin; niacin arising from dietary niacin coenzymes or tryptophan; vitamin A arising from dietary vitamin A or carotenoids. In such cases it is often difficult to define the relative contributions of the two (or more) sources, whose efficacy may vary independently under different conditions.

2. A wide variety of substances, particularly drugs and xenobiotics, can alter the absorption, disposition, or metabolism of individual nutrients in various different ways. Some drugs may have wide ranging general effects (such as purgatives, diuretics, antidiuretics, inducers of microsomal drug oxidation enzymes); others may have more specific effects on certain nutrients (e.g. folate antagonists). Many of these interactions are only partly mapped at the present time, for instance the interactions of antiepileptic drugs, antimalarials, antibiotics, etc. with specific nutrients are only partially understood. The effect of smoking on nutrient status (major effects on vitamin C and carotene levels) could be considered a special case of xenobiotic interactions, and alcohol, likewise, has a variety of effects on nutrient status indices. Clearly, with the increasing use of drugs in human medicine, drug–nutrient interactions are becoming of increasing significance in modulating the relationship between nutrient intakes and status.

3. Gender, physiological stage (pregnancy, lactation) and age can affect not only the true requirements for nutrients, but also their distribution between body compartments, and hence the performance of certain (e.g. enzyme and metabolic pathway) indices, in ways that may complicate the intake–status index relationships. Long term adaptations to very low or very high intakes may disturb the 'natural' relationships between intake and status indices. These are encountered more frequently for mineral nutrients than for vitamins.

Table 7.5. Chemical changes, interactions, and *de novo* synthesis, which may affect the availability of nutrients in food

Nutrient	Process	Effect	Possible sources of variation
Carotenoids	Cleavage to retinol in the mucosa	Conversion to vitamin A	Amount of carotenoids, vitamins A and E, fat and possibly protein, in the diet
Vitamin A esters	De-esterification by lipases	Conversion to free retinol	May affect availability of vitamin A in infants
Vitamin K	Synthesis of menaquinones by intestinal flora	Significant contribution to vitamin K status	Suppressed by certain oral antibiotics
Thiamin	Destruction by thiaminases	Losses	Food preparation methods; raw fish
Thiamin and niacin	Interactions with mycotoxins	?Reduced availability	Mycotoxin contamination of foods, especially rice
Folate	Removal of polyglutamyl side chain	Increased availability	Varies with food preparation methods, and probably also between individuals
Vitamin B_{12}	Release from protein-bound forms in food. Adsorption to salivary haptocorrins and gastric intrinsic factor	Greatly enhanced availability	Essential for adequate absorption; failure of intrinsic factor typically results in pernicious anaemia. Affected by several abnormal medical conditions, which tend to increase with age
All multivalent metal ions	Interaction with phytate and other organic polyanions in food	Usually diminished availability	Balance between animal and plant foods; levels of dietary protein and other enhancers of absorption

Table 7.5. (continued)

Nutrient	Process	Effect	Possible sources of variation
Calcium	Induction of calcium-binding protein by vitamin D	Enhanced absorption	Determinants of vitamin D status (sunlight; diet sources); determinants of hormone balance; specific disease states
Iron	Interactions with chelating or reducing agents, e.g. ascorbate, protein, etc.	Enhanced absorption	Meal composition. Absorption also controlled by body stores, limiting excessive absorption
Zinc, copper	Interactions with protein, etc.	Enhanced absorption	Competition between metal ions and interaction of each metal with food chelators
Lipids	Cis to trans isomers	Reduced availability	Heating and hydrogenation of oils in formation of margarines
Protein	Maillard reaction; protease inhibitors in legumes	Reduced availability; reduced absorption	Food preparation methods

4. Disease processes may upset these relationships, and again produce potentially misleading changes. For instance, any substance that is affected by changes in acute-phase protein status in the bloodstream will show alterations during infection and inflammation, that do not reflect either changes in intake or changes in general tissue nutrient status. The increase in plasma ferritin level during the acute phase reaction, for example, does not reflect iron status in the way that the ferritin levels do in a healthy subject. Retinol-binding protein is a negative acute-phase reactant, which therefore decreases in concentration in plasma during inflammation and infection. Such changes have often not been recognized, and low retinol concentrations have been incorrectly interpreted as 'poor' vitamin A status, i.e. diminished body stores.[14] Buffy coat vitamin C levels become reduced during the leukocytotic response to infection because the normal balance between white cell populations in the bloodstream is temporarily altered. Table 7.6 lists some of these changes, which can clearly have a major effect on normal intake–status index relationships, and thus confuse interpretation. Disease processes that affect the intestine or kidneys will clearly affect nutrient absorption and renal excretion respectively; diseases affecting the liver may likewise affect the metabolism of nutrients and of their plasma binding proteins; diseases of the immune system may also have profound effects on nutrient balance. Some nutrients (eg. vitamin C and vitamin E) appear to be destroyed at a rate that is at least partially determined by their involvement in tissue-protective reactions and these, in turn, may be affected by diseases, especially those in which oxidative processes play an important part. However, the quantitation of such effects remains poorly defined. Diseases that affect nutrient status may, of course, be either inherited or acquired, and of these a proportion may be ameliorated by high intakes of the nutrients affected, e.g. where there is impaired absorption, impaired transport or impaired conversion to the active metabolite (cofactor, etc.). Such 'nutrient-responsive errors of metabolism', which occur both for vitamins (e.g. pernicious anaemia, due to impaired absorption of vitamin B_{12}) and minerals (e.g. acrodermatitis enteropathica, due to impaired absorption of zinc) naturally represent gross departures from the 'normal range' of intake–status relationships. Their correct and early diagnosis can be critical, both for the attainment of adequate nutritional status and also for the prevention of irreversible degenerative damage in certain tissues. Another type of interaction that can affect the relationship between nutrient intake and status indices is exemplified by glucose-6-phosphate dehydrogenase deficiency, which virtually abolishes the increase in activation coefficient of glutathione reductase during riboflavin deficiency in subjects with this enzyme deficiency. It appears that, when a genetic abnormality increases the demand by the red cell, the organism can override the normal redistribution of cofactor. Table 7.6 lists some examples both of inborn errors and of other disease states

Table 7.6. Some examples of disease states that may affect nutrient status indices independently of intake

Disease	Nutrient indices that may be altered (usually lowered)
Pernicious anaemia	Vitamin B_{12} (secondary effect on folate)
Vitamin-responsive metabolic errors	Usually B-vitamins (e.g. vitamins B_{12}, B_6, riboflavin, biotin, folate)
Tropical sprue	Vitamins B_{12} and folate (local deficiencies); protein
Steatorrhoea	Fat-soluble vitamins, lipid levels, energy
Abetalipoproteinemia	Vitamin E
Thyroid abnormality	Riboflavin, iodine, lipid levels, energy
Diabetes	Possibly vitamin C, zinc, and several other nutrients, lipid levels
Infections, inflammation, acute phase reaction	Vitamin C, vitamin A, and several other nutrients, lipids, protein, energy
Measles, upper respiratory tract infections, diarrhoeal disease	Especially vitamin A, lipid levels, protein
Renal disease	Increased retention or increased loss of many circulating nutrients, lipid levels, protein
Cystic fibrosis	Especially vitamin A, lipid levels, protein
Various cancers	Lowering of vitamin indices
Acute myocardial infarction	Lipid levels affected for about 3 months
Malaria, haemolytic disease, hookworm, etc.	Iron, vitamin A, lipid
Huntington's chorea	Energy
Acrodermatitis enteropathica; various bowel, pancreatic or liver disease	Zinc, lipid levels, protein
Hormone imbalances	Mineralocorticoid, parathyroid hormone, thyrocalcitonin (effects on the alkali metals and calcium), lipid levels affected by oral contraception and oestrogen therapy

that affect nutrient status independently of intake. Such a list obviously cannot be comprehensive because of the wide range of potential inter-actions between functional derangement and nutrient index values.

7.2 MARKERS OF DIETARY INTAKE: INORGANIC NUTRIENTS

7.2.1 Sodium and potassium

There is tight homeostatic control of the blood levels of sodium and potassium, and blood levels do not therefore reflect dietary intake except at the extremes of deficiency or excess that are associated with acute clinical signs.

The urinary excretion of sodium is generally a good indicator of dietary intake[11,15] and the same is true for potassium, but with a somewhat larger and more variable excretion via the faeces.

In health, urine is the major route of excretion of sodium and potassium. Faecal excretion of sodium is minimal, in the order of 2–4 mmol per day.[16,17] In temperate climates it is assumed that skin losses are minor, so that on an average basis, 24-hour urine excretion of sodium can be shown to account for 95–98 per cent of dietary intake when this is directly analysed rather than calculated from food tables. However, the within-person variability in sodium excretion is in the order of 30 per cent and substantial numbers of observations are needed to gain precision in the overall mean for individuals.[18,19] This low level of precision, together with the difficulty of ensuring complete 24-hour urine collections, accounts for some of the poor agreement between individual estimates of diet and indi-vidual estimates of urine sodium excretion. Table 7.7 shows that correlation

Table 7.7. Estimates of dietary intake of sodium and potassium in comparison with 24-hour urine excretion

Days of collection	Urine	Na	K	Number and sex of subjects (reference)
Analysed diet				
28	28	0.76	0.82	28 M,F[16]
28	7	0.81	0.49	8 F[166]
3	3	0.31	0.56	9 M,F[15]
Calculated diet				
7	7	0.42	0.23	8 F[166]
3	3	0.04	0.40	9 M,F[15]
6	1	0.61	0.62	55 M,F[167]
7	1	0.25	0.26	794 M[21]
7	1	0.36	0.26	834 F[21]

coefficients are generally in the order of 0.4 for short periods of observation. At least 7 days of observation of both urine and diet are needed before reported correlation coefficients of 0.8 emerge. This is as predicted by Liu and Stamler,[19] who suggested that at least eight 24-hour urine collections were needed to achieve a diminution of the true correlation coefficient by less than 10 per cent. Not unexpectedly, comparisons between calculated intakes of sodium and urine excretion show poorer agreement than comparisons with direct analysis.

With the exception of the data of Holbrook,[16] where good correlations between urinary excretion and dietary intake were obtained for both sodium and potassium based on 28 days of collection, Table 7.7 shows that the agreement between diet and urine is less good and more variable with fewer days of collection. The within person variation in potassium excretion is in the order of 24 per cent, and compared with sodium, faecal losses constitute a greater proportion of dietary intake, from 5–13 mmol per day in western populations, or 11–15 per cent of the dietary intake.[16,18,20] The faecal loss may vary between different populations depending on faecal weight, so that up to 30 per cent of the dietary intake may be lost by this route in South African populations.[17] As with sodium, when only single 24-hour urine collections are available and dietary intake is calculated rather than analysed, the agreement between the two values is particularly weak, with correlation coefficients in the order of 0.3–0.4.

Other factors also contribute to the poor agreement between 24-hour urine excretion and dietary intake. The difficulties of obtaining complete collections have been mentioned, and the PABA marker has been developed for the purposes of validating dietary assessments with 24-hour urine estimations of nitrogen (see section 7.4.2). When used to validate 24-hour urine specimens for estimation of sodium excretion in blood pressure studies, regression coefficients were larger in the subgroup of individuals whose 24-hour collections were classified as complete by the PABA technique than in the analysis of the group as a whole.[22] Heavy perspiration in non-adapted individuals could detract further from the closeness of the relation between intake and excretion, and secretion into breast milk of approximately 7.8 mEq (180 mg) sodium and approximately 12.8 mEq (500 mg) potassium per litre, is also a significant diversion. Severe and prolonged diarrhoea causes major losses.

Replacement of 24-hour urine collections with overnight or casual urine specimens in epidemiological studies has been extensively discussed. Values for 24-hour excretion extrapolated from 8-hour collections have been used to assess group compliance with study protocols in low salt intervention studies in hypertension.[23] Liu and Stamler suggest that full 24-hour specimens are necessary for estimation of individual sodium and potassium output, and estimated the correlation between mean 24-hour urine sodium excretion and true mean overnight sodium excretion to be

0.72. They suggest that multiple measurements of the sodium/potassium to creatinine ratios might be feasible for assessing the relation between blood pressure and electrolyte excretion.[19] Correlations between overnight, random, and true electrolyte excretion seems to vary in different populations; Ogawa found correlations in the order of 0.8 between overnight and 24-hour collections[24] whereas Yamori found the greatest agreement (correlation coefficients in the order of 0.8) for evening collections, with less good agreement between overnight and 24-hour collections (correlation coefficient 0.6).[25]

7.2.2 Calcium, phosphorus, and magnesium

These alkaline earth metals are less completely absorbed than the alkali metals and, although the net amount of them that is absorbed virtually equals the amount excreted in the urine for a subject in balance, the prediction of intakes from the amount in the blood or excreted in the urine can only be approximate and into broad categories. This is because the percentage of calcium that is absorbed varies between from about 70 per cent at very low intakes, to about 30 per cent at daily intakes of 2 g in adults.[26] At intakes below 200 mg/day the subject is generally in negative balance, i.e. urinary excretion exceeds absorption, and above this break-point there is a linear increase, albeit with considerable scatter.[26] Much of this scatter is due to a major dependence of calcium excretion on salt and protein intake. There is a strong homeostatic control of plasma calcium levels and the amount in plasma is not generally a useful predictor of intake, although there are, of course, transient increases following meals or supplements.

The extent of absorption of dietary magnesium is similar in magnitude to that of dietary calcium, i.e. around 50 per cent of intake and, like calcium, the plasma level is held remarkably constant,[27,28] although the mechanism of this homeostasis is not well understood. Thus, urinary magnesium is the best available, although approximate and poorly-validated, index of dietary intake.

The absorption of phosphorus from the diet is normally around 50–70 per cent, rising to around 90 per cent when the intake is low, or is from a 'good' source, such as human milk.[29] The absorbed phosphorus must be renally excreted at balance, so the amount in the urine should generally be a fairly good reflection of recent intake. However, there are several unavailable forms of phosphorus (e.g. phytates) that can complicate this relationship.

7.2.3. Iron

Iron is not excreted to any significant extent in the urine and therefore there have to be alternative ways of ensuring that tissue overload cannot occur, especially as iron is potentially a very toxic element. The main way that this is achieved is by strictly limiting the extent of absorption to the amount that is required either for replacement (mainly the net requirement for haemoglobin synthesis), or for storage.

In addition to the control that is exerted upon intestinal absorption according to the subject's existing iron load, there is also a wide variation in the availability of different types of dietary iron, which is further complicated by potential interactions with other food components.[30] Thus, a fairly constant amount (approximately 25 per cent) of haem iron in food is absorbed, but absorption of non-haem iron may very between 1 and 40 per cent, even in individuals with similar iron status, depending on the dietary amounts of protein, ascorbate, and other acids that enhance absorption, and of phytates and certain types of fibre or protein that may inhibit it. The overall result is that none of the conventional indices of iron status (serum iron, per cent saturation or transferrin, serum ferritin, or free erythrocyte porphyrin) can yield an entirely satisfactory estimate of iron intakes, at least on an individual basis. The best of the available indices, at reflecting a wide range of long term intakes on a population basis, is serum ferritin, because this can reflect iron overload as well as iron deficiency. However, raised serum ferritin levels can also result from situations (i) where haemoglobin synthesis is inhibited (e.g. by lead poisoning); (ii) by the acute phase reaction; and (iii) in liver damage associated with iron overload; so that it needs to be interpreted with care. Very low serum ferritin levels, coupled with raised erythrocyte protoporphyrin levels and a low percent saturation of transferrin, are diagnostic of a long term insufficiency of intake. However, as noted above, this only implies insufficiency of available iron, not necessarily of total dietary iron. Similarly, low haemoglobin levels may reflect low dietary iron, but many other factors, including low intakes of vitamin B_{12}, folic acid, helminthic infestation, haemoglobinopathies, and a variety of diseases will reduce circulating haemoglobin, and higher iron intakes above the levels required for adequate haemoglobin formation will not be reflected in raised haemoglobin levels.

7.2.4 Zinc, copper, and other trace metals

Although a small part of the dietary intake of zinc is excreted in the urine, the amount in this compartment has not proved very useful, either for measuring status or for predicting intakes. At intakes typical of Western diets (7–15 mg/day) the percentage absorption of dietary zinc measured by tracer studies is around 50–70 per cent, but most of this is re-excreted via the intestine, and only 5–10 per cent appears in the urine.[31] Serum zinc is a poor indicator of status, and an equally poor indicator of intake, although it can probably distinguish between the extremes of intake for population groups. The zinc content of specific white cell types may prove better indicators of long term status, but these seem unlikely to prove to be much better markers for intake. As with iron, the total amount of zinc in a diet is poorly correlated with the amount that is utilizable by the body. Apart from the faecal index, status indices for transition elements tend to reflect the biological availability, rather than the total amounts in the diet.[32] Food table values rarely distinguish between total and available amounts of nutrients such as zinc and iron in foods, and this represents a further bar to accurate prediction. Measurements of zinc status based on hair or nail clipping analysis do not correlate well with zinc intake or other measures of zinc status.

What has been written above about zinc and iron is also true, in general terms, about the other trace metal nutrients: copper, manganese, chromium, molybdenum, vanadium, etc. There are no biochemical markers for these metals to reflect their intakes accurately. Even the measurements of status and of human requirements remains very difficult, and the search for markers here is in its earliest stages. A recent study by Gallagher *et al.*[33] compared interindividual variation between biochemical status indices for calcium, copper, iron, magnesium and zinc, and also compared mean values of these indices between two groups of women with different long term intakes. Little, if any, discernible effect of dietary intake on the biochemical index values was observed.

In studies of the relationship between copper intake and tissue markers, both the copper-dependent enzyme superoxide dismutase in erythrocytes,[34] and the copper–protein complex caeruloplasmin in serum,[35] have been shown to be associated with copper intake. Unfortunately, both of these markers may be influenced by non-dietary factors,[36] although superoxide dismutase seems the more reliable, in spite of a difficult assay. Measurements of copper in hair and urine (a minor excretory route) are of little value in assessing either copper intake or status.

7.2.5 Iodine, selenium, and other anionic elements

Of the electronegative elements, the halide ions (chloride, fluoride, and iodide) may exhibit the best reflection of intakes, because a very high proportion of the intake appears rapidly in the urine. Provided that renal clearance is normal and that other routes of removal, mainly perspiration and breast milk, are allowed for, the urinary content virtually equals intakes for these substances, so they do accurately reflect intakes over the short term.

The relationship between selenium intake and biochemical markers is reasonably good, although somewhat less close than is the case for halides. Urine is the major route of excretion and provides a reasonable marker of intake.[37] Plasma levels reflect intake to a degree provided the range of variation is large; red cell selenium or glutathione peroxidase activity are markers of medium term status and therefore of longer term intakes. Hair and toe-nail levels have been employed as long–term status indicators and are thus alternative possibilities, although contamination of hair samples by shampoos must be controlled for.

Non-dietary factors such as age, smoking, and alcohol use are associated with reduced levels of markers, but the extent to which this may reflect reduced intakes is not clear. Important interactions between selenium-dependent enzyme systems and other components of the body's antioxidant defences (for example vitamins E, C, and β-carotene) may necessitate a broader examination of these factors in studies assessing the effects of selenium on disease risk.

Free sulphate in the diet is freely absorbed and freely excreted in the urine. Sulphur in other forms, such as amino acids, sulphated polysaccharides, etc, is generally converted to sulphate during turnover and is excreted via the urinary pathway, so that urinary sulphate should provide information about intake. However, little direct confirmation exists.

7.3 MARKERS OF DIETARY INTAKE: VITAMINS

7.3.1 Retinol and carotenoids (vitamin A)

Retinol   Vitamin A is a fat-soluble vitamin and the name is used to include retinol and its metabolites and the provitamin A carotenoids, the most important of which is β-carotene. The vitamin is essential for numerous metabolic processes, particularly vision, growth, cellular differentiation, reproduction, and immunity. The latter function in particular has attracted much attention recently because studies have suggested that even mild deficiency may be clinically important and responsible for much of the morbidity in Third World countries.[14] Carotenoids are present in vegetables and fruits and provide more than 90 per cent of Third World vitamin A requirements; retinol is only present in foods of animal origin.

It was estimated from available evidence about two decades ago that, of the dietary carotenoids in a Western diet, an average of one-sixth of the β-carotene and one-twelfth of the other dietary carotenoids are converted to vitamin A in the intestinal mucosa.[38] This is, of course, an approximation, which undoubtedly varies considerably between individuals and different food types. Thus, carotenoids in oily solution or in fruit juices such as mango are more efficiently utilized than carotene in carrots—the 'typical' carotenoid source in Western diets. With the recent increase in interest in carotenoids for their intrinsic properties, independent of conversion to vitamin A, there is bound to be a resurgence in interest in their dietary availability. As the amount ingested increases, from typical dietary levels towards pharmacological intakes, the percentage absorbed falls sharply, but the total amount absorbed continues to increase.

The two main biochemical markers of vitamin A that need to be considered are plasma retinol and the 'relative-dose-response' (RDR) test,[39] both of which reflect only the lowest segment of the intake scale on a long term basis. In Western countries, where vitamin A deficiency is now very rare, dietary intake of this vitamin is only a very minor determinant of its plasma levels. This was demonstrated in the recent survey of UK adults,[21] in which the cross-sectional correlation between vitamin A intakes and plasma vitamin A was non-significant for women, and explained only 1 per cent of the variance in plasma vitamin A for men (Table 7.8). The RDR test is believed to be more informative at intermediate status and intake levels[39] but it is more difficult to perform and has not been used for normal Western populations.

Ninety per cent of the body's vitamin A is stored in the liver, 9 per cent in other tissues, and 1 per cent is present in the plasma. Furthermore, retinol present in the plasma is homeostatically controlled and only represents that in the liver at the two extremes. Plasma retinol is very low when the liver is virtually exhausted but when there is 10 to 30 μg retinol/g liver, plasma retinol rises to a plateau that remains relatively constant until the liver becomes saturated at 300 μg/g.[40] Therefore, plasma retinol concentrations below 0.70 μmol/l are regarded as borderline vitamin A status and those below 0.35 μmol/l as deficient.[41] (see Table 7.9).

It is widely accepted that plasma retinol below 0.35 μmol/l is associated with low liver reserves and clinical signs of deficiency, although malaria infection and acute-phase reaction may also result in low plasma values without associated clinical signs of deficiency.[14,42–44] In contrast, it is advised that the so-called borderline category, 0.35–0.70 μmol/l, should be regarded with caution because such values may be associated with inadequate protein intake, parasitic infestation, liver disease, and other conditions.[40,41,45]

Measurements of retinol are done on a lipid solvent extract of plasma using HPLC,[46–48] and both retinol and carotenes are stable in stored plasma/serum provided samples are not haemolysed and are handled with appropriate care. The temperature of storage should be −50°C or below if stored beyond 6 months but −20°C is satisfactory for 3–6 months.[8,49]

Retinol is transported in plasma in a 1:1 molar combination with retinol binding protein (RBP). Competitive protein binding and other techniques can be used to measure RBP but the only advantage may be slightly greater stability of the protein over retinol in plasma over long periods of storage.[40]

Relative dose response (RDR)

The control of retinol transport by RBP has provided the basis of a functional test for retinol stores. In vitamin A deficiency, there is continued

Table 7.8 Cross-sectional correlations between dietary intake of nutrients and biochemical indices (markers) in the UK adult study (Gregory et al.)[21]

Nutrient (in food)[a]	Biochemical index[b]	No. of subjects (M/F)	Correlation coefficients	
			Male	Female
			r (P)	r (P)
Iron	Haemoglobin	788/821	−0.04 (NS)	−0.02 (NS)
Iron	Serum ferritin	793/689	0.02 (NS)	0.04 (NS)
Folate	Red cell folate	745/673	0.22 (<0.01)	0.18 (<0.01)
Vitamin B_{12}	Serum vitamin B_{12}	825/755	0.11 (<0.01)	0.10 (<0.01)
Carotenes	Plasma β-carotene	880/902	0.20 (<0.01)	0.38 (<0.01)
Carotenes	Plasma α-carotene	880/902	0.41 (<0.01)	0.43 (<0.01)
Retinol	Plasma vitamin A	881/906	0.10 (<0.01)	0.01 (NS)
Vitamin E	Plasma vitamin E	881/906	0.20 (<0.01)	0.14 (<0.01)
Vitamin E	Plasma tocopherol/cholesterol	856/773	0.29 (<0.01)	0.27 (<0.01)
Riboflavin	Erythrocyte glutathione reductase activation coefficient	874/888	−0.23 (<0.01)	−0.31 (<0.01)

[a] Data given refer to nutrients from food sources only, calculated from 1 week of weighed intake data per subject. The publication includes some additional information relating to all sources, including supplements.
[b] One blood sample from each subject collected after, but not necessarily immediately after, the completion of the diet record (not necessarily a fasting sample). NS, not significant.

Table 7.9. Criteria for assessment of fat-soluble vitamin status in adults for the recommended methods

Vitamin	Measurements	Level of risk			References
		High Risk	Medium Risk	Acceptable	
Retinol (vitamin A)	Plasma retinol (μmol/l)	<0.35	0.35–0.70	>0.7	40, 45, 62
	Relative dose response, (percent change)	>20		<20	40
Cholecalciferol (vitamin D)	plasma 25-hydroxychole-calciferol (nmol/l)	<12.5 (<25.0*)	12.5–25.0	>25	61, 62
Tocopherol (vitamin E)	α-tocopherol: cholesterol (μmol/mmol)	<2.22		>2.22	68, 70
Phylloquinone (vitamin K)	Clotting time (seconds)	>26	13–26	11–13**	45, 81

* Higher risk threshold suggested for subjects who are housebound or similarly restricted during late summer months.
** Recommended clotting time to standardize the wide variety of conditions that exist.[45]

synthesis of RBP, which remains in the liver as apoRBP. The RDR is like a loading test, in that a blood sample is taken and a loading dose of retinol is given followed by a second sample of blood after 5 h. The effects differ from the conventional loading test in that the plasma response is greatest in deficient subjects. The presence of apoRBP in the deficient liver readily combines with the incoming retinol and emerges into the plasma. If the preloading concentration of retinol is increased by more than 20 per cent, this indicates a deficient liver retinol below 20 μg/g. There is very little increase in plasma retinol in the person with normal vitamin A status.

This method has the disadvantage of needing two blood samples and a 5 h wait in between. A modification to this has been proposed, in which the load of retinol would be replaced by dehydroretinol and a single blood sample drawn after a set interval. Dehydroretinol is not normally present in the diet and therefore, using HPLC techniques to separate the two isomers, its concentration could be expressed as the percentage of the total of the two isomers. Initial experiments in both rats and humans appear promising,[50] and this technique may therefore be useful for assessing subclinical retinol deficiency in epidemiological studies.

Thus, the prediction of vitamin A intakes from biochemical indices is possible only in the very broad terms of distinguishing long term deficient intakes from those that are 'adequate'. Another category where blood vitamin A levels become informative is that of excessive intakes and potential toxicity.[51] In lactating women, breast milk vitamin A levels reflect status rather more clearly than blood levels,[52] but the relationship is still not sufficiently precise to be able to predict intakes, except in very broad categories.

Carotenes The only biochemical marker that is currently used for carotenoids is the plasma concentration, which reflects short to medium term intakes over a wide range. Interindividual variation in the plasma response was found to be 'substantial' in one recent supplementation study.[53] However, Romieu et al.[54] observed a significant cross-sectional correlation between dietary carotene intake and plasma β-carotene levels ($r = 0.38–0.43$) in a group of non-smoking North Americans, and a similar correlation between intake and plasma carotenoids was seen in the recent UK study of adults[21] (Table 7.8). Evidence from a study by Tangney et al.[55] indicated that plasma β-carotene was sensitive to intake but remained relatively constant within individuals, so that it reflected fairly long term habitual intakes.

There is currently considerable interest in carotenes as antioxidants, but until a physiological requirement for substances with this property can be identified, the adequacy or otherwise of these substances in the blood cannot be assessed. All the carotenoids in blood have similar structures and may have similar antioxidant properties. If antioxidant function does prove to be of biological relevance, then the non-provitamin A carotenoids in blood, e.g. lutein[56] may be the more useful markers of dietary intake or status because the rate of conversion of the provitamin A carotenoids can influence their levels in blood. Lutein is as common as β-carotene in most fruits and vegetables.[57] Furthermore, the sex differences noticed with the provitamin A carotenoids do not seem to be as obvious in the non-provitamin A carotenoids.[58,59]

7.3.2 Vitamin D

Following the conversion of 7-dehydrocholecalciferol to vitamin D_3 in the skin, or absorption of dietary vitamin D_3 in the gut, the vitamin is stored in the body fat or metabolized in the liver to 25-hydroxy-cholecalciferol (25-OHD). 25-OHD circulates in the blood as the main active reservoir, or is metabolized to one or other of the dihydroxy metabolites by the kidney or excreted in the bile. The 1,25-dihydroxy-cholecalciferol (1,25-OHD) is the active metabolite of vitamin D and maintains calcium levels in the blood, but its levels are influenced by serum calcium, parathyroid hormone, and other D metabolites. Both the 1,25-and 25-OHD metabolites can be used to measure vitamin D status, but the higher plasma concentrations and greater stability of the latter make it the better option. Plasma 25-OHD concentrations thus tend to reflect the availability of vitamin D in the body [60] whereas 1,25-OHD reflects the metabolic need. In deficiency, 1,25-OHD concentrations are low but on supplementation with vitamin D will rise into the normal range, whereas 25-OHD concentrations will remain low until tissue reserves accumulate. 25-OHD is thus a marker of medium to long term vitamin D availability from both dietary and endogenous sources, and it can be measured directly by HPLC.

Those factors that might influence exposure to sunlight (time of the year, habit of dress, mobility, season, age, gender, etc.) should be considered when interpreting 25-OHD results. There is far less endogenous synthesis of vitamin D during the winter than the summer months at higher latitudes, so there are pronounced seasonal fluctuations in plasma 25-OHD in all age groups, and particularly the elderly. Thus, Lawson *et al.*[61] showed that in elderly people in the UK, a strong cross-sectional relationship existed between winter dietary intakes of the vitamin and winter 25-OHD levels because the sunlight contribution was small ($r = 0.55$; $p < 0.02$; $n = 23$), whereas in the summer there was no significant relation between intake and plasma 25-OHD, but the latter was then strongly related to an 'outdoor score', i.e. to sunlight exposure ($r = 0.62$; $P < 0.01$). Thus, there should be a reasonable prediction of broad categories of intake from measurements of plasma 25-OHD in those who are only minimally exposed to sunlight or to other UV light sources, for a period of several months. Persons who restrict their exposure to sunlight need to achieve minimum stores of vitamin D during the summer months to maintain them through the winter. The threshold of 'risk' in such people should be the level associated with osteomalacia (below 12.5 nmol/l) plus a 'safety margin'. Thus, for persons whose potential sunlight exposure is adequate, marginal concentrations of 25-OHD will be 12.5–25 nmol/l but in the elderly, particularly in the latter part of the summer months, such levels would be considered a high risk.[61,62] (Table 7.9).

Other factors that may affect vitamin D status at the lower end of the intake scale include the increased turnover of the vitamin that may occur in people eating typical Asian diets, which are very low in calcium and high in cereals.[63] Vitamin D levels in breast milk from unsupplemented mothers are very low but they do respond markedly to high level supplementation.[64] Thus, both plasma and breast milk levels of vitamin D and its metabolites will detect excessive intakes, and thus potential toxicity, in human subjects. Very low vitamin D intakes by some breast fed infants have been associated with rickets or biochemical deficiency; a broad correlation between intake and marker level also exists in this vulnerable age group.

7.3.3 Vitamin E (α-tocopherol)

Vitamin E consists of eight naturally-occurring chromanols made up of four tocols and four tocotrienols. α-Tocopherol has the highest biological activity and is the least resistant to oxidation. Furthermore it is the predominant form of the tocopherols in animal and human tissues, but is not always the one which is most abundant in foods.[65] α-tocopherol is present in a wide variety of different foods but the largest proportion in human diets comes with dietary fat. A large number of biological and chemical methods are available to measure vitamin E[66] but liquid chromatography is the most relevant to the nutritionist measuring vitamin E status. Unfortunately, however, none of the methods currently available will reliably assess the intake of vitamin E in unsupplemented diet for the reasons described below.

Although dietary vitamin E exhibits some relation to blood tocopherol levels over a wide range of intakes, so that vitamin E supplements have a reasonably predictable effect on individuals' plasma, red cell or white cell vitamin E levels,[67] the predictive power of all the biochemical indices for individual intakes in supplemented diets is only moderate, as can be seen in the weak relationship between intakes and plasma levels in the recent UK adult study[21] (Table 7.8). Here, variations in intake explained only 4 per cent of the variance in total plasma vitamin E, or about 7 per cent of the variance in the tocopherol:cholesterol ratio (which is considered to be a better reflection of status (see below).[68] This weak correlation is partly because the absorption of the vitamin is incomplete and variable (between 20 and 80 per cent in published studies), and partly because the extent of absorption declines with increasing amounts per meal. A further complication is the variable biological activity of different members of the tocopherol family.[69]

α-Tocopherol in the blood The measurement of vitamin E status is commonly made by measuring the concentration of tocopherol circulating in the plasma, where values less than 11.6 μmol/l are generally accepted as indicating vitamin E deficiency.[45]

However, tocopherol circulates in the blood predominantly with the low density lipoprotein fraction, and it was pointed out several years ago that vitamin E was closely correlated with total lipid in the blood.[70] Blood lipids comprise mainly cholesterol, triglycerides, and the phospholipids, and vitamin E correlates best with the cholesterol fraction.[68] The molar cholesterol:vitamin E ratio is approximately 200:1 and is found in plasma samples from healthy persons in Third World and developed countries.[71] In addition, a molar ratio of 200:1 for polyunsaturated fatty acid to tocopherol is found in membranes and microsomes of highly oxygenated tissues of heart and lung and the *in vitro* antioxidant efficiency of vitamin E is of a similar order.[72]

We have therefore suggested that the vitamin E:cholesterol ratio is more biologically relevant than vitamin E alone as a marker of vitamin E status.[68,71] Its use prevents the over-estimation of vitamin E deficiency in Third World countries, it enables comparisons between Western countries with different plasma lipid levels[73] and enables comparisons between different age groups within a community.[21,74] Very few persons fall below the high risk threshold of 2.2 μmol α-tocopherol/mmol cholesterol.[68] Furthermore, the assay only requires the additional measurement of cholesterol to standardize the results.

Functional tests of vitamin E status The antioxidant properties of vitamin E are believed to protect biological membranes against oxidant damage. This feature was used by Horwitt *et al.*[75] to develop the hydrogen peroxide haemolysis test (erythrocyte stress test) to assess the vitamin E status by the ability of red cells to resist oxidant damage. The hydrogen peroxide haemolysis procedure must be performed in a standardized manner with caution exercised with regard to sample handling, time lapse between sample collection and test, preparation of reagents, incubation temperatures, etc.[45,75,76] Unfortunately, the method lacks specificity[77] and many workers have reported difficulties. Where simultaneous estimations of blood tocopherol and the red cell peroxide haemolysis test have been done, the results suggest that appreciable haemolysis is rarely observed if plasma tocopherol is greater than 11.6 μmol/1. Unfortunately, this agreement between the results of the two tests is only a reflection of the tocopherol concentration in the blood and does not necessarily reflect the vitamin E status of other tissues in the body.[45]

A modification of the peroxide test has recently been suggested in which malonaldehyde (MDA) generated by exposure of red cells to peroxide is measured instead of haemolysis.[76] The authors claim that MDA production more accurately reflects vitamin E deficiency as documented by plasma vitamin E or E:lipid ratios. However, as many features of the MDA and haemolysis tests are common, the MDA procedure suffers from most of the limitations of the hydrogen peroxide haemolysis test.

Platelet vitamin E has also been examined as an index of vitamin E status.[77] α-Tocopherol inhibits platelet aggregation and both deficiencies and excess of α-tocopherol have been shown to alter platelet function. Vatassery *et al.*[77] found that platelet α-tocopherol concentrations did not correlate with plasma lipids and reported a linear relationship between platelet α-tocopherol and supplements of DL-α tocopherol up to 1800 IU/ day. They suggested these results indicated that platelet α-tocopherol was a better indicator of vitamin E status than plasma measurements. The first point is worth further investigation but supplementary vitamin E also produces a linear response in plasma concentrations in short term experiments.

Currently, the most useful measurement of vitamin E status is the plasma α-tocopherol:cholesterol ratio (Table 7.9).

7.3.4 Vitamin K

The major dietary form of vitamin K is phylloquinone, derived mainly from plant sources. Its absorption is variable and incomplete because it depends on solubilization within intestinal micelles containing bile salts and the products of pancreatic lipolysis.[78] The development of adequate assay procedures for the very small amounts of vitamin K that are found in human plasma has been achieved only recently, and the limited evidence available suggests a partial, but not very strong relationship with dietary phylloquinone.[79,80] The picture is further complicated by synthesis of vitamin K (menaquinones) in the gut, which may contribute as much as 50 per cent of the total vitamin K in the body. Certainly little evidence exists to suggest that plasma vitamin K can do better than define a very broad classification of group intakes.

The major criterion for assessing the adequacy of vitamin K status in adults is the maintenance of plasma prothrombin concentrations in the normal range (1.2–1.8 μmol/l). Prothrombin levels are mostly estimated using tests that determine clotting (prothrombin) time[81] but prothrombin levels can now be measured directly by radioimmunoassay.[82] It has been suggested that the ratio of non-carboxylated:carboxylated prothrombin in plasma may be a useful indicator of marginal vitamin K deficiency in individuals who have not yet developed defects in blood clotting.[83] The measurement of abnormal prothrombin by radioimmunoassay and its disappearance following injection of vitamin K is also used as a measure of vitamin K status and is claimed to be a 1000-fold more sensitive than prothrombin time.[84] Its use in patients with chronic gastrointestinal disease and/or resection revealed one-third with evidence of deficiency. Abnormalities of vitamin K-dependent decarboxylation are also present in patients with cirrhosis, acute hepatitis, and hepatocellular carcinoma but these do not respond to vitamin K.

Most people have a diet nutritionally adequate in vitamin K_1 plus an unknown amount of K_2 from micro-organisms in the gut.[83] The group with most evidence of prolonged clotting times is the elderly.[85] Seventy-five per cent of more than 1000 hospitalized elderly had abnormal prothrombin times, but most of these were associated with anticoagulant therapy or hepatic damage.

Low plasma prothrombin levels are also found in newborn infants and, because breast milk contains little vitamin K, intramuscular injections of phylloquinone have been recommended to prevent haemorrhagic disease of the newborn, although there are some reservations about this.[86] The very small amounts of vitamin K that are present in breast milk are sensitive to major changes in maternal intake of the vitamin[64,87] but these variations have not yet been refined to permit them to predict intakes. Since it is the young breast fed infant who is most clearly at risk of developing vitamin K deficiency, it will probably be within the area of lactational and breast milk vitamin K nutrition that future efforts will be concentrated.

7.3.5 Thiamin (Vitamin B_1)

Thiamin deficiency is closely associated with the consumption of milled rice, which is why the deficiency disease beri-beri has been commonly associated with South-East Asian countries. However, thiamin is present in a wide variety of foods and it is restriction in food choice that commonly precipitates the disease.

As with most of the water-soluble vitamins, there is no recognizable store of thiamin in the body and the only reserve is that part of the thiamin pool that is functionally bound to enzymes within the tissues. A characteristic urinary excretion pattern has been demonstrated for thiamine (and also riboflavin and vitamin B_6)[88] in which an initially slow rise with increasing intakes is followed by a rapid rise at relatively high intakes, after saturating the main tissue compartments and reaching the urinary excretion threshold. Although none of these vitamins exhibits a complete recovery of intake in the urine, even at relatively high intakes, because intestinal absorption becomes the limiting factor, it is nevertheless possible to predict intake fairly precisely at high intakes, at least on a population basis. On an individual level, variations in absorption efficiency tend to blur this relationship. It depends, of course, on the chemical form of the vitamin present in the diet, on the transit time through the gut region of maximum absorptive capacity, etc. Moreover, excretion is increased by infection and exercise[89] and in situations of negative nitrogen balance, although not to the same extent as riboflavin.[90]

Twenty-four-hour urine collections, and dietary intakes, are both tedious and difficult to achieve, and methods to use both shorter timed (4–6 h) and random urine samples were developed. The thiamin:creatinine ratio is useful for the interpretation of random samples[45] (Table 7.10 and Fig. 7.1) while loading doses of 1–5 mg thiamin administered orally or intramuscularly, and coupled with the measurement of urinary thiamin over 4 or 24 hours, have been used to make the urinary measurement of thiamin more indicative of tissue saturation. Different workers have suggested that if the proportion of urinary thiamin is below 20 per cent of the administered dose in the subsequent 24 hours, then thiamin deficiency is indicated.[91] However, these two techniques fail to provide continuous quantitative markers of thiamin intake for epidemiological purposes. Measurement of urinary excretion below 0.5 mg/1000 kcal (4200 kJ) deviates from linearity in relation to intake and loses sensitivity; and percentage excretion of an administered dose above 20 per cent says little about the degree of deficiency. A combination of the two techniques may help to develop a scheme for classifying individual intakes into broad categories, but problems remain in epidemiological studies regarding the collection of urine samples.

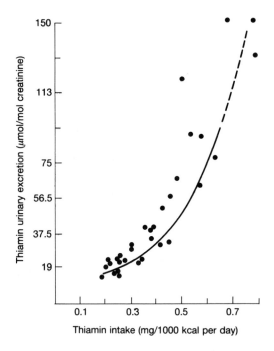

Fig. 7.1. Thiamin intake and urinary excretion. Data collected in the National Nutrition Surveys by the Interdepartmental Committee on Nutrition for National Defence.[190]

Table 7.10. Criteria for assessment of water-soluble vitamin status in adults for recommended methods

Vitamin	Measurement Blood	Measurement Urine	High risk	Medium risk	Acceptable	References
Thiamin	RBC thiamin nmol/l		<90	90–132	132–284	97, 168
		thiamin: creatinine µmol/mol	<10.1	10.1–24.5	>24.5	45
Niacin		NMN: creatinine mmol/mol	<0.4	0.4–1.3	1.3–3.9	109
Pyridoxine	Pyridoxal 5'-phosphate nmol/l		<10.0	10.0–20.0	20.0–165	62,118, 169
Folate	RBC folate mmol/l		<0.23	0.23–0.34	>0.34	45, 62, 123
	plasma folate nmol/l		<6.8	6.8–13.4	>13.4	45, 62, 123
Vitamin B_{12}	serum vitamin B_{12} pmol/l		<74	74–147	>147	45, 62, 125
Ascorbate	plasma ascorbate µmol/l		<6.0	6.0–17.0	>17.0	45, 62, 170
	Buffy layer ascorbate pmol/ 10^6 WBC		<40	40–86	>86	62, 171
	Ascorbate load 15 mg/kg body wt		<14 µmol/l plasma ascorbate at 3 h		>14 µmol/l plasma ascorbate at 3 h	172

The newer method for assessment depends on the reactivation of the cofactor-depleted red cell enzyme transketolase *in vitro*. This is sensitive over a lower range of intakes, from the 'deficient' to the 'moderate intake' range. While it is possible to 'titrate' deficient individuals with varying amounts of the vitamin *in vivo*, and to observe a fairly close correlation between intakes and status indices, it is also clear that the magnitude of the biochemical response to a given intake varies considerably between individuals. This will limit the accuracy of prediction of individual (long term) intakes from the status index values. For example, thiamin intakes in the elderly in the UK did not correlate well with the results of the transketolase test.[13] Thus, while values of the transketolase activation coefficient (TKL-AC) above 1.25 are indicative of thiamin deficiency (see Table 7.2), and those near 1.0 suggest that intakes are sufficient to saturate tissues, the values in between suggest a low to moderate intake, but the correlation of TKL-AC and intake within this range may be poor.[92–94] Furthermore, a combination of a TKL-AC below 1.25 and low TKL activity may indicate chronic thiamin depletion. However, there is some question about the stability of haemolysate TKL activity unless storage at $-70°C$ is possible.[62,95,96]

Direct analysis by HPLC of thiamin diphosphate (TPP), the form in which thiamin coenzyme is mainly found in red blood cells, offers an alternative assay to the TKL-AC. While the range of sensitivity is not greater than with TKL-AC, the reliability of the assay is, and hence its usefulness is improving.[97]

7.3.6. Riboflavin (Vitamin B$_2$)

Riboflavin is present in meats, cereals, and vegetables, but the richest dietary source is dairy products. Consequently, riboflavin intakes are generally lower in milk-free diets, and hence riboflavin deficiency occurs in many parts of the tropics.[5,98–101]

Urinary riboflavin was the first method to be used extensively for the assessment of riboflavin status.[102,103] As with thiamin, there is a linear relationship between intake and excretion at levels of riboflavin intake in excess of dietary requirements.[38] However, when riboflavin intake falls below tissue requirements there are adaptive improvements in the utilization of riboflavin coenzymes that reduce riboflavin excretion; the sensitivity of the assay is also reduced.

The intersection of the excretion curves produced by dietary intakes of riboflavin, below and above the amounts required to saturate the tissues is very marked.[38] However, the optimal amount required to saturate tissues depends upon protein intake being adequate and the subject being in positive nitrogen balance. Thus, infections or drugs that induce a breakdown of tissue protein will increase urinary excretion.[9] Thus, the measurement of urinary riboflavin is of limited usefulness in situations where low protein intake or chronic infection is common.

As with thiamin, there is a red cell enzyme (glutathione reductase) that is dependent on a cofactor derived from riboflavin. This gives rise to the erythrocyte glutathione reductase stimulation test (activation coefficient) or EGRAC. The measurement is like that of total red cell riboflavin, in being a measure of tissue saturation and long term riboflavin status. However, it has the advantage of being stable and extremely sensitive and can be easily made on finger-prick samples.[98] The test appears to be independent of age and sex.

The test is sensitive only at low levels of riboflavin intake, and does not correlate particularly well with values of intake over a wide range. Thus, there was a low correlation between long term riboflavin intakes and several repeated measurements of EGRAC in elderly UK subjects.[12] And in the recent UK adult study[21] (Table 7.8) correlation coefficients between −0.13 and −0.31 were observed between riboflavin intakes and the glutathione reductase index.

EGR activity can be influenced by fluctuations in circulating riboflavin when nutritional status is poor. For example, there is evidence that riboflavin released from the tissues during negative nitrogen balance may give rise to an apparent improvement in status. Bates *et al.*[100] reported a fall in EGRAC values in pregnant Gambian women associated with a fall in body weight during the rainy season (i.e. an apparent improvement in riboflavin status, although other factors suggested that malnutrition increased). Others have shown similar changes in EGRAC (in sick children) that reversed on treatment.[101] Furthermore, EGRAC measurements are rapidly reduced by riboflavin supplementation.[99]

Measurements of EGRAC between 1.00 and 1.30 represent more or less complete saturation of the tissues with riboflavin[99,104] and are obtained in young men on daily intakes of 1.5 mg riboflavin.[105] However, in young women, Belko *et al.*[106] found that amounts of riboflavin between 1.2 and 2.4 mg were required to maintain EGRAC values in this range. EGRAC values of 1.2–1.4 indicate borderline status and were obtained in pregnant women on 1.5 mg in the Gambia and Cambridge.[100] Values around 1.5–2.5 are found in populations consuming minimal intakes of riboflavin, together with evidence of clinical deficiencies.[100,107,108] The EGRAC is thus a useful measure to classify subjects into broad categories of intake, but its sensitivity becomes poorer as dietary intakes of riboflavin approach the levels that correspond to tissue saturation.

7.3.7 Niacin (Vitamin PP)

Niacin is present in large amounts in most cereals and can also be synthesized from the essential amino acid tryptophan and so deficiencies are uncommon. However, maize is an exception, because the niacin is present in a bound form and is unavailable if the food preparation does not include some form of hydrolysis. The niacin deficiency disease pellagra became common in southern Europe and north Africa following the introduction of maize from the New World and was responsible for a tremendous death toll in the southern states of the USA following the social and economic upheaval of the American Civil War.[109]

An Indian variety of sorghum known as jowar has also been linked with pellagra[110] and it was pointed out that jowar contains a high content of leucine, which may interfere with tryptophan metabolism by creating an amino acid imbalance. Other workers have also found evidence that leucine interferes with the metabolism of tryptophan, particularly when niacin intake is low.[111]

The most sensitive method for the determination of niacin, niacinamide and closely related compounds in serum, urine, food, tissues, etc. is by microbiological methods.[112] Chemical methods are far less sensitive and require extensive purification.

The most sensitive indicator of niacin status in experimental animals is the tissue concentrations of the NAD(P) coenzymes. In man, it has been suggested that whole blood NAD(P) may serve the same purpose but, while the method is sufficiently sensitive to use finger-prick samples, the coenzymes are too labile (10–30 s) for the method to be practical.[109]

The principal urinary metabolite of nicotinamide, and hence the coenzyme NAD(P), is N'-methylnicotinamide (NMN) and this substance forms the basis of the most widely used method of assessing niacin nutritional status.[113] The method has high sensitivity and reproducibility.[112] NMN is measured on a timed urine sample or expressed in terms of the creatinine concentration in random samples.

There is also a second urinary metabolite, N'-methyl-2-pyridone-5-carboxamide (2-pyridone) that is more severely reduced in marginal deficiency than NMN and virtually ceases several weeks before the appearance of clinical signs of deficiency. It has been suggested that a more precise measure of niacin status can be obtained by measuring the ratio of 2-pyridone to NMN.[114] This overcomes the problem of timed urine collections but, at the present time, methods to analyse 2-pyridone are still somewhat unsatisfactory.[109]

The excretion of NMN expressed as mmol/mol creatinine in random samples of urine is technically simple and a useful guide to niacin status (Table 7.10). The sensitivity of the index in relation to total intake of niacin equivalents (niacin + tryptophan/60) is better at the margins of adequacy and below than it is at higher intake.

7.3.8 Pyridoxine (Vitamin B₆)

Pyridoxine is widely available in foods of vegetable and animal origin, the range of intake is wide, and deficiencies are rare. The requirement for vitamin B_6 is linked to protein intake, and its role in amino acid metabolism.

Several biochemical markers are currently used for vitamin B_6 (plasma pyridoxal phosphate levels (PLP), red cell transaminase activation, and urinary excretion of B_6 degradation products). Although plasma pyridoxal phosphate levels have gained some popularity, recent studies[115,116] suggest that there is unlikely to be a strong interindividual correlation between B_6 intakes and index levels and that many confounding factors exist, including recent dietary intake, prolonged fasting concomitant with the release of PLP from glycogen phosphorylase,[117] and conditions associated with a raised plasma alkaline phosphatase that can hydrolyse PLP to pyridoxal (PL), a second major vitamer in blood.[118] Incomplete availability of some dietary (e.g. glycosylated) forms of vitamin B_6 imposes a further complication.

In vitamin B_6 deficiency, the erythrocyte transaminase activation coefficient allows the increase in the catalytically inactive apoenzyme of various PLP-dependant enzymes to be evaluated. It has been shown that two enzymes in erythrocyte lysates, alanine (ALT) and aspartate (AST) aminotransferase (Table 7.2) can be used to assess the degree of PLP unsaturation. ALT is considered the more sensitive but AST is more active and more frequently used.[119] Like other activation coefficients, the test is most sensitive at and below marginal intakes (Table 7.2), and is less valuable for ranking individuals with higher (more normal) intakes.

Two metabolic loading tests have been developed to assess vitamin B_6 status. In the tryptophan load test, the potentially rate-limiting enzyme kynureninase is especially sensitive to vitamin B_6 depletion. The excretion of kynurenic and xanthurenic acids is measured before and after the loading dose of tryptophan. However, there are many factors that interfere with this test[120] and its usefulness is very restricted.

In contrast, the methionine load test is less frequently used but there are no reports of artifacts. Three enzymes are involved and, in vitamin B_6 deficiency, a test dose of methionine results in an abnormal accumulation and excretion of homocysteine, cystathionine, cysteine, and cysteine-sulphinic acid and a reduced excretion of taurine.[121] Both of these tests require the collection of timed urine samples, a disadvantage from the epidemiological standpoint.

The concentration of urinary metabolites also reflects recent dietary intake of the vitamin rather than the underlying state of tissue reserves.[122] 4-pyridoxic acid is the main metabolite of PLP and there is some evidence that catabolism increases with age.[45] Loss of sensitivity of the marker at low intakes is problematic.

As with the other B vitamins, there is no single marker for intake with equal sensitivity at all levels of dietary intake, and the use of two or more markers for the same nutrient, if feasible, may help to bridge some of the discontinuities. For thiamin, riboflavin, and pyridoxine especially, the red cell vitamin concentrations seem potentially more useful indices of dietary intake than plasma levels, but their value as markers of intake for individuals has yet to be demonstrated.

7.3.9 Folate

Folate deficiency is one of the more frequently occurring vitamin deficiencies found in Western populations. Folate is necessary for purine and pyrimidine synthesis and actively growing tissue raises folate requirements, e.g. in pregnancy and infancy. Vegetables are the most important dietary source of folate but, since folate is easily oxidized, the freshness and vitamin C content influence the folate content. Folate metabolism is also intimately linked with vitamin B_{12} status, which must therefore be considered in interpreting folate measurements (see below).

The most useful tests of folate status are measurements of folate concentrations in serum and red cells. Because folic acid is susceptible to oxidation, suitable antioxidants (e.g. 1.0 per cent sodium ascorbate) must be added to stabilize folate in samples during collection and storage. Red cell folate is a better measure of long term status because it reflects body stores at the time of red cell synthesis, while serum concentrations reflect recent dietary intake (see Table 7.10).[123] However, because of the chemical and biological complexity of the dietary folates, and the wide variety of factors that determine their bioavailability,[21] only broad categories of intake can be predicted, e.g. for population groups. Experience with the elderly UK subjects[124] shows that their red cell folate levels were more closely related to their dietary folate intake than was plasma folate. This appears to confirm the suggestion that red cell folate measures long term integrated status. In the UK adult study[21] (Table 7.8) the correlation (r) between dietary folate and red cell folate ranged from 0.18 to 0.22, due in part to the relatively short term measure of intake, and in part due to the lack of specificity in the food assay for available forms of folate.

For a complete picture of folate status, both serum and red cell folate should be measured, together with serum vitamin B_{12}, to exclude any involvement of that vitamin in folate metabolism.

In vitamin B_{12} deficiency the metabolism of folate intermediates is blocked, serum folate is normal or high, but red cell folate is low because the deficiency also blocks the tissue uptake of folate.[125,196]

In recent years, radioassay kits have superseded microbiological assays in the measurement of folate. The former are simpler to perform and are not affected by antibiotics. However, the affinity for folate monoglutamate of the binding proteins used in different commercially available kits can vary enormously.[126] A radioassay that makes a good comparison between microbiological assay for folate in red cells has also been described.[127]

An alternative measure of folate status utilizes formiminoglutamate

(FIGLU), a product of histidine metabolism that is normally metabolized by formiminotransferase to 5-formiminotetrahydrofolate. Excretion of FIGLU in folate deficiency is elevated in urine and is particularly elevated following a histidine load.[128] The assay is specific for folate deficiency but offers no advantage over serum or red cell folate assays. Similarly, macrocytic anaemia may indicate folate deficiency but again, these measurements provide no information on the continuum of intake above the levels needed to prevent signs of anaemia from appearing.

7.3.10 Cyanocobalamin (Vitamin B$_{12}$)

Vitamin B$_{12}$ is only present in foods of animal origin, therefore people who are most likely to be at risk of this deficiency are those living wholly on vegetable foods. However, absorption of this vitamin depends upon a binding protein secreted in the stomach. Hence, old age, hypochlorhydria, gastrectomy, and pernicious anaemia, which all influence the production of this protein, can give rise to an absorptive vitamin B$_{12}$ deficiency. Thus, markers of dietary intake may lose their sensitivity in these circumstances.

Vitamin B$_{12}$ influences the metabolism of folate—apparently by starving the tissues of formyl tetrahydrofolate. When vitamin B$_{12}$ status is poor, serum folate may be normal or high, but erythrocyte folate low, because vitamin B$_{12}$ is also necessary for uptake of folates by tissue.[196]

Vitamin B$_{12}$ status can only be estimated from serum levels, not from red cell levels (Table 7.10). Although in normal subjects dietary vitamin B$_{12}$ is considered to possess good bioavailability, the correlation between dietary intake and serum levels is generally not very strong ($r = 0.09$–0.12 in the UK adult study,[21] Table 7.8). One possible reason for this is that body stores of B$_{12}$, which are mainly in the liver, are generally large in comparison with daily intakes, so that the amount in the diet only affects circulating levels very slowly; i.e. it is a long term marker. When serum B$_{12}$ concentrations fall below 90 pmol/l, the liver concentration is below the normal range [125] and serum B$_{12}$ concentrations between 110 and 147 pmol/l (microbiological assay), are indicative of deficiency. In practice, this index seems incapable of defining individual intakes accurately and can only define group intakes in very broad categories relating to levels of deficiency. A marker for the full range of dietary intakes has yet to be described.

7.3.11 Vitamin C

Of all the vitamins, vitamin C exhibits possibly the strongest and most significant correlation between intake and biochemical indices, so that its intake can be predicted with moderate precision from the wide range of biochemical values that are encountered within the population of a

Western country, e.g. the UK. Basu and Schorah[129] reviewed the quantitative relationships between vitamin C intakes, plasma vitamin C and leucocyte vitamin C. Plasma levels exhibit a characteristic S-shaped curve, with the steepest change in plasma levels between about 30 and 90 mg intake per day for adults (Fig. 7.2). Below 20 mg/day intake, most of the vitamin enters the tissues, and little is therefore available to circulate. Above 60–70 mg/day there is a marked renal threshold effect, with the excess of the circulating vitamin then being excreted in the urine. Thus, urine vitamin C

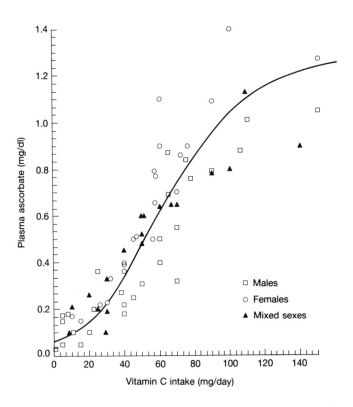

Fig. 7.2. *Relationship between group mean values of plasma ascorbate and levels of vitamin C intake, from published studies.* Data have been compiled from Basu and Schorah[129] and some more recently published studies; each data point represents a group of individuals of varying magnitude and composition, and assay procedures have also varied between different studies, so that the composite picture obtained is intended to give a generalized over-view of the published data, not a precise relationship. There is a clear tendency for women to exhibit higher plasma ascorbate levels for a given intake, than men. Individual studies have recently explored this relationship.[13,185–189] (0.2 mg/dl ≡ 11.4 μmol/l)

is a potential marker for high intakes, although chemical instability is a potential problem, as well as the individual variability of the renal threshold. Amounts in the buffy coat do not exhibit the lower threshold effect that plasma and urine levels do, and hence provide a more sensitive measure of lower intakes (Table 7.10), but the assays require more blood, are time-consuming, and are sometimes difficult to interpret for other reasons (e.g. leucocytosis during infection or surgery.[130–132]). The long term study of elderly men and women living at home in the UK[13] demonstrated a reasonably close relationship between vitamin C intakes and plasma or buffy coat levels. The confounding non-dietary influences here included a clear sex difference and an effect of smoking, both of which are well established influences on vitamin C status.[129,133] The closest temporal correlation was between the biochemical index value and the seven days of intake (estimate) immediately preceding the blood sample (Fig. 7.3). Longer periods of estimation were less relevant because of periodic fluctuation,

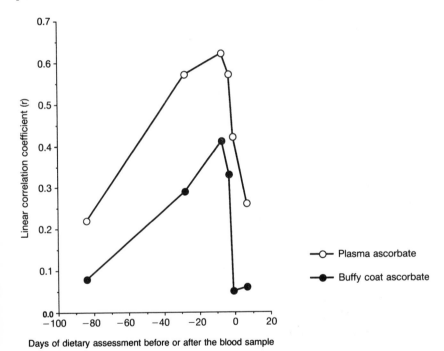

Fig. 7.3. Within-subject correlations between intake and plasma or buffy coat vitamin C levels in healthy elderly men and women. Tabulated values from Table 7.4 of Bates *et al.*[13] are here presented graphically to illustrate the observation that maximum values for the positive correlation between estimated vitamin C intakes and either of the two biochemical index values were obtained when the dietary estimates extended for 7 days before the blood sample collection in each case.

both in intake and in status; shorter periods were less well correlated, probably because of inaccuracies in the short term dietary measurements and medium term buffering of plasma levels by the tissue pools. This analysis provided an indication of the time scale over which such biochemical markers of intake might be validated in the future.

A study of controlled vitamin C supplementation in Gambian lactating women[134] has further illustrated the strength of association between biochemical indices of vitamin C and its intake. This study provided a 'calibration curve' whereby the intake in a group of subjects could be predicted from the biochemical index values. Breast milk vitamin C was also found to be a potentially useful index in the low to moderate range of intakes, a conclusion that confirms that of other published studies.[64]

Brubacher[135] has shown that children exhibit a steeper relationship between their vitamin C indices and their dietary intake than adults. Thus age effects, plus the effects of gender, smoking,[136] and of infection[137,138] and other metabolic stresses on the intake:marker relationship, imply that any 'calibration curve' will only be valid for one particular population group; therefore the latter (as well as the assay and diet assessment procedures) must be precisely specified. With this proviso, estimate of vitamin C intakes or of status indices can often provide a useful categorization of individuals into risk categories (either within a country such as the UK, or within a region such as Europe) that are strongly predictive of certain types of disease susceptibility. In a nutrition survey of the elderly in the UK[139] a comparison between one week of intake data and a single leucocyte ascorbate measurement yielded correlation coefficients $r = +0.49$ for men and $+0.36$ for women; both were significant at $P < 0.001$.

The measurement of vitamin C presents certain problems because of its instability. The most common substances used to stabilize ascorbate are trichloracetic acid and metaphosphoric acid and, in the writers' experience, plasma extracts stored at $-20°C$ are stable for at least 7–8 weeks, and for 3–6 months at $-70°C$. More recently it was shown that dithiothreitol (DTT) is an effective stabilizing reagent over a wide pH range[140] and, as ascorbate stored in the presence of this reagent is stable for more than 1 year at $-80°C$, this technique is appropriate for the preparation and use of quality control material.[141] If samples cannot be processed immediately, then whole blood stored up to 8 hr at $4°C$ in the dark before processing shows minimal changes in plasma ascorbate[142] but blood can also be collected directly into a solution of DTT without causing coagulation. Thus, any ascorbate oxidation is prevented during the process of blood collection, red cell removal or the subsequent storage of plasma.[141]

While stabilizing ascorbate, DTT converts any dehydroascorbate (DHA) to the reduced form, thus the presence or absence of DTT in plasma prior to the addition of the protein precipitant can be used to measure DHA by difference.[143] Until recently, the commonest methods for measuring ascorbate have been colorimetric[143] or fluorimetric.[144] Liquid chromatography in conjunction with electrochemical detection improves selectivity and sensitivity by at least two orders of magnitude in comparison with colorimetric methods[141] making the measurement of ascorbate in 50 μl plasma easily attained.

7.4 MARKERS OF DIETARY INTAKE: LIPIDS, PROTEIN, DIETARY FIBRE, AND ENERGY

7.4.1 Lipids

Lipids are broadly defined as substances that can be extracted from biological materials with fat solvents, consisting primarily of esters or potential esters of fatty acids. There are many different types of lipids that can be described in animals and plants. They may be divided into (i) simple lipids such as fatty acids, neutral fats (mono-, di-, and triacylglycerols) and waxes (esters of fatty acids); and (ii) complex lipids such as ceramides, phosphoglycerides plasmalogens, sphingolipids, glycolipids, sterols, and sterol esters.

The main lipids in human plasma are cholesterol, cholesteryl esters, triglycerides (triacylglycerol), phospholipids, and non-esterified fatty acids. Lipids are also structural components of cell membranes; here they are found in a molar ratio of 1:1 between phospholipid and free cholesterol. Short-chain fatty acids are water-soluble, but other lipids are insoluble in water, and to be carried in the bloodstream they need to be coated with a hydrophilic layer, made of phospholipids and proteins. The protein moiety is composed of several specific proteins (apolipoproteins). These complexes are termed lipoproteins and may be subdivided on the basis of their particle size and density (Table 7.11). The lipid composition of these lipoproteins differs substantially: chylomicrons are mainly triglyceride; VLDL is mainly triglyceride with phospholipid, cholesteryl esters and protein; the most common lipid in LDL is cholesteryl esters; and the major component in HDL is protein.

The vast majority of fat in the diet is triglyceride (TG), which is made up of glycerol and three fatty acids. In the process of digestion, fats are emulsified by bile salts in the small intestine and hydrolysed by intestinal and pancreatic lipases into di- (10 per cent) and monoglycerides (40 per cent) and fatty acids and glycerol (50 per cent). About 70 per cent are immediately resynthesized to TG, enter the lacteals as chylomicrons, pass into the lymphatic system and eventually enter the general circulation. Short-chain fatty acids are absorbed via the hepatic portal system. The rate of absorption is affected by transit time. When split from the glycerol moiety in the liver and other tissues, fatty acids enter the bloodstream as

Table 7.11 Properties and composition of human serum lipoproteins

	Chylomicrons	VLDL	LDL	HDL$_2$	HDL$_3$
Density (g/ml)	0.93–1.006	0.95–1.006	1.019–1.063	1.063–1.125	1.125–1.21
Molecular weight	$0.4–30 \times 10^6$	$5–10 \times 10^6$	$2–3 \times 10^6$	3.6×10^5	1.75×10^5
Diameter (Å)	750–6000	250–750	170–260	60–140	40–100
Components (% wt of total lipoprotein)					
Phospholipids	6–9	16–20	24–30	24–30	22–25
Free cholesterol	1–3	4–8	9–12	2–5	2–3
Cholesteryl ester	3–6	9–13	28–30	16–20	10–13
Triglycerides	82–86	50–60	7–11	4–5	4–5
Protein	1–2	8–11	20–22	41–50	55–58
Apoprotein (g/100g)					
A-I	33.0	0.9	0.8	58.7	64.9
A-II	Trace	0.2	0.4	10.0	25.6
A-IV	14.0	ND	ND	ND	Trace
B-48	5.0	Absent	Absent	Absent	Absent
B-100	Absent	25.0	95.0	3.0	Absent
C	32.0	55.0	2.0	13.0	5.0
D	ND	ND	Trace	2.0	4.0
E	10.0	15.0	3.2	3.0	1.0

Modified from Edelstein,[173] ND, no data.

components of lipoproteins, and are oxidized, incorporated into membranes and other structures, or stored in adipose tissues via albumin.

Because lipids are found in all cell membranes, it is theoretically possible to measure lipid levels in any of these membranes. However, lipids are commonly measured in serum, plasma, or components of blood (red cells and white cells such as neutrophils, eosinophils, basophils, lymphocytes, and monocytes and platelets). Individual fatty acids can be measured in the cholesteryl ester, phospholipid or TG fractions of plasma or serum, or as free fatty acids. The turnover of the different cells from which the fatty acids are derived may reflect different time frames of dietary intake: platelets may reflect days and red cells months, although there is some exchange between membranes and plasma lipids throughout the life of the cell. It is probably desirable to assess fatty acids in specific compartments of the plasma rather than using a total plasma estimate. However, van Houwelinger *et al.*[145] showed that the per cent linoleic acid in total plasma lipid was as good an indicator of dietary intake as the proportion in phospholipid and cholesteryl esters. The measurement of total serum fatty acid composition is far less time consuming and can be applied to a large number of samples.[146]

The composition of fats can also be measured in adipose tissue and these levels probably reflect usual intake over several years. Adipose tissue fatty acid composition is a good indicator of linoleic acid intake but not of n-3 fatty acids.

In many studies, lipids and lipoprotein fractions are studied as outcome variables in their own right. For example, there is a vast literature on the dietary influences on cholesterol and fatty acid levels. In this chapter we are only focusing on the measurement of lipids as markers of dietary intakes, although much of the evidence for the relationship between dietary intake and tissue levels comes from studies that have sought to modify tissue levels by dietary modification. It is worth noting that, within a population, variations in plasma cholesterol may reflect genetic variation more than differences in fat intake, which show a real but small influence.[147]

Depending on the purpose of the study, different lipid fractions will be appropriate. The principle of a marker is that it is just that, a marker of intake. As with any measurement, the objective will be to measure that marker with required validity. In experimental studies the objective is to use the marker to confirm the dietary intake and to check compliance during the study. For example, in studies looking at the effects of changing the type or amount of fat in the diet on blood pressure, dietary intake can be assessed and related to levels in various plasma and blood cells or sampled in tissues depending on the time frame of the study. The marker needs to be sensitive to change within the time frame of the study. There is little point measuring change in adipose tissue fatty acids in a study lasting only several weeks. It may also be important that the marker does not change too much. For example, free fatty acids in plasma will be affected by what has just been eaten, and may not reflect the levels of fat incorporated in cell membranes. Platelets will be appropriate for short term trials (e.g. for assessing eicosapentaenoic acid,[148] whereas red cells may not be (although red cells may be better for docosahexaenoic acid). Fat biopsies may provide the most appropriate measure for very long studies.

Assessment of lipids (fatty acids in particular) is most commonly undertaken in experimental studies where the investigator aims to modify dietary fat intake and assess the effects on either short or long term outcome measures predictive of heart disease, for example, blood pressure and serum lipids (total cholesterol or lipoproteins).

Non-functional tests of fatty acid and cholesterol status are most commonly used, such as concentrations in blood or cell membranes. At the lower limits of intake (i.e. to assess essential fatty acid status) it is also necessary to measure the derivatives of linoleic and alpha-linolenic acid, and plasma phospholipids are favoured because of the high rate of turnover.[149] While there are functional tests of lipid turnover and balance, these are not widely used in epidemiological studies and will not be discussed here. However, it is likely that, in metabolic ward studies, these functional tests will become more common.

Factors affecting lipid levels in general   Many factors influence blood lipid levels in general. Apart from the obvious dietary factors, intakes of carbohydrates (including non-starch polysaccharides), energy, alcohol and smoking may alter lipid levels. Obesity, exercise, stress, sex hormones, and pregnancy have all been reported to affect lipid levels, given an unaltered dietary intake. It has been well demonstrated that, in malnourished children, cholesterol, triglycerides, and free fatty acid levels are affected in different ways depending on the degree of fatty liver change. In children with kwashiorkor, cholesterol and TG levels may be lowered, whereas in marasmic children levels may be lowered, normal or raised. Other disease states also affect lipid levels (see Table 7.6) and lipid levels may be lowered for several months after an acute myocardial infarction.

This list is not exhaustive and the main point is to consider the effect that the health of the subject could have on their lipid levels and also on the way they may respond to change.

It is important to consider the other factors in the diet and lifestyle of the subjects that may affect the lipid levels measured in the body. And it is necessary to consider the possibility of the effects of *de novo* synthesis when assessing the relationship between intake and tissue levels.

Applicability of lipid measurements in epidemiological studies   To date there no markers of total fat intake. Recent work by Weinberg *et al.*[150] demonstrates that apoA-IV levels change rapidly with changes in dietary fat intake and can be used to monitor *changes* in fat intake in the short term (days or weeks). In the long term, apoA-IV stabilizes in relation to the new dietary fat intake level and loses its value as a measure of total fat intake until a new change is introduced.

With rapidly advancing technologies it is becoming more and more feasible to measure lipids in serum, cells, and tissues in both observational and experimental studies. However, it is important to ensure that all samples are collected following a strict protocol. In multicentre trials it is still advisable for all assays to be done blind in one centre. Ease of collection of samples, and effects on subject compliance, may also influence the choice of methods to be used. While there have been several recent observational studies that have collected adipose tissues samples, in a general population it is likely that a request for a fat biopsy will reduce the participation rate.

Measuring fatty acids in various cell compartments represents a very useful way to check on dietary compliance, provided that the tissue being used has been shown to be sensitively related to dietary levels and that the within-subject variability is within reasonable bounds (5 per cent). It is often assumed that a level of fat derived from a tissue is a more reliable marker of intake than a level derived from a dietary questionnaire or recording technique. This may not always be the case, although the assertion either way is quite difficult to assess.

From an epidemiological point of view, in terms of measuring lipids as markers of intake, it is important to consider how the fatty acids and cholesterol that are taken into the body are handled by the body, and to consider how the availability of substrates necessary to transport the lipids (proteins, etc.) may influence the levels measured in the blood or in tissues. It is beyond the scope of this section to discuss all these issues, but they should be borne in mind when the relationship between dietary intake and tissue levels are being assessed.

Fatty acids   The simplest division of fatty acids is on the basis of whether they are saturated or unsaturated. Unsaturated acids have one or more double bond in the carbon chain, whereas saturated fatty acids have no double bond. Most naturally occurring fatty acids are straight-chain saturated or unsaturated acids containing an even number of carbon atoms. However, certain fish oils have an odd number of carbon atoms. Animal cells cannot form linoleic acid or linolenic acid, and these, together with oleic acid, are precursors for the biosynthesis of individual families of polyunsaturated fatty acids.

Fatty acids can be further classified on the basis of the number and location of the double bonds in the chain. For example, linolenic acid is designated 18:3n–3, which means that it has 18 carbons in the chain, three double bonds and that the first double bond is three carbons from the terminal methyl carbon. This basic structure is given for the main fatty acids in the diet in Table 7.12. Broadly, there are four groups of fatty acids in terms of the position of the first double bond, n3 (for example, 18:3n–3), n6 (18:2n–6 linoleic acid), n7 (16:n–7 palmitoleic) and n9 (18:1n–9 oleic). Because of the double bonds in the molecule it is possible that unsaturated fatty acids can exist as either the cis or trans isomer. They have different properties, and changes from cis (the most common isomer) to trans in food processing may influence the metabolic activity and fate of the fatty acid.

The composition of the fatty acid profile is usually expressed as a relative percentage of the total (although a measure that reflected absolute levels of intake would obviously be preferred). Using relative levels, if one fatty acid increases, logically, others must go down, and it is therefore not possible to differentiate the absolute effect from the relative effect.

Up to 400 individual peaks representing different fatty acids on a chromatograph have been identified. However, in the human diet the major fatty acids are oleic (about 36 per cent), palmitic (22 per cent), linoleic (16 per cent), stearic (10 per cent) and linolenic (1 per cent) (Table 7.12).

Fatty acids may be extracted from a large variety of cells, membranes, or tissues in the body. The levels measured in different tissues may be used to indicate dietary intakes in the short term (hours, e.g. plasma triglycerides), medium term (several days, e.g. cholesteryl esters and phospholipids in red cells), slightly longer (weeks, e.g. red cells membranes or platelets) or longer term (months or years, e.g. adipose tissue), depending on the nature of the study proposed. There has been a rapid expansion of interest in the effects of fatty acid modification on blood lipid levels. A review of studies published over the last year shows that across the range of fatty acids in the diet (including longer chain fatty acids from fish oils) and in studies that aim to modify fatty acid intake by dietary manipulation, fatty acid levels measured in blood and other tissues reflect the dietary levels. However, as Table 7.12 shows, in subjects following typical unchanged diets, the relative percentage of fatty acids varies from tissue to tissue, because there is competition between the n-3 and n-6 fatty acids. It is therefore important to have baseline assessments in each tissue level against which to compare change, and not to assume that levels will be comparable across tissues.

Despite differences in laboratories and methods used, there seems to be reasonably good agreement between studies in the relative proportions of fatty acids measured within the same tissue or plasma lipid fraction. As mentioned elsewhere, there should always be a strict protocol for the collection of samples to minimize bias. The prime concern should be on internal validity in experimental studies that modify diet. It is recommended that blanks and an internal reference standard are always used to check on quality control.

Table 7.12 Composition of fatty acids in various tissues

Level of fatty acid (%)	Palmitic (16:0)*	Palmitoleic (16:1n-7)	Stearic (18:0)	Oleic (18:1n-9)	Linoleic (18:2n-6)	Linolenic (18:3n-6)	Arachidonic (20:4n-6)	Docosahexaenoic (22:6n-3)
Usual diet	22	3	10	36	16	1	1	Trace
Total Serum Lipids	17–21	3	6–8	18–22	30–34	0.3–0.5	6–9	1–2
Serum Lipid Fractions								
Cholesteryl esters	12	4	1	20	50	7	8	0.5
Phospholipids	27	1	11	9	23	0.2	9	1.2–2.2
Triglycerides	24	6	3	38	20	1.2	2	0.4
Diglycerides	29	3	6	36	13	0.7	0.7	NS
Phosphotidylcholine	27	1	18	9	31	0.2	10	3
Free fatty acids	25	5	10	39	1.6	0.7	1	0.3
Red Blood Cells								
Phospholipid	21–25	NS	14–23	13–20	6–9	NS	13–15	NS
Phosphatidylcholine	39	NS	11	15	24	NS	5	NS
Phosphatidylethanolamine	19	NS	8	17	7	NS	19	NS
Platelets	NS	NS	NS	NS	9	NS	21	NS
Neutrophils								
Adipose tissue	19	8	4	47	12–16	NS	NS	NS
Cheek cells	23	7	20	37	8	NS	NS	NS

Fatty acid

* Number of carbon atoms:number bonds; n, position of first double bond from terminal methyl carbon; NS, not stated. Compiled from references,[173–184].

Table 7.13. Summary of methods used to measure lipids*

Lipid	Methods
Fatty acids	Separate lipid fractions by i Thin layer chromatography (TLC) ii Tubular thin layer chromatography iii TLC, flame ionization detector iv Silica cartridges
	Once in separate fractions measure fatty acid methyl esters i Gas–Liquid chromatography (with column) (GC or GLC) ii High performance liquid chromatography (HPLC) iii Mass spectrometry (usually with GC) (MS/GC) analysed by electron impact ionization mode or soft ionization technique
Cholesterol	i Enzymatically (directly in plasma, H_2O_2 formed is measured spectrophotometrically) ii Colorimetrically (hydrolysis then extraction)
Triglycerides	i Enzymatically (NADH measured spectrophotometrically) ii Chemical (isolated by chromatography after extraction)
Lipoproteins	i Ultracentrifugation ii Precipitation iii Adsorption iv Gel filtration v Affinity chromatography vi Electrophoresis vii Immunochemical Subfractions sometimes calculated by subtraction using formula LDL = Total cholesterol (Serum TG/2.2 − HDLC) or LDL = Total cholesterol − HDLC + VLDLC VLDL = Plasma TG/5
Phospholipids	i Colorimetrically (after lipid extraction and oxidation)
Apolipoproteins	i Immunoassay (radio, electro, radial) ii Immunonephelometry iii Enzyme-linked and fluorescence immunoassays

* Method mentioned first is the most commonly cited at time of writing.

The methods used for measuring fatty acids (Table 7.13) are reasonably standardized, although developments in this area are rapid (see Christie[151] for details). The methods listed in Table 7.13 are those that are cited most commonly in the recently published literature. At present, most centres following extraction of samples use gas liquid chromatography (GC or

GLC) with a column. The HPLC system appears to work well for more simple fatty acid mixtures and can separate geometric isomers. It also has advantages in analysing polymeric, oxidized, less volatile, very polar, and heat labile components that cannot be separated by GLC. At the present time, for complex mixtures of fatty acids from animal organs and marine oils, the separation of the more polyunsaturated fatty acids is more difficult with HPLC than with GLC. Sample collection and storage needs careful attention (see Thompson[152]).

Cholesterol The cholesterol that is taken into the body, together with endogenous production (up to twice the dietary intake), is carried in various lipoproteins. It is possible, therefore, to measure a total cholesterol level ignoring the distribution within lipoproteins, or to measure lipoprotein specific levels. The relationship between dietary cholesterol and total and lipoprotein levels of cholesterol is complex and appears to vary across the range of cholesterol intake. Because the low density lipoproteins contain the most cholesterol, LDL levels correlate most closely with total cholesterol levels. As indicated in Table 7.13, various formulae have been proposed to describe the relationship between fat intake and serum cholesterol levels. It is clear that dietary cholesterol is not the only determinant of serum cholesterol, and consideration must be given as to the effects of the type of fat in the diet and intakes of other nutrients or factors, such as dietary fibre. There is a vast literature on the effects of diet on serum cholesterol and a discussion of these data is beyond the scope of this chapter.

A summary of the methods most commonly used to measure serum cholesterol and the lipoproteins is given in Table 7.13. Fasting blood samples are not required, but consideration needs to be given as to how the samples are processed and stored.[152] Blood samples should be collected and processed in the same way for all subjects in the study. Total cholesterol is stable once frozen for a reasonably long time, however HDL is more susceptible to degradation and for this assay, serum should be stored at −70°C.

7.4.2 Protein

24-hour urine nitrogen 24-hour urine nitrogen is the most well known biological marker, with individual results from published metabolic studies where dietary intake is kept constant over prolonged periods of time showing a fair correlation between daily nitrogen intake and daily urine nitrogen excretion. Its use depends on the assumption that subjects are in nitrogen balance, there being no accumulation due to growth or repair of lost muscle tissue, or loss due to starvation, slimming or injury. This was appreciated as early as 1924, when it was suggested that actual protein intake, as assessed from 24-hour urine excretion, was far lower than the recommended level.[153]

The apparent accuracy of 24-hour urine nitrogen as a biological marker has led to the suggestion that it be used to validate estimates of protein intake from various dietary survey methods.[154] In 1980, Isaksson summarized a number of studies carried out by his group that showed that estimates of protein intake obtained from 24-hour recalls of food intake were low when compared with the urine nitrogen, but those estimated from diet histories and food records were in good agreement with the urine values.[154] Van Staveren also found agreement between 24-hour urine nitrogen and diet history estimates of protein intake.[155] However, these comparisons were only intended on a group basis, because only one or two 24-hour urine collections were obtained from each individual. Other early comparisons between average urine nitrogen and dietary intake have been summarized elsewhere.[11,156] In general, there is poor agreement between individual estimates of usual protein intake, and the 24-hour urine nitrogen output.

The previously reported poor agreement between protein intake and urinary nitrogen may have been due to incomplete urine collections, too few days of collection, or extrarenal losses.

Urine collections may not have been complete

Earlier studies used creatinine to check on the completeness of urinary collection. Creatinine excretion is dependent upon both creatinine intake, primarily from meat in the diet, and creatinine production, which is proportional to fat-free mass. Where diets vary considerably within individuals, especially in their meat content, creatinine excretion is not a reliable marker of completeness. Where collections are known to be complete, within-subject variability of urinary creatinine has been shown to be of the order of 10 per cent, similar to that for urinary nitrogen.[18,157] Between-subject variation in creatinine excretion is about 23 per cent in a mixed population, again similar to total nitrogen.[18]

Para-amino benzoic acid (PABA) has recently been used to check on the completeness of urinary collections.[158] The method consists of three tablets of 80 mg PABA, taken with meals, which is quantitatively excreted within 24 hours so that single 24-hour collections containing less than 85 per cent of the PABA marker can be classified as unsatisfactory, either because the tablets have not been taken, or because one or more specimens were omitted from the collection. Tables 6.5 and 6.6 show that there is a systematic difference, particularly in urea and total nitrogen between collections that are deemed complete by the PABA method and ones that contain less than 85 per cent of the PABA marker. Omission of such a marker, will, therefore, cause underestimation of 24-hour urine nitrogen or urea output, and contributes to the poor agreement between estimates of usual intake, diet, and estimates of 24-hour urine output.

Too few days of recording intake or excretion to be able to characterize an individual

The estimation of the relationship between intake and output depends on the variability of the measures used. Daily variation is such that on any one day an individual is not likely to be in balance, therefore measurements of intake and output are required over several days to characterize the relationship within an individual with reasonable reliability. Table 7.14 shows that expected correlations between daily intake and output are in

Table 7.14. Comparison of 24-hour* urine N output and dietary N intake with different numbers of observations[158]

	Single day diet and urine	8 days urine 18 days diet	28 days urine 28 days diet
Correlation coefficient	0.47	0.95	0.99
Urine N as percentage of diet N average	81	81	81
Coefficient of variation	24	5	2

* All 24-hour urine collections verified for completeness.

the region of 0.5 when a single day's data are used, with a low estimate of precision giving a coefficient of variation of 24 per cent. When eight days of urine collections and 18 days of dietary observations are available, the correlation improves to 0.95, and the coefficient of variation falls to 5 per cent. Several 24-hour collections, validated for their completeness, are therefore required to make accurate comparisons with dietary intake data, the exact number depending on the reliability required. With an average coefficient of variation of 13 per cent in urine nitrogen excretion, eight days of collection will estimate nitrogen output to within 5 per cent.

Extrarenal losses

These losses also vary from individual to individual. In a carefully controlled balance study, where faecal, urinary, skin, and blood losses were measured, it was shown that urine nitrogen underestimated intake at higher levels of protein intake and overestimated at lower levels if a constant factor for faecal and skin losses was used.[158]

Urea, other markers of protein intake Urine urea is a constant proportion (85 per cent) of total nitrogen excretion when individuals are consuming normal mixed western diets and are in overall nitrogen balance.[18] It can therefore replace the estimation of total nitrogen in these circumstances and is considerably easier to analyse. As a proportion of total nitrogen intake, 24-hour urine urea nitrogen is 70 ± 7 per cent and urea plus creatinine nitrogen is 73 ± 7 per cent of the habitual diet when eight 24-hour collections are obtained.[158]

Due to the difficulty of obtaining complete 24-hour collections, and the lack of reliability using one collection, replacement with partial collections has been investigated. Yamori et al.[25] obtained 24-hour collections split into four time periods from 16 volunteer medical students and the variation of urea and creatinine in relation to the full 24-hour period is shown in Table 7.15 together with the correlation coefficients between separate samples and the complete 24-hour urine collections. Values for overnight

Table 7.15. Partial collections in relation to 24-hour urine collections.

Time of urine Collection	Daily variation in 24-hour*		Correlation with 24-hour	
	Urea N	Urea/Creatinine Ratio[25]	Urea N	Urea/Creatinine Ratio[24,25]
Morning	101 (34)	103 (33)	0.63	0.72
Afternoon	122 (36)	111 (39)	0.72	0.50
Evening	114 (44)	106 (44)	0.78	0.81
Overnight	74 (27)	86 (29)	0.76	0.81
24-hour	100 (26)	100 (23)		

* Mean (SD) of all samples, converted so that the mean values in the 24-hour samples equals 100[25].

collections in relation to full 24-hour collections obtained from 21 men and women aged 19 to 65 years from the study of Ogawa[24] are also shown.

From this, it would seem that overnight collections contain both less urea and a lower urea to creatinine ratio than other collections, whereas afternoon values are higher. Correlation coefficients are of the same order for both evening and overnight collections. It is possible that the proportion of constituents in partial collections varies, as indicated by the relatively large standard deviations in Table 7.15, probably depending on the timing of diet and main meal consumption. This is probably also true of different populations, so that it is not possible to make general statements of the utility of partial collections, other than that they are less accurate than full 24-hour collections for estimating protein intake. The possibility of increasing validity by repeat partial collections requires investigation in subsamples of the population of interest (Greene and Bingham, unpublished).

As a marker of sulphur amino acid intake, urinary sulphate was also measured by Yamori and colleagues.[25] Correlation coefficients ranged from 0.28 for morning urines versus 24-hour, to 0.72 for evening urine, with no improvement from adjustment to creatinine. Correlation co-efficients were 0.84 for urinary sulphate to creatinine ratio in overnight versus 24-hour urines in the study of Ogawa.[24] Ogawa also measured 3-methyl histidine as a marker of muscle protein and found a correlation coefficient of 0.76 between overnight and 24-hour collections. Although 3-methyl histidine is specific for muscle protein,[159] it is comparatively difficult to analyse and is not specific for diet because it is also released from lean body tissue and endogenous variations occur from factors such as body size and the amount of exercise taken. Creatinine and 3-methyl histidine have been used in experimental studies as checks on dietary compliance. In this situation the objective is not to relate intake precisely to output, as in a metabolic ward study, but as a rather crude check on whether the subjects have followed dietary instructions. In this situation both of these markers have been shown to be useful in, for example, checking on compliance in subjects changing from an omnivore diet to a vegetarian diet.[160]

7.4.3 Dietary fibre (non-starch polysaccharides)

Faecal weight is known to increase in response to an increase in dietary fibre consumption, there being a linear response of an average 5 g increase in faecal weight for every 1 g of non-starch polysaccharides (NSP) consumed.[161] However, the measurement of faecal weight is fraught with problems and is unacceptable to the general public, particularly when an attempt is made to gain valid estimates. Valid estimates require obser-vations of at least 5-day collections on individuals because there is great day to day variation in stool size and frequency. For accurate work, the collections also need to be validated for completeness using inert markers, such as radio-opaque plastic pellets taken by mouth.[162] Even when this is done, the relationship on an individual basis is poor, due largely to unexplained individual biological variation in both transit time and stool weight, even when constant diets are consumed.[162] On a group basis, collection of a single stool from each individual may either over or under estimate 24-hour faecal weight, depending on the frequency of daily bowel habit.

Other suggested markers for NSP consumption include faecal neutral detergent fibre (NDF),[163] but quantitative estimates again require stool collections. Also, the estimate is unlikely to represent total dietary NSP because the majority of NSP is fermented in the large bowel, and little NDF remains in faeces.[162] Indices of fermentation, such as breath methane and hydrogen production, may be a feasible approach and are presently being investigated (McKeown and Bingham, unpublished).

7.4.4 Total energy

There are no quantitative markers for carbohydrate and fat consumption and an estimate of total energy intake cannot, therefore, be obtained by usual means. Isaksson has suggested that an estimation can be made for groups of subjects from 24-hour urine nitrogen, because the contribution of protein to total energy intake is constant for groups of subjects.[154] The doubly-labelled water technique measures energy expenditure and interferes minimally with free-living subjects' routine.[164] In the absence of weight gain or loss, the fact that intake equals expenditure allows estimates of dietary intake to be validated (see section 8.4.1). However, the technique is too expensive for use in most types of epidemiological study (about £350 per subject for the isotope alone).

Metabolic rate calculated from body weight (see Table 6.8, section 6.5.1) can be used as an index of total energy intake of groups of individuals, assuming that the ratio of total energy expenditure (and therefore intake when body weight is stable) to basal metabolic rate is 1.6 on average in sedentary individuals.[165] The ratio for individuals is far less certain (see section 6.5.1).

7.5 SUMMARY

Validation of biochemical markers as predictors of dietary intake of nutrients (as distinct from the development of biochemical indices for the estimation of status) is currently at an early and rather unsatisfactory stage of evolution. There are many interlocking factors to be taken into account and different conclusions for different nutrients.

For the minerals, there exist a small group of alkali metals and halide ions whose short term intakes appear to be quite well predicted by the measurements of urinary excretion levels, provided that the completeness of urinary collections can be properly validated. For another group of minerals (alkaline earth metals, phosphate, probably sulphur and selenium) urinary excretion rates can provide a fairly good general estimate of intakes when other dietary factors are reasonably constant, but a number of interactions may affect the relationship, especially in free-living people. For the remaining minerals, especially the transition elements, urinary excretion is a minor route that does not reflect dietary intakes, and the best that can be hoped for is a very broad classification of long term population group intakes, obtainable from a variety of markers in the bloodstream. For most purposes, their predictive power would be considered inadequate.

There are few instances of very close agreement between intake and biochemical markers for the vitamins, although broad categories of intake for population groups and sometimes for individuals can be achieved in certain cases. However, each vitamin must be considered separately, as few generalizations can be made about this entire category, or even about the subgroupings, such as fat-soluble vitamins, B-vitamins, etc.

For those vitamins for which urinary excretion is a major route of excess-disposal, e.g. vitamin C and certain B-group vitamins, the level of intake in the short term can be assessed moderately well in the moderate to high intake range by the level of urinary excretion, even though absorption is not quantitative. At the other end of the time and intake scale, red cell enzyme activation coefficients generally reflect long term intakes in the low to medium, but not the high, intake range. The same tends to be true of red or white cell concentrations of vitamins, in those cases where measurement is both feasible and sensitive to intake. Plasma nutrient levels usually have a complex relationship with intakes, comprising both a short term turnover component reflecting recent dietary intake and one or more long term components, reflecting body stores and the flux between them. They can, in some instances, provide a useful reflection of intake over a limited range (e.g. plasma vitamin C), but in other cases they are so heavily influenced by controlled production of binding proteins (e.g. for plasma retinol), that the intake:marker relationship is limited to a narrow band within the deficient range. Where vitamins arise from a variety of dietary or non-dietary sources (e.g. niacin, vitamins A and D), the amount present in all the internal compartments will reflect the total amount that is made available from all sources, not just the preformed vitamin in the food. Variations in bioavailability are especially important, as much for the vitamins as for trace elements, and this may be affected by speciation (e.g. folate polyglutamates that are incompletely available), by specific interactions (e.g. vitamin B_{12} with intrinsic factor), by conversion during absorption (e.g. carotenoids to vitamin A) and many other processes. Thus, the amounts entering the body are seldom a simple reflection of the amount present in the diet. In addition, some of the vitamin content of the food may be destroyed by the gut flora or by other (chemical) processes in the gut. In contrast, vitamin K and certain B-vitamins may be produced and made available in useful amounts by the gut flora. Disease processes, drugs and xenobiotics, and physiological variations between individuals, will inevitably alter the 'normal' diet–marker relationships. It is probably for these reasons that biochemical indices have only infrequently been used as markers of dietary intake. However, if intake cannot be estimated directly, or if bioavailability rather than total nutrient intake is required, then biochemical markers may give very valuable information.

For lipids, markers of usual intake are limited to the analysis of the proportions of fatty acids in serum or plasma, in cell membranes, and in adipose tissue. While the blood compartments offer opportunities to examine these proportions over several time periods, ranging from hours to months, and adipose tissue may reflect diet over even long periods, there are no biochemical markers available at the moment that allow for an assessment of absolute intakes. Such markers would need to be widely distributed in known concentrations in all forms of dietary fat and to be excreted or stored quantitatively without major metabolic change. Alternatively, a functional metabolic marker that is associated with the quantity of fat either absorbed or metabolized is required. Additionally, there are numerous factors (e.g. dietary fibre intake, alcohol consumption, smoking, etc.) that are likely to influence the way in which fat is absorbed or metabolized, and these will be reflected in the measures that are used to distinguish one subject from another and should, in theory, be taken into account when attempting to rank or categorize individuals. At the moment, all that is available are markers that indicate the proportions, but not the absolute intakes, of dietary fats. And for the longer term markers, such as per cent linoleic acid in adipose tissue, little is known about how metabolic processes that differ between individuals influence the dietary time period reflected by the measurement.

For protein, the relationship between intake and urinary excretion of the marker is closer than for virtually all other nutrients (except perhaps sodium), assuming that the subject is in balance. The principal drawback from the epidemiological point of view is the necessity to collect multiple 24-hour urine samples, the completeness of which has to be verified. The use of shorter (e.g. overnight or casual) repeat specimens requires further investigation. Pursuance of these objectives opens the possibility of having a marker for the completeness of diet recording or reporting generally, as the level of agreement between validated urinary excretion of nitrogen and estimates of intake based on food composition tables (corroborated by duplicate diet analysis) is good. This approach to assessing the completeness of records underlies some of the recent work comparing energy intake and expenditure using doubly-labelled water, but the high costs of this technique make it unsuitable for widespread use in nutritional epidemiological studies. A low-cost technique based on nitrogen excretion from short term urine specimens offers an attractive alternative. There is an urgent need to develop low-cost biochemical markers for the assessment of dietary fibre and energy intake for use in epidemiological studies.

REFERENCES

1. Whitehead, T. P. (1977). In *Quality control in clinical chemistry*. Wiley, New York.
2. Glatzle, D., Weber, F., and Wiss, O. (1968). Enzymatic test for the detection of riboflavin deficiency. NADPH-dependent glutathione reductase of red blood cells and its activation by FAD *in vitro*. *Experimentia*, **24**: 1122.

3. Beutler, E. (1969). Effect of flavin compounds on glutathione reductase activity; *in vivo* and *in vitro* studies. *J. Clin. Invest.*, **48**: 1957–66.

4. Garry, P. J. and Owen, G. M. (1976). An automated flavin adenine dinucleotide-dependent glutathione reductase assay for assessing riboflavin nutriture. *Am. J. Clin. Nutr.*, **29**: 663–74.

5. Thurnham, D. I. and Rathakette, P. (1982). Incubation of NAD(P)H$_2$: glutathione oxidoreductase (EC.1.6.4.2) with flavin adenine dinucleotide for maximal stimulation in the measurement of riboflavin status. *Br. J. Nutr.*, **48**: 459–66

6. Thurnham, D. I. and Flora, P. S. (1988). Stability of individual carotenoids retinol and tocopherol in stored plasma. *Clin. Chem.*, **34**: 1947.

7. Matthews-Roth, M. M. and Stampher, M. T. (1984). Some factors affecting the determination of carotenoids in serum. *Clin. Chem.*, **30**: 459–61.

8. Craft, N. E., Brown, E. D., and Smith, J. C. (1988). Effects of storage and handling conditions on concentrations of individual carotenoids, retinol, and tocopherol in plasma. *Clin. Chem.*, **34**: 44–8.

9. Bro-Rasmussen, F. (1958). The riboflavin requirement of animals and man and associated metabolic relations (parts 1 and 2). *Nutr. Abstr. Rev.*, **28**: 1–23, 369–86.

10. Horwitt, M. K. (1986). Interpretations of requirements for thiamin, riboflavin, niacin, tryptophan and vitamin E plus comments on balance studies and vitamin B$_6$. *Am. J. Clin. Nutr.*, **44**: 973–85.

11. Bingham, S. A. (1987). The dietary assessment of individuals; methods, accuracy, new techniques and recommendations. *Nutr. Abstr. Rev.*, **57**: 705–42.

12. Rutishauser, I. H. E., Bates, C. J., Paul, A. A., and Black, A. E. (1979). Long-term vitamin status and dietary intake of healthy elderly subjects: 1. Riboflavin. *Br. J. Nutr.*, **42**: 33–42.

13. Bates, C. J., Rutihauser, I. H. E., Black, A. E., Paul, A. A., Mandal, A. R., and Patnaik, B. K. (1977). Long-term vitamin status and dietary intake of healthy elderly subjects. 2. Vitamin C. *Br. J. Nutr.*, **42**: 43–56.

14. Thurnham, D. I., (1989). Vitamin A deficiency and its role in infection. *Trans. Roy. Soc. Trop. Med. Hyg.*, **83**: 721–3.

15. Schachter, J., Harper, P. H., Radin, M. E., Caggiula, A. W., McDonald, R. H., and Diven, W. F. (1980). Comparison of sodium and potassium intake with excretion. *Hypertension*, **2**: 695–9.

16. Holbrook, J. T., Patterson, K. Y., Bodner, J. E., Douglas, L. W., Veillon, C., Kelsay, J. L., Mertz, W., and Smith, C. (1984). Sodium and potassium intake in adults consuming self selected diets. *Am. J. Clin. Nutr.*, **40**: 786–93.

17. Barlow, R. J., Connell, M. A., and Milne, F. J. (1986). A study of 48 h faecal and urinary electrolyte excretion in normotensive black and white South African males. *J. Hypertension*, **4**: 197–200.

18. Bingham, S., Williams, R., Cole, T. J., Price, C. P., and Cummings, J. H. (1988). Reference values for analytes of 24 h urine collections known to be complete. *Ann. Clin. Chem.*, **25**: 610–19.

19. Liu, K. and Stamler, J. (1984). Assessment of sodium intake in epidemiological studies on blood pressure. *Ann. Clin. Res.*, **16**: 49–54.

20. Bingham, S., Goldberg, G., Coward, W. A., Prentice, A. M., and Cummings, J. H. (1989). The effect of improved physical fitness on basal metabolic rate *Br. J. Nutr.*, **61**: 155–173.

21. Gregory, J., Foster, K., Tyler, H., and Wiseman, M. (1990). *The Dietary and Nutritional Survey of British Adults.* HMSO, London.
22. Elliot, P., Forrest, R. D., Jackson, C. A., and Yudkin, J. S. (1988). Sodium and blood pressure. *J. Hum. Hypertension,* **2:** 89–95.
23. Forster, J. I. Jeffery, R. W., Van Natta, M., and Pirie, P. (1980). Hypertension trial. *Am. J. Clin. Nutr.,* **51:** 253–7.
24. Ogawa, M. (1986). Feasibility of overnight urine for assessing dietary intakes of sodium, potassium, protein in field studies. *Jap. Circ. J.,* **50:** 595–600.
25. Yamori, Y., Kihara, M., Fujikawa, J., Soh, Y., Nara, Y., Ohtaka, M., Horie, R., Tsunematsu, T., Note, S., and Fukase, M. (1982). Dietary risk factors for stroke and hypertension in Japan. *Jap. Circ. J.,* **46:** 933–8.
26. Nordin, B. E. C. and Marshall, D. H. (1988). Dietary requirements for calcium. In B. E. C. Nordin, (ed). *Calcium in Human Biology.* pp. 447–471. ISLI Human Nutrition Reviews, Springer-Verlag, London.
27. Lowenstein, F. W. and Stanton, M. F. (1986). Serum magnesium levels in the United States 1971–1974. *J. Am. Coll. Nutr.,* **5:** 399–414.
28. Quamme, G. A. (1980). Renal handling of magnesium: drug and hormone interactions. *Magnesium,* **5:** 248–72.
29. Life Sciences Research Office. (1981). Effects of dietary factors on skeletal integrity in adults: calcium, phosphorus, vitamin D and protein. *Fed. Am. Soc. Exp. Biol.,* Bethesda, MD.
30. FAO (1988). *Requirements of vitamin A, iron, folate and vitamin B_{12}.* Report of a joint FAO/WHO expert consultation. FAO Food and Nutrition Series, No. 23.
31. King, J. C. and Turnlund, J. R. (1989). Human zinc requirements. In C. F. Mills, (ed.). *Zinc in Human Biology,* pp. 335–50. ILSI Human Nutrition Reviews, Springer-Verlag, London.
32. Sandstrom, B. (1989). Dietary pattern and zinc supply. In C. F. Mills, (ed.). *Zinc in Human Biology,* pp. 351–63. ISLI Human Nutrition Reviews, Springer-Verlag, London.
33. Gallagher, S. K., Johnson, L. K., and Milne, D. B. (1989). Short-term and long-term variability of indices related to nutritional status I: Ca, Cu, Fe, Mg and Zn. *Clin. Chem.,* **35:** 369–73.
34. Varry, R., Castillo-Duran, R., Fisberg, M., Fernandez, N., and Valenzuela, A. (1985). Red cell superoxide dismutase activity on an index of human copper nutrition. *J. Nutr.,* **115:** 1650–5.
35. Delves, H. T. (1976). The microdetermination of copper in plasma protein fractions. *Clin. Chim. Acta.,* **71:** 495–500.
36. Solomons, N. W. (1985). Biochemical, metabolic, and clinical role of copper in human nutrition. *J. Am. Coll. Nutr.,* **4:** 83–105.
37. Robinson, Jr, Robinson, M. E., Levander, O. A., and Thomson, C. D. (1985). Urinary excretion of selenium by New Zealand and North American human subjects on differing intakes. *Am. J. Clin. Nutr.,* **41:** 1023–31.
38. WHO. (1967). *Technical Report Series No. 362. Requirements of Vitamin A, Thiamine, Riboflavin and Niacin.* Report of a Joint FAO/WHO Expert Group. Geneva.
39. Flores, H., Campos, F., Aranjo, C. R. C., and Underwood, B. A. (1984). Assessment of marginal vitamin A deficiency in Brazilian children using the relative dose response procedure. *Am. J. Clin. Nutr.,* **40:** 1281–9.

40. Olson, J. A. (1984). Serum levels of vitamin A and carotenoids as reflectors of nutritional status. *J. Nat. Cancer. Inst.*, **73**: 1439–44.
41. World Health Organization. (1976). In *Vitamin A deficiency and xerophthalmia*, WHO Technical Series No. 590. Geneva.
42. Thurnham, D. I., Singkamani, R., Kaewichit, R., and Wongworapat, K. (1990). Influence of malaria infection on peroxyl-radical trapping capacity in plasma from rural and urban Thai adults. *Br. J. Nutr.*, **64**: 257–71.
43. Thurnham, D. I., Kwiatkowsky, D., Hill, A. V. S., and Greenwood, B. M. (1990). The influence of malaria on plasma retinol. *Int. J. Vit. Nutr. Res.*, 60, 184.
44. Reddy, V., Bhaskaram, P., Raghuramulu, N., Milton, R. C., Rao, V., Madhusudan, J., and Radha Krishna, K. V. (1986). Relationship between measles, malnutrition and blindness: a prospective study in Indian children. *Am. J. Clin. Nutr.*, **44**: 924–30.
45. Sauberlich, H. E., Dowdy, R. P., and Skala, J. H. (eds). (1974). *Laboratory tests for the assessment of nutritional status.* CRC Press, Florida.
46. Bieri, J. G., Brown, E. D., and Smith, J. C. Jr. (1985). Determination of individual carotenoids in human plasma. *J. Liq. Chromatogr.*, **8**: 473–84.
47. Milne, D. B. and Botnen, J. (1986). Retinol, α-tocoperol, lycopene, and α-and β-carotene simultaneously determined by isocratic liquid chromatography. *Clin. Chem.*, **32**: 874–6.
48. Thurnham, D. I., Smith, E. and Flora, P. S. (1988). Concurrent liquid-chromatographic assay for retinol, α-tocopherol, β-carotene, α-carotene, lycopene and β-cryptoxanthin in plasma, with tocopherol acetate as internal standard. *Clin. Chem.* **34**: 377–81.
49. Thurnham, D. I., and Flora, P. S. (1988). Stability of individual carotenoids retinol and tocopherol in stored plasma. *Clin. Chem.* **34**: 1947.
50. Tanum Ihardjo, S. A., Furr, H. C., Erdman, J. W. Jr, and Olson, J. A. (1990). Use of the modified relative dose response (MRDR) in rats and its application to humans for the measurement of vitamin A status. *Eur. J. Clin. Nutr.* **44**: 219–24.
51. Bauernfeind, J. C. (1984). The safe use of vitamin A. A report of the International Vitamin A Consultative Group (IVACG). The Nutrition Foundation, New York.
52. Wallingford, J. C. and Underwood, B. A. (1986). Vitamin A deficiency in pregnancy, lactation and the nursing child. In Bauernfeind J. C. (ed.) *Vitamin A Deficiency and its Control*, pp. 101–52. Academic Press, London.
53. Dimitrov, N. V., Meyer, C., Ullrey, D. E., Chenoweth, W., Michelakis, A., Malone, W., and Boone, C. (1988). Bioavailability of β-carotene in humans. *Am. J. Clin. Nutr.*, **48**: 298–304.
54. Romieu, I., Stampfer, M. J., Stryker, W. S., Herandez, M., Kaplan, L., Sober, A., Rosner, B., and Willett, W. C. (1990). Food predictors of plasma β-carotene and α-tocopherol: validation of a food frequency questionnaire. *Am. J. Epid.* **131**: 864–76.
55. Tangney, C. C., Shebelle, R. B., Raynor, W., Gale, M., and Betz, E. P. (1987). Intra- and inter-individual variation in measurements of β-carotene, retinol and tocopherols in diet and plasma. *Am. J. Clin. Nutr.*, **45**: 764–9.
56. Thurnham, D. I. (1989). Lutein, cholesterol and risk of cancer. *Lancet*, ii: 441–2.

57. Heinonen, M. I., Ollilainen, V., Linkola, E. K., Varo, P. T., and Koivistoinen, P. E. (1989). Carotenoids in Finnish foods: vegetables, fruits and berries. *J. Agric. Food Chem.*, **37**; 655–9.
58. Thurnham, D. I. and Flora, P. S. (1988). Do higher vitamin A requirements in men explain the difference between the sexes in plasma provitamin A carotenoids and retinol. *Proc. Nutr. Soc.*, **47**: 181A.
59. Ito, Y., Ochiai, J., Sasaki, R., Otani, M., and Aoki, K. (1990). *Serum concentrations of carotenoids in healthy persons aged 7–86 years*. Ninth International Symposium on Carotenoids, Abstract 151.
60. Haddad, J. G. and Chyu, K. J. (1971). Competitive protein binding radioassay for 25-hydroxycholecalciferol. *J. Clin. Endocinol.* **33**: 992–5.
61. Lawson, D. E. M., Paul, A. A., Black, A. E., Cole, T. J., Mandal, A. R., and Davie, M. (1979). Relative contributions of diet and sunlight to vitamin D state in the elderly. *Br. Med. J.*, **3**: 303–5.
62. Thurnham, D. I. (1985). Interpretation of biochemical measurements if vitamin status in the elderly. In J. Kemm (ed.). *Vitamin deficiency in the elderly*. pp. 46–67. Pergamon Press, London.
63. Clements, M. R. (1989). The problem of rickets in UK Asians. *J. Hum. Nutr. Dietet.*, **2**; 105–16.
64. Bates, C. J. and Prentice, A. (1988). Vitamins, minerals and essential trace elements. In P. N. Bennett (ed.). *Drugs and human lactation*. pp. 433–93. Elsevier, London.
65. Bauernfeind, J. (1980). Tocopherols in foods. In L. J. Machlin (ed.). *Vitamin E, a comprehensive treatise*. pp. 99–169. Dekker, New York.
66. Desai, I. D. (1980). Assay methods. In L. J. Machlin (ed.). *Vitamin E, a comprehensive treatise*, pp. 67–98. Dekker, New York.
67. Lehmann, J., Rao, D. D., Canary, J. J., and Judd, J. T. (1988). Vitamin E and relationships among tocopherols in human plasma, platelets, lymphocytes and red blood cells. *Am. J. Clin. Nutr.*, **47**: 470–4.
68. Thurnham, D. I., Davies, J. A., Crump, B. J., and Situnayake, R. D. and Davis, M. (1986). The use of different lipids to express serum tocopherol: lipid ratios for the measurement of vitamin E status. *Ann. Clin. Biochem.*, **23**: 514–20.
69. Diplock, A. T. (1985). Vitamin E. In A. T. Diplock (ed.). *Fat-soluble vitamins, their biochemistry and applications*. pp. 154–224. Technomic Publications Co, Lancaster, PA.
70. Horwitt, M. K., Harvey, C. C., Dahm, C. H., and Searcy, M. T. (1972). Relationships between tocopherol and serum lipid levels for the determination of nutritional adequacy. *Ann. N. Y. Acad. Sci.*, **203**: 223–36.
71. Thurnham, D. I. (1990). Antioxidants and pro-oxidants in malnourished populations. *Proc. Nutr. Soc.*, **49**: 247–59.
72. Fukuzawa, K., Tokumura, A., Ouchi, S., and Tsuka, H. (1982). Antioxidant activities of tocopherols in Fe^{2+}-ascorbate-induced lipid peroxidation in pecithin liposomes. *Lipids*, **17**: 511–13.
73. Gey, K. F. (1986). On the antioxidant hypothesis with regard to arteriosclerosis. *Bibliotheca. Nutritio. et Dieta (Basle)*, **37**: 53–91.
74. Per Haga, M. D., Ek, J., and Kran, S. (1982). Plasma tocopherol levels and vitamin E/β-lipoprotein relationships during pregnancy and cord blood. *Am. J. Clin. Nutr.*, **36**: 1200–4.

75. Horwitt, M. K., Harvey, C. C., Duncan, G. D., and Wilson, W. C. (1956). Effects of limited tocopherol intake in man with relationship to erythrocyte haemolysis and lipid oxidation. *Am. J. Clin. Nutr.*, **4**: 408–19

76. Cynamon, H. A. and Isenberg, J. N. (1987). Characterization of vitamin E status in cholestatic children by conventional laboratory standards and a new functional assay. *J. Ped. Gastroenterol. Nutr.*, **6**: 46–50.

77. Vatassery, G. T., Krezowski, A. M., and Eckfeldt, J. H. (1983). Vitamin E concentrations in human blood plasma and platelets. *Am. J. Clin. Nutr.*, **37**: 1020–4.

78. Shearer, M. J., McBurney, A., and Barkham, P. (1974). Studies on the absorption and metabolism of phylloquinone (vitamin K) in man. *Vit. Horm.*, **32**: 513–42.

79. Mummah-Schendel, L. L. and Suttie, J. W. (1986). Serum phylloquinone concentrations in a normal adult population. *Am. J. Clin. Nutr.*, **44**: 686–9.

80. Suttie, J. W., Mummah-Schendel, L. L., Shah, D. V., Lyle, B. J., and Greger, J. L. (1988). Vitamin K deficiency from dietary vitamin K restriction in humans. *Am. J. Clin. Nutr.*, **47**: 475–80.

81. Quick, A. J. (1970). *Bleeding Problems in Clinical medicine.* WB Saunders & Co., Philadelphia.

82. Blanchard, R. A., Furie, B. C., Kruger, S. F., Waneck, G., Jorgensen, M. J., and Furie, B. (1983). Immunoassay of human prothrombin species which correlate with functional coagulation activities. *J. Lab. Clin. Med.* **101**: 242–55.

83. Olson, J. A. (1987). Recommended dietary intakes (RDI) of vitamin K in humans. *Am. J. Clin. Nutr.*, **45**: 687–92.

84. Krasinski, S. D., Russell, R. M., Furie, B. C., Kruger, S. F., Jacques, P. F., and Furie, B. (1985). The prevalence of vitamin K deficiency in chronic gastrointestinal disorder. *Am. J. Clin. Nutr.*, **41**: 639–43.

85. Hazell, K. and Baloch, K. H. (1970). Vitamin K deficiency in the elderly. *Gerontol. Clin. (Basel)*, **12**: 10–17.

86. Golding, J., Paterson, M., and Kinlen, L. J. (1990). Factors associated with childhood cancer in a national cohort study. *Br. J. Cancer*, **62**: 304–8.

87. von Kries, R., Shearer, M., McCarthy, P. T., Haug, M., Harzer, G. and Gobel, U. (1987). Vitamin K_1 content of maternal milk: influence of the stage of lactation, lipid composition and vitamin K supplementation given to the mother. *Paed. Res.*, **22**: 513–17.

88. Gibson, R. S. (1990). *Principles of nutritional assessment.* Oxford University Press.

89. Reinhold, J. G., Nicholson, J. T. L., and Elsom, K. O. (1944). The utilization of thiamin in the human subject: the effect of high intake of carbohydrate or of fat. *J. Nutr.*, **28**: 51–62.

90. Consolazio, C. F., Johnson, H. L., Krzywicki, H. J., Daws, T. A., and Barnhart, R. A. (1971). Thiamin, riboflavin, and pyridoxine excretion during acute starvation and calorie restriction. *Am. J. Clin. Nutr.*, **24**: 1060–7.

91. Ziporin, Z. Z., Nunes, W. T., Powell, R. C., Waring, P. P., and Sauberlich, H. E. (1965). Excretion of thiamine and its metabolites in the urine of young adult males receiving restricted intakes of the vitamin. *J. Nutr.*, **85**: 287–96.

92. Iber, F. L., Blass, J. P., Brin, M., and Leevy, C. M. (1982). Thiamin in the elderly—relation to alcoholism and to neurological degenerative disease. *Am. J. Clin. Nutr.*, **36**: 1067–82.

93. Vir, S. C. and Love, A. H. G. (1979). Nutritional status of institutionalised and non-institutionalised aged in Belfast, Northern Ireland. *Am. J. Clin. Nutr.*, **32:** 1934–47.
94. Vir, S. C., Love, A. H. G., and Thomson, W. (1980). Thiamin status during pregnancy. *Int. J. Vit. Nutr. Res.*, **50:** 131–40.
95. Puxty, J. A. H., Haskew, A E., Ratcliffe, J. G., and McMurrey, J. (1985). Changes in erythrocyte transketolase activity and the thiamine pyrophosphate effect during storage of blood. *Ann. Clin. Biochem.* **22:** 423–7.
96. Anderson, S. H. and Nicol, A. D. (1986). A fluorimetric method for measurement of erythrocyte transketolase activity. *Ann. Clin. Biochem.*, **23:** 180–9.
97. Baines, M. (1985). Improved high performance chromatographic determination of thiamin diphosphate in erythrocytes. *Clin. Chim. Acta.*, **153:** 43–8.
98. Thurnham, D. I., Migasena, P., and Pavapootanon, N. (1970). The ultramicro glutathione reductase assay for riboflavin status: its use in field studies in Thailand. *Mikrochim. Acta.*, **5:** 988–93.
99. Thurnham, D. I., Migasena, P., Vudhivai, N., and Supawan, V. (1972). The effect of riboflavin supplementation on the urinary hydroxyproline index in a resettlement village in rural Thailand. *Br. J. Nutr.*, **28:** 99–104.
100. Bates, C. J., Prentice, A. M., Paul, A. A., Sutcliffe, B. A., Watkinson, M., and Whitehead, R. G. (1981). Riboflavin status in Gambian pregnant and lactating women and its implications for recommended daily allowances. *Am. J. Clin. Nutr.*, **34:** 928–35.
101. Bamji, M. S., Bhaskaram, P., and Jacob, C. M. (1987). Urinary riboflavin excretion and erythrocyte glutathione reductase activity in preschool children suffering from upper respiratory tract infections and measles. *Ann. Nutr. Metab.*, **31:** 191–6.
102. Horwitt, M. K., Hills, O. W., Harvey, C. C., Liebert, E., and Steinberg, D. L. (1949). Effects of dietary depletion of riboflavin. *J. Nutr.*, **39:** 357–73.
103. Horwitt, M. K., Harvey, C. C., Hills, O. W., and Liebert, E. (1950). Correlation of urinary excretion of riboflavin with dietary intake and symptoms of ariboflavinosis. *J. Nutr.* **41:** 247.
104. Glatzle, D., Korner, W. F., Christellar, F., and Wiss, O. (1969). Method for the detection of biochemical riboflavin deficiency. *Int. J. Vit. Nutr. Res.*, **40:** 166–83.
105. Tillotson, J. A. and Baker, E. M. (1972). An enzymatic measurement of the riboflavin status in man. *Am. J. Clin. Nutr.*, **25:** 425–31.
106. Belko, A. Z., Obarzanek, E., Kalkwarf, H. J., Rotter, M. A., Bogusz, S., Miller, D., Hass, J. D., and Roe, D. A. (1982). Effects of exercise on riboflavin requirements of young women. *Am. J. Clin. Nutr.* **37:** 509–17.
107. Thurnham, D. I., Rathakette, P., Hambidge, K. M., Munoz, N., and Crespi, M. (1982). Riboflavin, vitamin A and zinc status in Chinese subjects in a high-risk area for oesophageal cancer in China. *Eur. J. Hum. Nutr.* **36C:** 337–49.
108. Low, C. S. (1985). Riboflavin status of adolescent southern Chinese: riboflavin saturation studies. *Eur. J. Clin. Nutr.* **39C:** 297–301.
109. Bender, D. A. and Bender, A. E. (1986). Niacin and tryptophan metabolism: the biochemical basis of niacin requirements and recommendations. *Nutr. Abs. Rev. (Ser. A)*, **56:** 695–719.
110. Gopalan, C. and Srikantia, S. G. (1960). Leucine and pellagra. *Lancet*, **i:** 954–7.

111. Bender, D. A. (1983). Effects of dietary excess of leucine on the metabolism of tryptophan in the rat: a mechanism for the pellagrogenic action of leucine. *Brit. J. Nutr.*, **50:** 25–32.

112. Hankes, L. V. (1984). Nicotinic acid and nicotinamide. In L. J. Machlin (ed.). *Handbook of Vitamins*, pp. 329–77. Dekker, New York.

113. Pelletier, O. and Brassard, R. (1977). Automated and manual determinations of N^1-methylnicotinamide in urine. *Am. J. Clin. Nutr.*, **30:** 2108–16.

114. De Lange, D. J. and Joubert, C. P. (1964). Assessment of nicotinic acid status of population groups. *Am. J. Clin. Nutr.* **15:** 169–74.

115. Manore, M. M., Vaughan, L. A., Carroll, S. S., and Leklem, J. E. (1989). Plasma pyridoxal 5-phosphate concentration and dietary vitamin B$_6$ intake in free-living, low-income elderly people. *Am. J. Clin. Nutr.* **50:** 339–345.

116. Vermaak, W. J. H., Ubbink, J. B., Barnard, H. C., Potgieter, G. M., Jaarsveld, H. V., and Groenewald, A. J. (1990). Vitamin B$_6$ nutrition status and cigarette smoking. *Am. J. Clin. Nutr.* **51:** 1058–61.

117. Black, A. L., Guirard, B. M., and Snell, E. E. (1978). The behaviour of muscle phosphorylase as a reservoir for vitamin B$_6$ in the rat. *J. Nutr.*, **108:** 670–7.

118. Thurnham, D. I., Singkamani, R., Situnayake, R. D., and Davis, M. (1986). Vitamin B$_6$ concentrations in patients with chronic liver disease and hepato-cellular carcinoma. *Br. Med. J.* **293:** 695.

119. Thurnham D. I. (1981). Red cell enzyme tests of vitamin status: do marginal deficiencies have any physiological significance? *Proc. Nutr. Soc.*, **40:** 155–63.

120. Bender, D. A. (1987). Oestrogens and vitamin B$_6$: actions and interactions. *Wld. Rev. Nutr. Diet.*, **51:** 140–88.

121. Park, Y. H., and Linkswiler, H. (1970). Effect of vitamin B$_6$ depletion in adult man on the excretion of cystathionine and other methonine metabolites. *J. Nutr.*, **100:** 110–16.

122. Lui, A., Lumeng, L., Aronoff, G. R., and Li, T. K. (1985). Relationship between body store of vitamin B$_6$ and plasma phosphate clearance: metabolic balance studies in humans. *J. Lab. Clin. Med.*, **106:** 491–7.

123. Herbert, V. (1967). Biochemical and haematological lesions in folic acid deficiency. *Am. J. Clin. Nutr.*, **20:** 562–9.

124. Bates, C. J., Fleming, M., Paul, A. A., Black, A. E., and Mandal, A. R. (1980). Folate status and its relation to vitamin C in healthy elderly men and women. *Age Ageing*, **9:** 241–8.

125. Rothenburg, S. P. and Cotter, R. (1978). Nutrient deficiencies in man: vitamin B$_{12}$. In M. Rechcigl Jr (ed.). *CRC Handbook Series in Nutrition and Food. Section E: Nutritional Disorders*, Vol. III, pp. 474–97. CRC Press, Florida.

126. Shane, B., Tamura, T., and Stokstad, E. L. R. (1980). A comparison of radioassay and microbiological methods. *Clin. Chim. Acta.*, **100:** 13–19.

127. Fuller, N. J., Bates, C. J., and Scott, K. J. (1983). A radioassay for folate in red cells. *Clin. Chim. Acta.*, **131:** 343–8.

128. Luhby, A. L., Cooperman, J. M., Teller, N., and Donnenfeld, A. M. (1958). Excretion of formimine glutamic acid in folic acid deficiency states. *J. Clin. Invest.*, **37:** 915.

129. Basu, T. K. and Schorah, C. J. (1982). *Vitamin C in health and disease*. Croom Helm, London.

130. MacLennen, W. J. and Hamilton, J. C. (1977). The effect of acute illness on leucocyte and plasma ascorbic acid levels. *Br. J. Nutr.*, **38**: 217–23.

131. Schorah, C. J., Habibzadeh, N., Hancock, M., and King, R. F. G. T. (1986). Changes in plasma and buffy layer vitamin C concentrations following major surgery: what do they reflect? *Ann. Clin. Biochem.*, **23**: 566–70.

132. Vallance, S. (1988). Changes in plasma and buffy layer vitamin C following surgery. *Br. J. Surg.*, **75**: 366–70.

133. Kallner, A. B., Hartman, D., and Hornig, D. H. (1981). On the requirements of ascorbic acid in man: steady state turnover and body pool in smokers. *Am. J. Clin. Nutr.* **34**: 1347–55.

134. Bates, C. J., Prentice, A. M., Prentice, A., Lamb, W. H., and Whitehead, R. G. (1983). The effect of vitamin C supplementation on lactating women in Keneba, a West African rural community. *Int. J. Vit. Nutr. Res.*, **53**: 68–76.

135. Brubacher, G. (1979). Relevance of a borderline vitamin deficiency in relation to the question of vitamin requirement. *Bib. Nutr. Diet.*, **28**: 176–83.

136. Pelletier, O. (1968). Vitamin C status in cigarette smokers and nonsmokers. *Am. J. Clin. Nutr.*, **23**: 520–4.

137. Sahud, M. A. and Cohen, R. J. (1971). Effect of aspirin ingestion on ascorbic acid levels in rheumatoid arthritis. *Lancet*, **i**: 937–8.

138. Manchanda, S. S., Khanna, S., and Lal, H. (1971). Plasma ascorbic acid as an index of vitamin C nutrition. *Ind. Paediatr.*, **8**: 184–8.

139. DHSS. (1972). *A nutrition Survey of the Elderly*. Report on health and social subjects No. 3. HMSO, London.

140. Okamura, M. (1980). Improved method for determination for L-ascorbic and L-dehydroascorbic acid in blood plasma. *Clin. Chim. Acta.*, **103**: 259–68.

141. Margolis, S. A. and Davis, T. P. (1988). Stabilization of ascorbic acid in human plasma, and its liquid-chromatographic measurement. *Clin. Chem.*, **34**: 2217–23.

142. Galan, P., Hercberg, S., Keller, H. E., Bellio, J. P., Bourgeois, C. F., and Fourlon, C. H. (1988). Plasma ascorbic acid determination: is it necessary to centrifuge and stabilize blood samples immediately in the field? *Int. J. Vit. Nutr. Res.*, **58**: 473–4.

143. Roe, J. H. and Keuther, C. A. (1943). The determination of ascorbic acid in whole blood and urine through the 2,4-dinitrophenyl hydrazine derivative of dehydroascorbic acid. *J. Biol. Chem.*, **147**: 399–407.

144. Deutsch, M. J. and Weeks, C. E. (1965). Microfluorimetric assay for vitamin C. *J. Assoc. Off. An. Chem.*, **48**: 1248–56.

145. van Houwelinger, A. C., Kester, A. D. M. and Hornstra, F. (1989). Comparison between habitual intake of polyunsaturated fatty acids from fish and their concentrations in serum lipid fractions. *Eur. J. Clin. Nutr.*, **43**: 11–20.

146. Lepage, G. and Roy, C. C. (1986). Direct transesterification of all lipid classes in a one step reaction. *J. Lipid Res.*, **27**: 114–20.

147. Sanders, T. A. B. and Roshanai, F. (1983). The influence of different types of n-3 polyunsaturated fatty acids on blood lipids and platelet function in healthy volunteers. *Clin. Sci.*, **64**: 91–9.

148. Sanders, T. A. B., Hinds, A., and Pereira, C. C. (1989). Influence of n-3 fatty acids on blood lipids in normal subjects. *J. Int. Med.*, **225**, Suppl. 1: 99–104.

149. Sanders, T. A. B. (1988). Essential and trans-fatty acids in nutrition. *Nutr. Res. rev.*, **1:** 57–78.

150. Weinburg, R B., Dantzker, C., and Patton, C. S. (1990). Sensitivity of serum apolipoprotein A-IV levels to changes in dietary fat content. *Gastroenterology*, **98:** 17–24.

151. Christie, W. W. (1989). Gas chromatography and lipids. The Oily Press, Ayr.

152. Thompson, G. R. (1990). *A handbook of hyperlipidaemia.* Current Science, Philadelphia.

153. Denis, W., Borgstrom, P. (1924). A study of the effect of temperature on protein intake. *J. Biol. Chem.*, **61:** 109–16.

154. Isaksson, B. (1980). Urinary nitrogen as a validity test in dietary surveys. *Am. J. Clin. Nutr.*, **33:** 4–12.

155. Van Staveren, W. A., de Boer, J. A., and Burema, J. (1985). Validity of the dietary history method. *Am. J. Clin. Nutr.*, **42:** 554–9.

156. Baghurst, K. I. and Baghurst, P. A. (1981). The measurement of usual dietary intake in individuals and groups. *Transactions of Menzies foundation*, **3:** 139–60.

157. Bingham, S. A. and Cummings, J. H. (1985). Urine nitrogen as an independent validatory measure of dietary intake: a study of nitrogen balance in individuals consuming their normal diet. *Am. J. Clin. Nutr.*, **42:** 1276–89.

158. Bingham, S. and Cummings, J. H. (1983). The use of 4-amino benzoic acid to validate the completeness of 24 h urine collections in man. *Clin. Sci.*, **64:** 629–35.

159. Young, V., Alexis, S., Balige, B., Munroe, H., and Muecke, W. (1972). Metabolism of administered 3 methyl histidine. *J. Biol. Chem.*, **247:** 3592–8.

160. Prescott, S. L., Jenner, D. A., Beilin, L. J., Margetts, B. M., and Vandongen, R. (1988). A randomised controlled trial of the effect on blood pressure of dietary non-meat protein versus meat protein in normotensive omnivores. *Clin. Sci.*, **74:** 665–72.

161. Cummings, J. H. (1986). The effect of dietary fibre of faecal weight and composition. In G. A. Spiller (ed.). *CRC handbook of dietary fibre in nutrition*, pp. 211–80. CRC Press, Florida.

162. Cummings, J. H. Jenkins, D. J. A., and Wiggins, H. S. (1976). Measurement of mean transit time of dietary residue through the human gut. *Gut*, **17:** 219–15.

163. Jacobsen, A., Newmark, H., Bright-See, E., McKeown Eyssen, G., and Bruce, W. R. (1984). Biochemical changes as a result of increased fibre consumption. *Nutr. Rep. Int.*, **30:** 1049–59.

164. Prentice, A. M., Coward, W. A., Davies, H., Murgatroyd, P., Black, A., Goldberg, G., Ashford, J., Sawyer, M., and Whitehead, R. G. (1985). Unexpectedly low levels of energy expenditure in healthy women. *Lancet*, **i:** 1419–22.

165. World Health Organization (1985). *Energy and protein requirements.* Technical Report Series 724. WHO, Geneva.

166. Clark, A. J. and Mossholder, S. (1986). Sodium and potassium intake measurements. *Am. J. Clin. Nutr.*, **43:** 470–6.

167. Caggiula, A. W., Wing, R. R., Nowalk, M. P., Milas, N. C., Lee, S., and Langford, H. (1985). The measurement of sodium and potassium intake. *Am. J. Clin. Nutr.*, **42:** 391–8.

168. Burch, H. B., Bessey, O. A., Love, R. H., and Lowry, O. H. (1952). The determination of thiamine and thiamine phosphates in small quantities of blood and blood cells. *J. Biol. Chem.*, **198:** 477.

169. Li, A. and Lumeng, L. (1981). Plasma PLP as an indicator of nutritional status: relationship to tissue vitamin B_6 content and hepatic metabolism. In J. E. Leklem and R. D. Reynolds (eds). *Methods in vitamin B_6 nutrition*, pp. 289–96. Plenum, New York.

170. Hodges, R. E., Hood, J., Canham, J. E., Sauberlich, H. E., and Baker, E. M. (1971). Clinical manifestation of ascorbic acid deficiency in man. *Am. J. Clin. Nutr.*, **24:** 432–43.

171. Windsor, A. C. W. and Williams, C. B. (1970). Urinary hydroxyproline in the elderly with low leucocyte ascorbic acid levels. *Br. Med. J.*, **1:** 732–3.

172. Dutra de Oliveira, J. E., Pearson, W. N., and Darby, W. J. (1959). Clinical usefulness of the oral ascorbic acid tolerance test in scurvy. *Am. J. Clin. Nutr.*, **7:** 630–3.

173. Edelstein, C. (1986). General Properties of Plasma Lipoproteins and Apolipoproteins. In A. M. Scanu and A. A. Spector (eds). *Biochemistry and Biology of Plasma Lipoproteins*, pp. 495–504. Marcel Dekker, New York.

174. Sacks, F. M., Rouse, I. L., Stampfer, M. J., Bishop, L. M., Lenherr, C. F., and Walther R. J. (1987). Effect of dietary fats and carbohydrate on blood pressure of mildly hypertensive patients. *Hypertension*, **10:** 452–60.

175. Melchert, H-U., Limasathayouat, N., Mihajlovic, H., Eichberg, J., Thefeld, W., and Rottka, H. (1987). Fatty acid patterns in triglycerides, oliglycerides, free fatty acids, cholesteryl esters and phosphatidylcholine in serum from vegetarians and non-vegetarians. *Atherosclerosis*, **65:** 159–66.

176. Heagerty, A. M., Ollerenshaw, J. D., Robertson, D. I., Bing, R. F., and Swales, J. D. (1986). Influences of dietary linoleic acid on leucocyte sodium transport and blood pressure. *Br. Med. J.* **293:** 295–7.

177. Berry, E. M., Hirsch, J., Most, J., McNamara, D. J., and Thornton, J. (1986). The relationship of dietary fat to plasma lipid levels as studied by factor analysis of adipose tissue fatty acid composition in a free-living population of middle-aged American men. *Am. J. Clin. Nutr.*, **44:** 220–31.

178. Kestin, M., Clifton, P., Belling, G. B., and Nestel, P. J. (1990). n-3 fatty acids of marine origin lower systolic blood pressure and triglycerides but raises LDL cholesterol compared with n-3 and n-6 fatty acids from plants. *Am. J. Clin. Nutr.*, **51:** 1028–34.

179. Heine, R. J., Mulder, C., Popp-Snijders, C., van der Meer, J., and van der Veen, E. A. (1989). Linoleic acid-enriched diet: long term effects on serum lipoprotein and apolipoprotein concentrations and insulin sensitivity in non-insulin dependent diabetic patients. *Am. J. Clin. Nutr.*, **49:** 448–56.

180. Delany, J. P., Vivian, V. M., Snook, J. Y., and Anderson, P. A. (1990). Effects of fish oil on serum lipids in man during a controlled feeding trial. *Am. J. Clin. Nutr.*, **5:** 477–85.

181. Phinney, S. D., Odin, R. S., Johnson, S. B., and Holman, R. T. (1990). Reduced arachidonate in serum phospholipids and cholesteryl esters associated with vegetarian diets in humans. *Am. J. Clin. Nutr.*, **51:** 385–92.

182. Glatz, J. F. C., Soffers, A. E. M. F., and Katan, M. B. (1989). Fatty acid

composition of serum cholesteryl esters and erythrocyte membranes as indicators of linoleic acid intake in man. *Am. J. Clin. Nutr.*, **49**: 209–76.

183. Schafer, L. and Overvad, K. (1990). Subcutaneous adipose-tissue fatty acids and vitamin E in humans: relation to diet and sample site. *Am. J. Clin. Nutr.*, **52**: 486–90.

184. McMurchie, E. J., Margetts, B. M., Beilin, L. J., Croft, K. D., Vandongen, R., and Armstrong, B. K. (1984). Dietary-induced changes in the fatty acid composition of human cheek cell phospholipids: correlation with changes in the dietary polyunsaturated/saturated fat ratio. *Am. J. Clin. Nutr.*, **39**: 975–80.

185. Garry, P. J., Goodwin, J. S., Hunt, W. C., and Gilbert, B. A. (1982). Nutritional status in a healthy elderly population: vitamin C. *Am. J. Clin. Nutr.*, **36**: 332–9.

186. Newton, H. M. V., Morgan, D. B., Schorah, C. J., and Hullin, R. P. (1983). Relation between intake and plasma concentration of vitamin C in elderly women. *Br. Med. J.*, **287**: 1429.

187. Newton, H. M. V., Schorah, C. J., Habibzadeh, N., Morgan, D. B., and Hullin, R. P. (1985). The cause and correction of low blood vitamin C concentrations in the elderly. *Am. J. Clin. Nutr.*, **42**: 656–9.

188. van der Jagt, D. J., Garry, P. J., and Bhagavan, H. N. (1987). Ascorbic acid intake and plasma levels in healthy elderly people. *Am. J. Clin. Nutr.*, **46**: 290–4.

189. Jacob, R. A., Otradovec, C. L., Russell, R. M., Munro, H. N., Hartz, S. C., McGandy, R. B., Morrow, F. D., and Sadowski, J. A. (1988). Vitamin C status and nutrient interactions in a healthy elderly population. *Am. J. Clin. Nutr.*, **48**: 1436–42.

190. Interdepartmental Committee on Nutrition for Defence (1963). In *Manual for nutrition surveys*. US Government Printing Office, Washington.

191. Fisher, M., Levine, P. H. Weiner, B. H., Johnson, M. H., Doyle, E. M., Ellis, P. A., and Hoogasian, J. J. (1990). Dietary n-3 fatty acid supplementation reduces superoxide production and chemiluminescence in a monocyte-enriched preparation of leukocytes. *Am. J. Clin. Nutr.*, **51**: 804–8.

192. Keys, A., Anderson, J. T., and Grande, F. (1965). Serum cholesterol response to changes in the diet. IV. Particular saturated fats in the diet. *Metabolism*, **14**: 376–87.

193. Hegsted, D. M., McGandy, R. B., Myers, M. L., and Stare, F. J. (1965). Quantitative effects of dietary fat on serum cholesterol in man. *Am. J. Clin. Nutr.*, **17**: 281–95.

194. Boyd, N. F., Cousins, M., Benton, M., Krivkov, V., Lockwood, G., and Tritchler, D. (1990). Quantitative changes in dietary fat intake and serum cholesterol in women: results from a randomized, controlled trial. *Am. J. Clin. Nutr.*, **52**: 470–6.

195. Whitehead, C. C. (1981). The assessment of biotin status in man and animals. *Proc. Nutr. Soc.*, **40**: 165–72.

196. Chanarin, I. (1990). *The megaloblastic anaemias*. Third edn. Blackwells Scientific Publications, Oxford.

8. The validation of dietary questionnaires

Michael Nelson

8.1 INTRODUCTION

The history of nutritional epidemiology is littered with the skeletons of discarded questionnaires. Why can there not be a single, all-purpose dietary assessment questionnaire which, once properly validated, could be shared by many workers? Why, apparently, are we all continually reinventing the wheel? This chapter addresses these questions and describes in detail the concepts and techniques essential to questionnaire validation. The matter of questionnaire design is discussed further in Chapter 1 (Appendix 2) and Chapter 6.

Epidemiological studies often require techniques of dietary assessment that are rapid and not labour intensive. At the same time, measurements of dietary variables must be as accurate as possible at the individual level. Questionnaires are usually devised in an attempt to strike a compromise between these conflicting demands and are often regarded as an effective 'short-cut' between speed and accuracy. However, to discover whether the measurements made using questionnaires are accurate, it is essential to compare them with measurements made using other, more intensive or invasive techniques of dietary assessment that have known validity. This process, known as 'validation', is a necessary step in the development of any questionnaire. It provides both information that may aid in the revision of a questionnaire, and evidence of the likely misclassification of individuals based on questionnaire responses. The latter is vital to the correct interpretation of estimates of disease risk in relation to diet, because a poor questionnaire may obscure diet–disease relationships that would become evident using more accurate techniques of dietary assessment. Using an unvalidated dietary questionnaire in nutritional epidemiology is equivalent to using uncalibrated equipment in the laboratory.

8.2 DEFINITIONS

8.2.1 Dietary questionnaire

The term 'dietary questionnaire' is defined as an interview schedule,[1] that is, a fixed series of questions, asked in the same order, regarding the frequency and/or amount of consumption of specific items of food and drink, including alcoholic beverages and dietary supplements, such as vitamin tablets or bran. The questions may be open ended (i.e. a verbatim response is recorded) or, more often, closed (the choice of responses is predetermined). The intention is typically to estimate the usual frequency and/or amount of consumption of foods or nutrients. This definition therefore includes:

1. Food Frequency Questionnaires (FQ)—simple questionnaires that focus on the frequency of consumption of particular foods.[2,3,4]

2. Food Frequency and Amount Questionnaires (FAQ).

The latter group includes questionnaires that aim to establish the intake of particular nutrients by asking about a limited number of food items which are the major sources of those nutrients;[5,6] comprehensive lists of foods, for each of which the respondent is asked to indicate usual frequency and amount of consumption, the intention being to estimate usual intake of a wide variety of nutrients;[7,8] and precoded food lists that are used by respondents to record current diet. Portion sizes are typically predetermined, using existing data on average portion sizes within the population.[9] Respondents may be given the opportunity to state the number or fraction of portions consumed. Aids such as household measures, food models, portion size models, and photographs are often used to help estimate portion sizes. Questionnaires may be administered by an interviewer, completed by the respondent without an interviewer, or administered interactively using a computer. The food codes associated with each food type are usually preassigned.

This definition of questionnaires would, strictly speaking, exclude 24-hour recall, diet history, and similar techniques in which the interview is unstructured or semistructured. In these techniques, the coding of responses will influence the estimates of food consumption or nutrient intake and constitutes an important additional source of error. However, the concepts of validation, discussed below, also apply to these techniques. A general discussion on the design of validation studies is given by Burema et al.[10]

8.2.2 Validity

Internal validity is an expression of the degree to which a measurement is a true and accurate measure of what it purports to measure (see 1.3.1). This implies that there should be an absolute standard against which the measurement can be compared; no such standard exists in nutrition. Because every measurement of dietary intake includes an element of bias (see Chapter 6), one can assess only the 'relative' or 'congruent' validity of measurement based on a questionnaire, comparing the results obtained with what are believed to be more accurate measures of food or nutrient intake. How to select an appropriate standard for comparison and how to interpret the measures of agreement are two of the principle themes of this chapter.

8.2.3 Reproducibility (repeatability, reliability)

Reproducibility (and its synonymous terms) indicates the extent to which a tool is capable of obtaining the same measurement when used repeatedly in the same circumstances. A measurement may have good reproducibility and yet have poor validity, but a measurement that has good validity cannot have poor reproducibility.

Because the diet of every individual varies on a daily, weekly and seasonal basis, the concept of 'the same circumstances' does not exist when trying to assess the reproducibility of a dietary questionnaire. A typical aim of many questionnaires is to assess 'usual' intake. Given this aim, if due consideration has been given to these time related factors when constructing a questionnaire, its reproducibility can, in theory, be assessed. In practice, subjects' weekly and monthly variations in diet are likely to influence their responses. Thus, the reproducibility assessed will be a combination of measurement error and within-subject variability.

8.3 THE CONTEXT OF VALIDATION

When deciding on the best method for validating a questionnaire, the purpose of the questionnaire and its frame of reference (e.g. time scale, type of study, etc.) must be clearly defined. The stated purpose of the questionnaire will dictate the techniques that are suitable for validation, and a clearly demarcated frame of reference will help to identify the important confounders of the validation process.

The purposes to which questionnaires may be put are as myriad as the questions posed by nutritional epidemilogy, but can be summarized under four major headings:

(1) current or past intake (8.3.1);

(2) food consumption or nutrient intake (8.3.2);

(3) determination of absolute or relative intakes of individuals (8.3.3);

(4) determination of group averages versus individual intake (8.3.4).

8.3.1 Current or past intake

The majority of validation studies have compared questionnaire estimates of food consumption or nutrient intake with more rigorous assessments of current or very recent diet. If the main purpose of the study in which the questionnaire is being used is to examine the relationship between current diet and disease, then such an approach to validation is satisfactory. More often, however, investigations of diet–disease relationships predicate an aetiological role for diet at some period in the past. The validation process then becomes much more difficult. If the questionnaire for dietary assessment asks about food consumption in the distant past then, in theory, validation requires a standard that was measured at the time to which the assessment relates. In practice, such standards are rare. Investigators are then faced with an unhappy choice: either to question subjects about past diet with no validation of the method, or to ask about current diet using a method that can be validated, and be forced to make a number of untestable assumptions about the way in which current and past diet are related. The latter is a particular problem in case-control studies, where the relationships between current and past diet may be different in the two groups because of the influence of the disease process on diet.

'Current or past intake' also begs the question about the time frame within which the validation process takes place. Questionnaires are often used to assess 'usual' intake over some specified period ('last month', 'over the last year', etc.). In theory, such questionnaire responses should be free of error attributable to within-subject variance. When questionnaire results are compared with short term records of diet (e.g. 7-day weighed intakes), then lack of agreement in ranking, for instance, can be attributed in part to the within-subject variance that is inherent in the more accurate standard. Alternatively, if the questionnaire is compared with a diet history, then questions concerning the accuracy of the history itself become important (see Chapter 6). These and other sources of error are discussed below under 'Factors affecting validation studies' (8.5).

8.3.2 Food consumption and nutrient intake

Abramson *et al.* in a study of the effect of diet on anaemia in pregnancy, validated a food frequency list (for assessing frequency of consumption of foods per week) by comparing the results with frequency data from a

30 min interview. While the interview itself may have been biased, the comparison was appropriate in that both techniques were addressing the question of usual frequency of consumption. The authors concluded that food frequency data was best suited to generating hypotheses, provided the sample under investigation was sufficiently heterogeneous.

Mojonnier and Hall[11] were interested in assessing adherence to prescribed diets in the National Diet-Heart study. The interviewer rated adherence 'subjectively' into four categories—excellent, good, fair and poor—based on her total knowledge of each patient's performance, and compared these with 'semiobjective' ratings of adherence based on 7-day recall and 7-day records of diet. All the ratings reflected frequency but not the amount consumed. There was better agreement of the 'subjective' ratings independently with the two 'objective' ratings than there was between the 'objective' ratings themselves. This illustrates the importance, particularly in food frequency validation studies, of the need to have so-called 'objective' measures that cover a sufficient time span to give results that are representative of individual habits. This also applies to questionnaires that measure patterns of food consumption (meal frequency, interval of consumption between meals or items, etc.), being aware of potential biases in the reporting or recording of consumption (as for sweets and alcohol, for instance).

Frequency data alone is too weak for many epidemiological purposes where quantity consumed is important in estimating exposure. Questionnaires that use frequency data with fixed portion sizes to estimate food consumption may 'over-standardize' consumption,[12] denying subjects the opportunity to describe their true diet. The agreement between questionnaire and standard is thus likely to be poor unless frequency itself is the overriding factor in estimating consumption. The selection of portion sizes is discussed further below, under 'Validation Techniques' (8.4).

If the aim of the questionnaire is to estimate nutrient intake, then the nutrient composition database used for calculation must be the same for both questionnaire and standard. The caveats above regarding the frame of reference must also be noted. Furthermore, the day to day variation in the intake of many nutrients will be less than for many foods, reducing the number of days for which diet need be recorded.

8.3.3 Absolute or relative intakes

In some circumstances, it may be sufficient simply to rank subjects according to food consumption or nutrient intake using questionnaire responses. For example, if the risk of heart disease was being assessed in relation to fifths of linoleic acid intake, then a questionnaire that ranked people correctly, but consistently measured only 75 per cent of linoleic acid sources in the diet, would fit the purpose. On the other hand, if the aim was to identify a dietary threshold for the intake of linoleic acid above which risk of heart disease decreased, then this type of relative measure of intake would not suffice, and the validation of the questionnaire would need to address both ranking and agreement with a standard that gave the best possible measure of absolute intakes. The different statistical techniques appropriate for these two types of analysis are discussed in section 8.6.

8.3.4 Group versus individual intakes

For comparisons between groups of people, a mean value for food consumption or nutrient intake may be sufficient. A questionnaire may therefore be adequate if the mean values rank the groups correctly or, if absolute intakes must be known, the means are close to the true intakes based on the standard. Validation may then be against any measure that provides an accurate mean value, such as 1-day records.[13] If, in addition, an estimate of variance within each group is required, then the standard must also be able to reflect this. If the questionnaire is assumed to provide an estimate of 'usual' intake, it can also, in theory, provide an estimate of between-subject variance, allowing for any variance that may be attributable to reproducibility. Thus, for purposes of validation of aggregate measures, it is still useful to be able to distinguish between-subject and within-subject variance in both the questionnaire and the standard. At least two observations using both measurements are needed from each subject for the within-subject component of the variances to be estimated.

8.4 TECHNIQUES OF VALIDATION

8.4.1 Choosing a standard

Current intakes The majority of validation studies have compared questionnaire results with a more 'accurate' measure of current diet. The choice of standard is a difficult one, and depends on the perceived validity of the standard itself. The two methods most widely adopted are the weighed inventory[14] and the full Burke diet history.[15] While neither of these techniques is able to measure diet without error (see Chapter 6), they are both highly reproducible within subjects and provide methods for assessment that can be used in large numbers of people and at reasonable costs. Moreover, they can be used (with appropriate attention to length of record or period of recall) to assess both food consumption (frequency and amounts) and nutrient intakes for a wide variety of foods and nutrients. An unusual standard used by Jain and co-workers[16] was a quantitative record of husband's food consumption kept over 30 days by their wives, but this technique limits validation to married couples, and it is not clear that husbands would be as effective recorders as wives if the women's intakes were under scrutiny. All of these techniques are generally better suited to the purpose than more accurate methods such as the doubly-labelled water technique[17] or balance studies.[18] While isotope and balance techniques have a role to play in validation, it is important to bear in mind that they are very expensive, can be used to validate only one nutrient at a time, and are far more time consuming than weighed inventory or history techniques.

Biochemical standards, such as urinary nitrogen excretion, adipose tissue fatty acid composition, or leucocyte ascorbic acid content also exist (see Chapter 7). While these measurements may be useful for describing the relationship between estimated intake and physiological endpoints, they do not, strictly speaking, constitute standards for validation of dietary assessment. There are three sources of error when comparing questionnaire results with biochemical standards:

(1) the difference between what is assessed by questionnaire and the true intake;
(2) the important stages of digestion, absorption, utilization, and metabolism, all of which bear on the biochemical measurement;
(3) the error associated with the biochemical assay itself.

These errors are likely to attenuate the association between estimated intake and biochemical measurement. This technique does not, therefore, enable the researcher to identify the component of error in estimating intake associated with the questionnaire alone. Poor agreement between a biochemical standard and estimated intake using a questionnaire does not necessarily indicate that the questionnaire has failed to assess intake correctly. Thus, such techniques can justify statements about a strong association between consumption and biochemical endpoints, but not about a lack of association.

In some circumstances biochemical validation may be the only technique available. For example, salt intake is only poorly assessed using standards that rely on food composition tables, and comparison of questionnaire scores on consumption of salty foods with seven consecutive measurements of urinary sodium excretion has proved useful.[5] The validity of a questionnaire on iodine intake where again, food composition data may be scanty, has been assessed against urinary iodine excretion.[19]

Past intakes   Selection of standards for past intakes involves identification of past dietary assessments that have used techniques sufficiently robust to provide valid data. Bakkum *et al.*[20] identified a group of subjects who had completed full diet histories 12–14 years earlier, against which they compared retrospective assessments of diet again based on diet histories. Byers and co-workers,[21] similarly, compared past diet histories with an abbreviated (47 food item) retrospective questionnaire. Van Leeuwen *et al.*[22] identified 7-day weighed inventories completed 4 years earlier for comparison with retrospective diet histories. In each of these studies, the interval of retrospective assessment was dictated by circumstances, but they all demonstrated that, for selected food items or nutrients, the ranking of subjects based on retrospective histories was closer to that recorded in the past than to ranking based on current intakes. Two other studies (Byers et al.[3] Lindsted and Kuzma[4]), using less rigorous past assessments of intake based on limited FAQs collected up to 25 years earlier, came to similar conclusions concerning retrospective assessments. However, in each of these studies the range of correlation coefficients was very wide, and the values for 'r' for similar food groups or nutrients vary widely between studies (Table 8.1). For example, recall of bread consumption amongst controls in Study 5 correlated only moderately with past intake ($r = 0.32$) whereas in Study 2, assessed over a similar time interval, the correlation

Table 8.1 Comparison of dietary assessments in the past with recalls of past diet. Correlation coefficients for foods and nutrients.

	1 r_S[a]	2 r	3 r	4 r_S	5 r_S Cases	Controls
	(79)	(175)	(323)	(46)	(117)	(99)
Food						
Meat	0.47	0.07	0.39	0.22	0.75	0.74
Vegetables	0.34	−0.01 to 0.36	0.41	0.41	0.20	0.25
Fruit	–	–	0.41	–	0.26	0.23
Milk	0.35	0.47	0.58	0.14	0.28	0.54
Bread	0.68	−0.04	0.51	0.44	0.22	0.32
Eggs	–	–	0.42	–	0.35	0.46
Tea	–	0.44	0.64	–	0.12	0.50
Coffee	0.67	0.52	0.71	–	0.60	0.61
Nutrient						
Energy	0.68	–	–	0.69	–	–
Protein	0.47	–	–	0.50	–	–
Fat	0.68	–	0.50	0.64	–	–
Dietary fibre	0.54	–	0.61	–	...	–
Vitamin A	–	–	0.61	–	–	–

[a] r_S: spearman rank correlation coefficient; r: pearson product moment correlation coefficient.
[1] Van Leeuwen et al.[22] 79 M+F 25–65; 7–day WI 1977 vs DH 1981.
[2] Byers et al.[3] 63 M, 112 F; 50–74 FAQ 1957–65 vs FAQ 1982.
[3] Byers et al.[2] 323 M+F; FAQ 1975–79 vs short FAQ 1984.
[4] Bakkum et al.[20] 46 M+F elderly; DH 1971–72 vs DH 1984–85.
[5] Lindsted and Kuzma,[4] 216 M+F; <82 FAQ 1960 vs short FAQ 1984.
DH, diet history; FAQ, food frequency and amount questionnaire; WI weighed inventory.

was -0.04. In these particular studies, the ability to assess nutrient intake in the past was better than the assessment of food consumption. It is interesting that the cases and controls in Study 5 seemed to be able to recall foods with similar levels of accuracy.

All these findings suggest that retrospective assessments are of value, but the investigator who chooses to use them without an appropriate past standard opens him- or herself to the dangers inherent in using any questionnaire that has not been properly validated, i.e. the true ranking of subjects may not be reflected in the observed rankings and the extent of the error in ranking remains unknown.

8.4.2 Validation procedures

The basic model of validation involves the comparison of a questionnaire against a standard of known validity. Having considered those factors that are involved in the design of the questionnaire itself (see Chapter 6), it is important to consider as a separate issue the design of the validation study.

Sequence of administration and frame of reference   Ideally, the questionnaire being validated should be administered prior to the assessment of the standard, for two reasons. The first is that subjects would normally, in the course of the main investigation in which the questionnaire was to be used, encounter the questionnaire independent of any other dietary assessment, and the validation procedure should mimic this. Secondly, the act of completing the work for the assessment of the standard may in itself draw respondents' attention to their diets. If the questionnaire was to be completed after the standard, subjects might attempt to recreate in their responses to the questionnaire the pattern of diet assessed for the standard. This might explain, for example, very high levels of agreement in the reported frequencies of food consumption between 7-day records and questionnaires completed either during or immediately after the recording period.[23] Stigglebout et al.[24] designed a questionnaire to assess 'usual' retinol and carotene intake over the previous year, and tested the effect of order of administration on questionnaire response when validating it against a full diet history (average interval between assessments was 25 days). The questionnaire responses agreed better with the diet history when the diet history was administered first (although the differences in response failed to reach statistical significance, possibly because of poor power at moderate sample size). A separate problem may be that a period of dietary assessment prior to completion of the questionnaire may draw the respondent's attention to aspects of their diet that they wish to modify, and there is the danger that an expression of the desired modification would find itself reflected in the questionnaire responses, independent of true intakes.

The question of sequence raises the issue of the frame of reference. Ideally, the period of assessment should be the same for both questionnaire and standard, i.e. one should compare like with like. As questionnaires are, by their nature, retrospective, it would therefore seem sensible to administer it after the standard. One can presume that eventually sufficient time will pass after measurement of the standard to allow a dietary assessment, which is not influenced by previous measurement procedures, using the questionnaire. This is probably of the order of a month or more, but then raises the further problem of deciding whether to ask the subject to recall diet that corresponds specifically to the period of assessment based on the standard, or simply to recall 'usual' diet, on the assumption that both the standard and the questionnaire relate to this concept. The choice is particularly important where seasonal effects may influence the pattern of food consumption relating to intake of nutrients such as vitamin C or carotene. Willett et al.[25] addressed these problems in one of the most extensive validation studies published, by asking 173 nurses to record diet by weighed inventory for one week, four times during the course of a year, and comparing the results with an FAQ administered once at the beginning and once at the end of the study. The second FAQ correlated better with the records than the first (correlations ranged from 0.33 to 0.73 compared with 0.18 to 0.53), suggesting that a learning process may have influenced the second set of responses.

In general, the frame of reference for validation should be dictated by the purpose of the questionnaire in the main study. If 'usual' diet is to be assessed, and seasonal influences are either not important or are taken into account when determining responses, then the questionnaire should be administered prior to the standard. Epstein and co-workers[26] administered a short questionnaire (for use in the Israel Ischaemic Heart Disease Study) using lay interviewers, and compared the results with Burke-type diet histories obtained by trained nutritionists between 4 and 30 days later. They reported good correlations between the two methods in a wide variety of samples when assessing intakes of energy, carbohydrate, protein, and fat (Table 8.2). However, the results were not consistent between subgroups and an important finding was that the strength of the correlation was directly proportional to the number of foods consumed (see section 8.5.9).

Basis for questionnaire design A difficulty arises when measurements derived from the standard are used in the design of the questionnaire. Numerous workers have, very sensibly, obtained detailed records or histories of diet from samples in the populations in which the intended questionnaire is to be used, in order to determine the key foods that contribute to nutrient intakes or that feature regularly in the diet. These foods are used as the backbone of the questionnaire. The investigators

Table 8.2. Correlation coefficients (Pearson r) between short and long FAQ estimates of nutrient intake (from Epstein et al. 1970[26]).

	Study group					
	A	B	D	E	L	M
Calories	0.65	0.50	0.58	0.82	0.62	0.73
Carbohydrate	0.70	0.31	0.48	0.81	0.49	0.57
Protein	0.52	0.42	0.69	0.80	0.53	0.57
Fat	0.63	0.46	0.24	0.66	0.56	0.81

A 25 M 20–39 years, North African
B 18 M 20–39 years, European
D 22 M 40+ years, North African, <5 years of school
E 24 M 40+ years, North African, ≥5 years of school
L 25 F 40+ years, North African
M 25 F + years, European

have then administered the questionnaire to the same group of subjects, and determined the validity (usually in terms of correlation coefficients) by comparing the questionnaire results with the standard. This procedure leads inevitably to an overstatement of validity. When questionnaires designed in this way have been re-evaluated in similar but independent samples drawn from the same population, the resulting correlation co-efficients have always, disappointingly, been lower.[27,28]

The questionnaire design, therefore, should be based upon as complete an assessment of usual diet in the population as is available, but the validation procedure should always be carried out in a sample that is representative of the population and independent of the samples used to provide the initial dietary profile.

8.5 FACTORS AFFECTING VALIDATION STUDIES

Many factors can potentially undermine the validation process, some of which have been alluded to in the previous section. Jacobs[29] suggests that the influence of these factors can be so great as to obscure completely any relationship between the questionnaire values and those based on the standard. Their potential influence must therefore be addressed compre-hensively if the value of a validation study is not to be lost.

It is equally important to remember that a questionnaire that has been validated in one setting may not have the same validity in another. The list of potential factors is long, and it may be necessary to undertake a new validation study to establish how the questionnaire performs in the new setting.

The precautions regarding questionnaire design and administration

(see section 6.9.3) concerning the day and time of questionnaire administration, interviewer training (minimizing observer bias, etc.) must, of
course, also apply to validation studies, even though they may not be listed
specifically below.

8.5.1 Gender

There is good reason to believe that women respond to questionnaires
differently from men. If a questionnaire validated in one sex is then used in
the other, one cannot say that the relationship between the questionnaire
responses and true intake is necessarily the same in both groups. This may
in part explain the failure in some studies to detect similar diet–disease
relationships in both sexes.[30,31] The corollary of this notion is that a validation study that includes both men and women must be analysed separately
by sex. The range of values across both sexes may yield a significant correlation coefficient, but when the data are analysed separately by sex, one
or the other may fail to reach statistical significance. For example, Figure
8.1 shows that the correlation coefficient for zinc intake assessed by questionnaire and by 16-day weighed inventory is $r = 0.43$ ($n = 52$; $P < 0.01$),
but when the results are analysed separately by sex, women show a much
higher correlation $r = 0.69$ ($n = 28$; $P < 0.01$) than men $r = 0.33$ ($n = 24$;
$P > 0.05$).[32] The number of subjects in this example is small and the 95 per
cent confidence intervals around the values for r for the two sexes in fact
overlap (i.e. there is no statistically significant difference in r between the
sexes), but the point is clearly illustrated. Statistical techniques for deter-

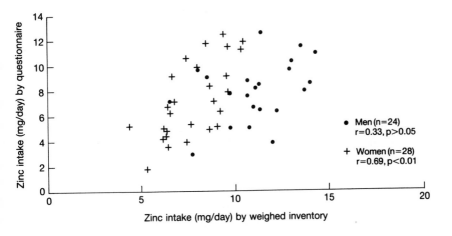

Fig. 8.1. Zinc intake (mg/day) estimated by questionnaire and by 16-day
weighed inventory in 24 men and 28 women aged 25–64 years, by sex.[32]

r=0.69, p<0.01   r=0.69, p<0.01

mining 95 per cent confidence intervals around correlation coefficients are given in the appendix.

8.5.2 Age

Adults between the ages of 18 and 64 do not generally show any consistent differences according to age in their ability to complete questionnaires satisfactorily. Outside this range, however, factors such as memory and conceptualization skills may have important influences on subjects' abilities to complete questionnaires successfully, and validity in these groups should be assessed separately.

8.5.3 Place

A questionnaire validated in Wales may perform quite differently in Scotland. This is a particular problem in multicentre studies (especially if more than one language is involved), as differences in the observed diet–disease relationships between centres may be in part due to differences in the way in which the questionnaires assess intake. Multicentre trials should try and ensure that the questionnaires being used perform in the same way in relation to true intake in all centres, or to assess differences in performance between centres.

8.5.4 Disease process

Many diseases, including vascular diseases and those of the gastrointestinal tract, may have a profound influence on food consumption, either through patients' awareness of dietary risk factors or changes in appetite and digestion. For example, dietary assessment by questionnaire in a case-control study may be substantially biased by the disease process in the cases. A questionnaire that has been validated only in subjects who are representative of the controls[33] may not, therefore, perform in the same way in the cases, and an attempt should be made to ensure that the quality of the responses is the same in both groups. This may only be feasible for hospitalized patients by comparing questionnaire results with those from a full diet history, because prospective techniques may not be an option. Care must be taken not to confound 'usual' diet with recall of the hospital diet.

8.5.5 Recency

Many case-control studies attempt to establish the aetiological role of diet by asking subjects to recall consumption in some period before the interview (6 months, a year, a number of years, or the period immediately prior to diagnosis in the cases). Several authors have reported a 'recency' effect, that is, the tendency for the recall of past diet to be influenced by recent consumption.[3,16,21,34] If the disease process has had a profound effect on diet, this influence will clearly be greater in cases than in controls.[16] This is very difficult to address as part of the validation process, because it is unlikely that the necessary standards for comparison, measured at the appropriate time period in the past, will exist for both cases and controls. An assessment of case-control differences in current diet may shed light on the ways in which recall of past diet may have been biased, but it does not assist in the assessment of the past diet *per se*, nor necessarily reflect the way that past diet may have influenced the disease process. One way around this problem is to assess the case-control comparison independently in a number of subgroups within the population who differ with regard to diet (e.g. social class groups). If the same pattern of differences between cases and controls can be seen in the different subgroups, this supports the credibility of the observed diet–disease relationship.

8.5.6 Social class and education

Questionnaires are often validated in groups of intelligent, highly motivated volunteers with non-manual occupations, producing good agreement with the standard. But if the questionnaires are then used in groups of patients that include many subjects from lower social classes, important unknown biases may influence estimates of consumption in these subgroups. Clearly, the sample in a validation study should include a sufficiently broad cross-section of the population, and analysis should control for social class or education.

8.5.7 Sequence and proximity of questionnaire and standard measurement

These factors have been discussed above (see section 8.4.2). It is worth re-iterating that the learning process associated with the measurement of the standard is likely to have a positive influence on the way in which subjects complete questionnaires, raising the level of agreement between the two measures. The assessment of a questionnaire's ability to measure 'usual' diet is thus best achieved by administering the questionnaire first and obtaining the standard measure subsequently. If the validation necessitates the administration of the questionnaire after the standard has been measured, then a minimum period of 3 or 4 weeks should elapse before the questionnaire is given.

8.5.8 Autocorrelation

This has been discussed above (see section 8.4.2). If a validation study is carried out in the same sample in which the food profile that provided the basis for the the questionnaire was initially measured, then the agreement between the questionnaire and the standard will be substantially greater than if the questionnaire and standard had been measured independently in another sample drawn from the same population.[28,35] This type of over-statement of agreement is analogous to that in which estimated intakes based on 3 days of diet record are correlated with the entire week's data from which the 3 days are drawn.[36]

8.5.9 Number of foods listed

In the same way that autocorrelation will lead to an overstatement of validity, the omission from an FAQ of foods that are frequently eaten or that are major contributors of nutrients will naturally reduce the accuracy of a questionnaire assessment and limit its validity.[37] Nomura et al.[38] also observed that it was more difficult to demonstrate agreement between repeat questionnaires (at 6 months and at 2 years) for items that were reportedly eaten less frequently than for those that were eaten frequently, although Kuzma and Lindsted [39] observed that the frequency of consumption of rarely eaten foods was also recalled accurately. Thus, one is more likely to select foods that are eaten frequently or very infrequently for inclusion in a questionnaire. In populations where the total number of foods eaten is small, it is probable that all of the major sources of nutrients for most subjects will be included. As the number of foods eaten increases and the variation in sources of nutrients between subjects becomes greater, the likelihood of misclassifying certain subjects because their food profile is different from the majority becomes greater and greater. This is reflected by the observation of Epstein et al.[26] that agreement between questionnaire and standard improved with an increasing number of foods reportedly consumed. Thus, those whose diets were similar to the selected profile were seen to have good agreement with the standard, while those whose diets differed and were presumably unable to find listed in the questionnaire the foods that contributed to their intakes showed poorer agreement with the standard.

Thus, it may be worthwhile to include in the questionnaire some foods that are eaten less frequently but that may be important contributors to nutrient intake in the diets of relatively few individuals. Choosing which foods to include in the questionnaire may therefore involve assessing the range of contribution that foods can make to the diets of individuals, rather than looking simply at the average contribution in the population as a whole. This is particularly important in multiracial societies in which the breadth of food choice may be especially wide,[40,41,42] but it can, of course, lead to exceptionally long lists of foods.[43]

8.5.10 Portion size

Two problems regarding portion size are particularly important. First, if the intention is to assess intake based on 'standard' portion sizes, allowing the respondent little or no opportunity to describe the amounts actually consumed, it is possible to inadvertently standardize out the true variation in intake.[44] This will naturally reduce the observed level of agreement between questionnaire and standard. Secondly, where a questionnaire is to be used in several groups whose dietary habits differ, a single set of standard portions may not reflect the true variation in portion size, as Tillotson et al.[45] observed in their study of Japanese men living in Japan, Hawaii, and California.

8.6 STATISTICAL TECHNIQUES AND INTERPRETATION

There are several techniques that can be used to determine the degree of agreement between two sets of measurements, and it is important to ask which aspect or aspects of validity are to be tested. Agreement can be expressed in terms of (i) group means (or medians); (ii) ranking; (iii) differences between mesurements within individuals.

8.6.1 Group means

In studies in which differences between groups are important (e.g. geographical correlation studies between estimated intake and disease prevalence in different regions[13,46]) validation should assess the ability of the questionnaire to reflect the group mean. These comparisons are best examined using t-tests. Yarnell et al.[7] compared the results of a short questionnaire to assess a wide variety of nutrient intakes against 7-day weighed records, and showed that in 119 men the questionnaire significantly underestimated the group mean for every nutrient except alcohol, in spite of the fact that the portion sizes used in the questionnaire were derived from the weighed intake data. The studies by Willett et al.[25] in nurses and by O'Donnell et al.[32] in adult men and women show similar findings (although the Willett questionnaire signficantly overestimated some nutrients). Yarnell and co-workers concluded that it is unlikely that 'a dietary questionnaire will completely replace the need for supplementary information by the use of more detailed dietary methods in epidemiological studies.'[7] However, this somewhat pessimistic conclusion does not consider the possibility of constant bias in the group means in different groups within the population. Any study that intends to use group means to rank groups must, of course, validate the questionnaire in each group separately. But if the ranking is consistent, then a questionnaire with a constant bias may be of use.

8.6.2 Ranking

The most common method of assessing the validity of questionnaires is to test the agreement in ranking of subjects between questionnaire and standard. Consistency of ranking is usually measured using the Pearson product-moment correlation coefficient (often on $\log_e$ transformed data to improve approximation to the normal distribution), although Spearman's and Kendall's correlation coefficients are also used.

As the purpose of most analytical nutritional epidemiological studies is to assess the relative risk of disease in relation to food or nutrient intake, the ability to separate subjects with high intakes from those with low intakes is paramount. Often, only the approximate level of intake need be known. For purposes of validation, then, the correlation would seem to be ideal, but there are important drawbacks to its use.

There are no hard and fast rules as to what constitutes a satisfactory level of correlation. No correlation will reach unity because both the sources of error in the questionnaire and the standard, and the true within-and between-subject variation in diet, preclude such a finding. Clearly, misclassification of subjects using the questionnaire increases as the correlation coefficient between questionnaire and standard falls. A bivariate normal model can be used to show the level of agreement between r and the correct ranking of subjects in the extreme thirds (see Table 3.1). The number of subjects correctly classified in the extremes of the distribution falls substantially as the values for r drop from 0.9 (over 80 per cent correctly classified) to 0.5 (60 per cent) to 0.1 (43 per cent). Few correlations in questionnaire validation studies reach 0.9, and many are below 0.5. The sensitivity of many questionnaires may thus be so low as to fail to demonstrate a diet–disease association (assuming one exists) because so many subjects are incorrectly classified. Thus, nutrients for which correlations reach statistical significance ($P < 0.05$) by virtue of large numbers of subjects in the validation study cannot necessarily be assessed adequately using the questionnaire being validated. It is also important to remember that the value for r reflects only the agreement between questionnaire response and standard, and that the relationship between true intake and questionnaire response may be better than at first appears. The following discussion illustrates some of the difficulties in assessing the value of validation studies based on correlation analysis, and explores ways in which these problems can be addressed.

In a study of three towns, in which 438 men and women aged 35–54 completed 24-hour records of diet followed three years later by a food frequency and amount questionnaire, statistically significant Spearman correlation coefficients varied from 0.15 ($P < 0.002$) for vitamin A to 0.36 ($P < 0.001$) for energy.[13] Mathematical modelling techniques were used to calculate the maximum correlation coefficient likely to be detected, accounting for diet record measurement error, FAQ measurement error, change in diet over time, and the likely within- to between-subject variance ratio. If it is assumed that there were no errors in either measurement and no change in diet, given the within- to between-subject variance ratio (taken from the literature), the highest detectable value would have been 0.34 for vitamin A and 0.6 for energy. Allowing for a 12 per cent measurement error in the diet record, 18 per cent error in the FAQ, and a 6 per cent average change in diet over time, the calculated correlations agreed well with those observed. Thus, the questionnaire seemed to be performing as well as could be expected. But if r^2 is taken to reflect the proportion of variance in ranking subjects according to recorded intake that is explained by the questionnaire, then only 13 per cent of the variation in recorded energy intake can be explained by the FAQ results, and only 2 per cent of the variation in vitamin A!

On the other hand, correctness of classification by fifths showed that almost two-thirds of subjects were classified by the questionnaire to within ± one quintile of their recorded intake. This seems reasonably good, and gives a much better impression of the value of the questionnaire for separating subjects into classes of intake than that based on r^2. It is possible to reconcile this apparent disparity by analysing the sources of error in more detail, and this will also shed light on the extent to which misclassification reduces the ability to detect significant diet–disease relationships.

Freudenheim and Marshall[47] have used mathematical modelling to demonstrate the extent to which the problem of misclassification (expressed in terms of correlation coefficients) can be addressed. If r_{12} is the observed correlation between questionnaire and standard, r_{1t} is the correlation between questionnaire and true intake and r_{2t} is the correlation between the standard and true intake, then $r_{12} = r_{1t} \times r_{2t}$, and $r_{1t} = r_{12}/r_{2t}$. If one assumes that the correlation between the standard and true intake is, in this instance, fairly modest (say $r_{2t} = 0.6$), then for the observed values for energy and vitamin A quoted above, r_{1t} would equal 0.6 and 0.25 respectively. The ratio of true to total variance for energy is $(r_{12})^2/(r_{2t})^2 = 0.36^2/0.6^2 = 0.36$, and for vitamin A, $0.25^2/0.6^2 = 0.17$, that is, 36 per cent of the variation in true energy intake and 17 per cent of the variation in true vitamin A intake is explained by the questionnaire. These values are an improvement upon the 13 per cent and 2 per cent quoted above, but the impact of this scale of error in being able to detect significant diet–disease relationships should not be underestimated. Freudenheim and Marshall have shown that a true median relative risk of 2.41 between lowest and highest fifths of intake is attenuated to 1.40 when the variance ratio is 0.18.[47] Thus, in this example one would be unlikely to detect an association of risk between diet and vitamin A intake at a level that would be regarded as important.

Table 8.3 shows correlation coefficients for a number of nutrients based on a variety of questionnaires. Several features stand out. First, there is no consistency in the strength of correlation for a given nutrient, except for

Table 8.3. Correlation coefficients between FAQ and 'standard' estimates of nutrient intake

	1	2	3	4	5	6	7	8	9	10 (a)	10 (b)	11	12
	(14)	(87)	(16)	(50)	(119)	(173)	(27)	(168)	(190)	(20)	(20)	(52)	(29)
Energy	0.74	0.34	0.43	0.63	0.30	–	0.67	0.57	0.45	0.56	0.29	0.35	0.50
Protein	0.80	–	0.32	0.60	0.41	0.18	0.60	0.53	–	0.42	0.42	0.43	–
Fat: total	0.94	0.36	0.53	0.58	0.34	0.27	0.76	0.51	–	0.59	0.08	0.39	0.59
SFA	0.85	0.40	0.50	0.51	0.31	0.31	0.74	0.56	0.56	0.60	0.12	–	0.58
PUFA	0.69	0.38[a]	0.27[a]	0.60[a]	–	0.31	0.74[a]	0.65	0.60	0.45	0.06	–	–
Cholesterol	–	0.42	0.61	0.47	–	0.46	0.67	0.54	–	–	–	–	–
Carbohydrate	–	–	–	–	0.27	0.48	0.60	0.60	–	0.55	0.48	0.35	–
Sugar	–	–	–	–	0.45	0.52	–	0.54	–	0.31	0.18	0.31	–
Dietary fibre	–	–	0.24	0.70	0.37	–	–	0.71	0.61	0.40	0.37	0.67	–
Alcohol	–	–	–	–	0.75	–	–	0.80	–	0.90	0.46	0.74	–
Vitamin A	–	–	–	–	–	0.21	0.63	0.41	0.40	–	–	0.31[b]	0.54[b]
Vitamin C	–	–	0.63	0.64	0.36	0.46	0.38	0.58	0.44	–	–	0.33	0.48

	1	2	3	4	5	6	7	8	9	10a	10b	11	12
Vitamin D	—	—	—	—	—	—	—	0.47	—	—	—	0.27	—
Vitamin E	—	—	—	—	—	—	—	0.64	0.53	—	—	0.39	0.45
Calcium	—	—	—	—	0.63	—	—	0.61	—	—	—	0.53	—
Iron	—	—	—	—	0.47	—	—	—	—	—	—	0.66	—
Percent energy from fat	—	—	—	—	—	—	—	0.38	0.38	—	—	—	—
P/S ratio	—	—	—	—	—	—	—	0.76	0.81	—	—	—	—

a based on log$_e$ transformed values

b retinol

1 Balogh et al., 1968 [48] 14 M 50–59; FAQ vs 7-day WI.

2 Morgan et al., 1978 [33] 87 F; DHQ vs 4-day diet record.

3 Jain et al., 1980 [14] 16 M 25–50; DHQ vs 30-day record by spouse.

4 Jain et al., 1982 [37] 50 F 40–59; DHQ vs DH interview at home.

5 Yarnell et al., 1983 [4] 119 M; FAQ vs 7-day WI.

6 Willett et al., 1985 [25] 173 F 34–59; FAQ vs 28-day WI.

7 Willett et al., 1987 [49] 27 M+F 20–54; FAQ vs 1-year diet record.

8 Pietinen et al., 1988 [5] 168 M 55–69; Food Use Questionnaire vs 24-day WI.

9 Pietinen et al., 1988 [50] 190 M 55–69; FAQ vs 24-day WI.

10 a) Boutron et al., 1989 [51] 20 M+F 30–79; FAQ (meals) vs 14-day WI.

    b) Boutron et al., 1989 [51] 20 M+F 30–79; FAQ (foods) vs 14-day WI.

11 O'Donnel et al., 1991 [32] 52 M+F 25–64; FAQ vs 16-day WI.

12 O'Brien and Nelson 1991 [52] 29 M+F 50–70; FAQ vs 7-day WI.

DH, diet history; DHQ, diet history questionnaire; FAQ, food frequency and amount questionnaire; WI, weighed food record.

alcohol, which is well correlated. There is more consistency in results within studies, suggesting that a questionnaire tends to be generally good or generally poor. Study 1 shows exceptionally good results, while studies 5 and 6 seem generally poorer than the others, yet the standard was based on weighed records in each case (7, 7, and 28 days, respectively), and there is no reason to believe why one group of subjects should perform so much better than another. The range of foodstuffs assessed was greater in studies 5 and 6 than in study 1, and the range of diets was probably much narrower in the former compared with the latter study. But in circumstances not dissimilar to study 6, Pietinen (studies 8 and 9) showed much better correlations, with the suggestion that the use of photographs is of some benefit in improving subjects' estimates of portion size and hence correlation with the standard. An excellent result was obtained by Willet et al.[49] (study 7) when questionnaire results were compared with a standard obtained from food records kept over an entire year, but one must then consider carefully the nature of subjects who would be willing to undertake such a study and that their ability to describe their food habits was perhaps better than most. Women do not seem generally better at describing their habits than men (as has often been stated), and the differences in study 11, although striking, do not reach statistical significance. (The method for calculating the 95 per cent confidence interval for r is given in the Appendix at the end of the chapter.) The diversity of these results emphasizes even more strongly the need to validate questionnaires in the population in which they are to be used.

An argument against using Pearson or Spearman correlation coefficients is that the null hypothesis assumes that there is no association between the two measures, but this seems unlikely when two techniques are used to measure the same variable. Lee[53] suggests that a better measure of association is the intraclass correlation r_I for interval measurements, or the Kappa statistic k for nominal (ordinal) measurements. This allows for a degree of association between two related measures, which is likely to arise by chance, and tends to give lower values than r.

Table 8.4 gives the results for a recent validation study of antioxidant vitamins carried out in 29 men and women aged 50–70 years.[52] The table shows mean intakes assessed by 7-day weighed record and by questionnaire, the within- to between-subject variance ratio (based on analysis of variance of the weighed records), Pearson (r_{12}) and intraclass (r_I) correlation coefficients, and corrections of the correlation coefficients for attenuation because the standard itself does not measure true intake.

One observes immediately that the questionnaire gives higher mean values for nutrient intake than the weighed records, the average difference for all nutrients except retinol being significantly greater than zero. The scale of the difference in relation to the mean is similar for energy and fat, and substantially greater for the vitamins, suggesting that there may be a

Table 8.4. Analysis of agreement between FAQ and 7-day weighed inventory (WI) estimates of energy and nutrient intake in 14 men and 15 women aged 50–70 years[52]

	WI	FAQ	Mean difference (FAQ–WI)	s_w^2/s_b^2	Pearson r	Intraclass r	r_{2t}	r_{1t}
Energy	1762	2163	400**	0.83	0.50	0.29	0.94	0.53
Fat: total	76.3	94.1	17.8**	1.29	0.59	0.41	0.92	0.64
SFA	25.9	31.9	6.0*	1.35	0.58	0.42	0.92	0.64
Retinol	912	1405	493	3.92[a]	0.54[a]	0.51[a]	0.80[a]	0.67[a]
β-carotene	2150	3223	1073**	4.28[a]	0.56[a]	0.39[a]	0.79[a]	0.71[a]
Vitamin A equivalents	1270	1943	673*	5.07[a]	0.49[a]	0.45[a]	0.76[a]	0.64[a]
Vitamin C	56	94	38***	2.43	0.48	0.16	0.86	0.55
Vitamin E	4.0	6.1	2.1***	1.44	0.45	0.05	0.91	0.49

[a] – based on $\log_e$ transformed values.

* $P < 0.05$; ** $P < 0.01$; *** $P < 0.001$.

r_{1t} correlation between questionnaire and true intake

r_{2t} correlation between weighed inventory and true intake.

scale of the difference in relation to the mean is similar for energy and fat, and substantially greater for the vitamins, suggesting that there may be a bias in the over-reporting of fruits and vegetables compared to other food groups. The Pearson correlation coefficients compare favourably with those shown in Table 8.3.

The intraclass correlation coefficient takes into account both the degree of correlation and the size of disagreement within pairs, and is calculated as $(s_b^2 - s_w^2)/(s_b^2 + s_w^2)$, where s_b^2 is the variance of the sum of the pairs of observations, and s_w^2 is the variance of the differences between pairs. As expected, all of the values for r_I are less than those for r. Those above 0.4 show what is regarded as good agreement, while values less than zero suggest that the differences within pairs are so great as to confound any meaningful ranking of subjects. The interpretation of r_I is sometimes difficult, because it is possible to have a questionnaire that correlates perfectly with the standard using Pearson's r, but which has a large variance of differences within pairs (s_w^2). Thus, if the assessment of ranking is the primary objective of the validation, then Pearson's r is a better measure, whereas if the aim is to assess the level of agreement between the measures, then the intraclass correlation may be more helpful.

An alternative method for assessing the extent of differences is to use the approach suggested by Bland and Altman[54] to plot the difference against the sum of each pair of observations. Like the intraclass correlation, this makes no assumption about which measure is better (this is left open to interpretation by the investigator) and assesses only the level of agreement. Figure 8.2 shows the plot for energy from the study by O'Brien and Nelson.[52] It can be seen that the 95 per cent confidence interval around the mean difference is wide and that, as a method for determining an individual's intake, the questionnaire would be likely to give rise to a substantial error. Moreover, there appears to be a trend suggesting that, as intake increases, the size of the difference between the measurements also increases. The two methods could not be regarded as interchangeable for the assessment of an individual's intake. Again, however, if the aim is to be able to distinguish those in the bottom part of the distribution of intakes from those in the top, then the confidence interval around individual values of intake based on the questionnaire would allow approximately 60 per cent of subjects to be correctly classified in the extreme thirds. This will naturally lead to an attenuation of the odds ratio calculation in a case-control study, and the true odds ratio will in all likelihood be higher (see Fig. 3.5).

Because neither the questionnaire nor the standard assesses true intake, the correlation of the two measures is inevitably an underestimate of the correlation of the questionnaire with the truth. The last three columns in Table 8.4 give correlations that are adjusted for this error. The value r_{2t} is the unobservable correlation between the 7-day weighed record data and the truth, calculated from the formula given in Nelson et al.[55]

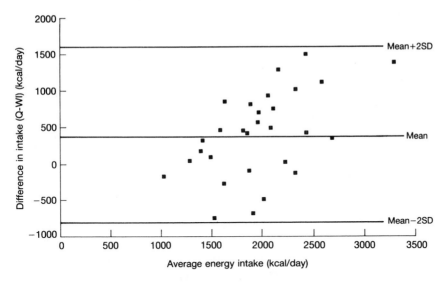

Fig. 8.2. Difference against mean of energy intake estimated by questionnaire and 7-day weighed inventory in 14 men and 15 women aged 50–70 years.[52]

$r = [d/(d + s_w^2/s_b^2)]^{0.5}$, where d is the number of days for which records were kept, s_w^2 is the within-subject variance and s_b^2 the between-subject variance. (This calculation assumes that the weighed record, day by day, is an unbiased measure of true intake, and addresses only the question of unreliability in the estimate of intake based on 7 days of record.) This value of r_{2t}, if divided into the observed r, gives r_{1t}, the likely correlation of the questionnaire with the truth. These values are all higher than the observed values, the greatest increase between r and r_{1t} occurring for nutrients such as retinol and carotene where the within- to between-subject variance ratio is high. This correction suggests that for all of the nutrients shown, up to 10 per cent more subjects would be correctly classified by thirds. It also implies that the correction for the relative risk calculation, if based in r_{1t} rather than r, would be less. The value for r_{1t} is the same as that obtained using the method suggested by Borrelli,[56] based on Liu et al.[57]

8.7 CONCLUSIONS

The external validity of measures of dietary exposure based on question-naires requires evaluation in order to:

1. Ensure that the measuring instrument used in nutritional epidemiologi-cal studies will allow the detection of diet–disease relationships, should they exist.

2. Determine the error associated with their use to facilitate the correct interpretation of disease risk in relation to diet.

Inadequate attention paid to validation may result in a substantial waste of resources and, more serious, the failure to observe the true relationship between diet and disease. The amount of resource that needs to be devoted to the validation process should not be underestimated at the initial design stages.

At the end of a validation study, there is always the (sometimes difficult) decision as to whether or not a questionnaire is felt to be satisfactory as a measuring instrument. There are no hard and fast rules as to what constitutes 'satisfactory', as it is usually dependent on the size and power of the study. Most investigators continue to use the questionnaire in the main study in the form used in the validation study, as the extent of the errors associated with its use are defined. To change the questionnaire could mean that the observed agreement between questionnaire and standard is altered, and the extent of the error is then unknown. Often, there is a difficult point of decision when, having evaluated a questionnaire, it is felt to be too insensitive to be of use. Three options are available:

(1) abandon the questionnaire and find an alternative method to assess the nutritional exposure;

(2) modify the questionnaire in order to overcome its apparent defects without re-evaluation;

(3) repeat the entire validation process with a revised questionnaire.

If the performance of the questionnaire in relation to the standard is really very poor, then the first option may be the most practicable. If no satisfactory alternative exists, then it may be better to cut one's losses at an early point and abandon the study until an appropriate measuring device can be found. Choosing the second option is a matter of judgement. If the flaws in questionnaire design that are responsible for the lack of agreement with the standard are very obvious, then it may be possible to modify the questionnaire in the likelihood that the changes will produce a better measuring instrument. However, the error associated with its use will then have to be estimated as the error based on the original validation study will no longer apply. It is worth bearing in mind, also, that disagreement between questionnaire and standard may not be due to a design fault in the questionnaire but to some factor in the calculation of nutrient intake (e.g. a faulty value in the food table that biases the results for questionnaire and standard in different directions). However, this option is safe only when design errors are obvious and should be adopted with great caution (and full acknowledgement in the final write-up!). The final option is usually outside the scope of the resources that have been allocated to the study, but in some circumstances (e.g. when there has already been a substantial investment in the project) may be a viable choice.

APPENDIX

Calculation of the 95 per cent confidence interval around a correlation coefficient.[58]

The correlation coefficient r is transformed to the variable z with a nearly normal distribution by the equation:

$$z = 0.5 \times [\log_e(1 + r) - \log_e (1 - r)]$$

and with the standard error (SE) given by:

$$\sigma_z = 1 / \sqrt{(n - 3)}$$

Since z is nearly normally distributed, the upper and lower 95 per cent confidence limits are given as:

$$\text{Upper limit} = z + 1.96 \text{ SE}$$
$$\text{Lower limit} = z - 1.96 \text{ SE}$$

The values for the upper and lower confidence limits can then be transformed back to the corresponding values of r using the equation:

$$r = (e^{2z} - 1)/(e^{2z} + 1)$$

so permitting the determination of the confidence interval. When the number of observations is small, the standard error is large in relation to z, and the confidence interval is wide (as in the illustration in Fig. 8.1). But if the validation study includes both sexes and is sufficiently large, then there is a greater likelihood of detecting significant differences in the correlation coefficient between sexes, which in turn may enhance the analysis of the disease risk in relation to diet.

REFERENCES

1. Moser, C. A. and Kalton, G. (1979). *Survey methods in social investigation.* Heinemann Educational, London.
2. Abramson, J. H., Slome, C., and Kosovsky, (1963). Food frequency interview as an epidemiological tool. *Am. J. Publ. Hlth.*, **53:** 1093–1101.
3. Byers, T. E., Rosenthal, R., Marshall, J. R., Rzepka, T. F., Cummings, K. M., and Graham, S. (1983). Diet history from the distant past: a methodological approach. *Nutr. Cancer*, **5:** 69–77.
4. Lindsted, K. D. and Kuzma, J. W. (1989). Long-term (24 years) recall reliability in cancer cases and controls using a 21-item food frequency questionnaire. *Nutr. Cancer*, **12(2):** 135–49.
5. Shepherd, R., Farleigh, C. A., and Land, D. G. (1985). Estimation of salt intake by questionnaire. *Appetite*, **6:** 219–33.
6. Nelson, M., Hague, G. F., Cooper, C., and Bunker, V. W. (1988). Calcium intake in the elderly: validation of a dietary questionnaire. *J. Hum. Nutr. Diet.* **1:** 115–27.
7. Yarnell, J. W. G., Fehily, A. M., Milbank, J. E., Sweetnam, P. M., and Walker, C. L (1983). A short questionnaire for use in epidemiological surveys: comparison with weighed dietary records, *Hum. Nutr. Appl. Nutr.* **37A(2):** 103–112.
8. Pietinen, P., Hartman, A. M., Haapa, E., Rasanen, L., Haapakoski, J., Palmgren, J., Albanes, D., Virtamo, J., and Huttunen, J. K. (1988). Reproducibility and validity of dietary assessment instruments. I. A self-administered food use questionnaire with a portion size picture booklet. *Am. J. Epid.*, **128:** 655–66.
9. Crawley, H. (1988). Food portion sizes. HMSO, London.
10. Burema, J., van Staveren, W. A., and van den Brandt, P. A. (1988). Validity and reproducibility. In Cameron, M. E. and van Staveren, W. A. (eds). *Manual on methodology for food consumption studies.* Oxford University Press, Oxford.
11. Mojonnier, L. and Hall, Y. (1968). The national diet–heart study—assessment of dietary adherence, *J. Am. Diet. Assoc.*, **52:** 288–92.
12. Hankin, J. H., Reynolds, W. E., and Margen, S. (1967). A short dietary method for epidemiologic studies. II. Variability of measured nutrient intakes. *Am. J. Clin. Nutr.*, **20(9):** 935–45.
13. Margetts, B. M., Cade, J. E., and Osmond, C. (1990). Comparison of a food frequency questionnaire with a diet record. *Int. J. Epid.*, **18:** 868–73.
14. Widdowson, E. M. (1936). A study of English diets by the individual method. Part I. Men. *J. Hyg.*, **36:** 269–92.
15. Burke, B. S. (1947). The dietary history as a tool in research. *J. Am. Diet. Assoc.*, **23:** 1041–6.
16. Jain, M., Howe, G. R., Johnson, K. C., and Miller, A. B. (1982). Evaluation of a diet history questionnaire for epidemiologic studies. *Am. J. Epid.*, **111:** 212–19.
17. Prentice, A. M., Coward, W. A., Davies, H. L., Murgatroyd, P. R., Black, A. E., Goldberg, G. R., Ashford, J., Sawyer, M., and Whitehead, R. G. (1985). Unexpectedly low levels of energy expenditure in healthy women. *Lancet*, **i:** 1419–22.

18. Fairweather-Tait, S. J., Johnson, A., Eagles, J., Ganatra, S., Kennedy, H., and Gurr, M. I. (1990). Studies on calcium absorption from milk using a double- and label stable isotope technique. *Br. J. Nutr.*, in press.

19. Nelson, M., Quayle, A., and Phillips, D. I. W. (1987). Iodine intake and excretion in two British towns: aspects of questionnaire validation. *Hum. Nutr. Appl. Nutr.*, **41A:** 187–92.

20. Bakkum, A., Bloemberg, B., van Staveren, W. A., Verschuren, M., and West, C. E. (1988). The relative validity of a retrospective estimate of food consumption based on a current dietary history and a food frequency list. *Nutr. Cancer*, **11:** 41–53.

21. Byers, T., Marshall, J., Anthony, E., Fielder, R., and Zielezny, M. (1987). The reliability of dietary history from the distant past. *Am. J. Epid.*, **125:** 999–1011.

22. Van Leeuwen, F. E., de Vet, H. C. W., Hayes, R. B., Van Staveren, W. A., West, C. A., and Hautvast, J. G. A. J. (1983). An assessment of the relative validity of retrospective interviewing for measuring dietary intake. *Am. J. Epid.*, **118:** 752–8.

23. Stefanik, P. A. and Trulson, M. F. (1962). Determining the frequency intakes of foods in large group studies. *Am. J. Clin. Nutr.* **11:** 335–43.

24. Stiggelbout, A. M., van der Giezen, A. M., Blauw, Y. H., Blok, E., van Staveren, W. A., and West, C. E. (1989). Development and relative validity of a food frequency questionnaire for the estimation of retinol and beta-carotene. *Nutr. Cancer*, **12:** 288–99.

25. Willet, W. C., Sampson, L., Stampfer, M. J., Rosner, B., Bain, C., Witschi, J., Hennekens, C. H., and Speizer, F. E. (1985). Reproducibility and validity of a semi-quantitative food frequency questionnaire. *Am. J. Epid.*, **122:** 51–65.

26. Epstein, L. M., Reshef, A., Abrahamson, J. H., and Biacik, O. (1970). Validity of a short dietary questionnaire. *Israel J. Med. Sci.*, **6:** 589–97.

27. Marr, J. W., Heady, J. A., and Morris, J. N. (1961). Towards a method for large-scale individual diet surveys. In *Proceedings of the 3rd international congress of dietetics*, pp. 85–91. London 10–14th July, Newman Books, London.

28. Hankin, J. H., Messinger, H. B., and Stallones, R. A. (1970). A short dietary method for epidemiologic studies. IV. Evaluation of questionnaire. *Am. J. Epid.*, **91:** 562–7.

29. Jacobs, D. R. Jr, Anderson, J. T., and Blackburn, H. (1979). Diet and serum cholesterol: do zero correlations negate the relationship? *Am. J. Epid.*, **110:** 77–87.

30. Kune, S., Kune, G. A., and Watson, L. F. (1987). Observations on the reliability and validity of the design and diet history method in the Melbourne colorectal cancer study. *Nutr. Cancer*, **9:** 5–20.

31. Kune, S., Kune, G. A., and Watson, L. F. (1987). Case-control study of dietary etiological factors: the Melbourne colorectal cancer study. *Nutr. Cancer*, **9:** 21–42.

32. O'Donnell, M. G., Nelson, M., and Wise, P. H. (1991). A computerised diet questionnaire for use in health education. I. Development and validation. *Br. J. Nutr.*, in press.

33. Morgan, R. W., Jain, M., Miller, A. B., Choi, N. W., Matthews, V., Munan, L., Durin, J. D., Feather, J., Howe, G. R., and Kelly, A. (1978). A comparison of dietary methods in epidemiologic studies. *Am. J. Epid.*, **107:** 488–98.

34. Rohan, T. E. and Potter, J. D. (1984). Retrospective assessment of dietary intake. *Am. J. Epid.*, **120:** 876–87.
35. Hankin, J. H., Rhoads, G. G., and Glober, G. A. (1975). A dietary method for an epidemiologic study of gastrointestinal cancer. *Am. J. Clin. Nutr.*, **28:** 1055–61.
36. Stuff, J. E., Garza, C., O'Brian Smith, E., Nichols, B. L., and Montandon, C. M. (1983). A comparison of dietary methods in nutritional studies. *Am. J. Clin. Nutr.*, **37:** 300–6.
37. Jain, M., Harrison, L., Howe, G. R., and Miller, A. B. (1982). Evaluation of a self-administered dietary questionnaire for use in a cohort study. *Am. J. Clin. Nutr.*, **36:** 931–5.
38. Nomura, A., Hankin, J. H., and Rhoads, G. G. (1976). The reproducibility of dietary intake data in a prospective study of gastrointestinal cancer. *Am. J. Clin. Nutr.*, **29:** 1432–6.
39. Kuzma, J. W. and Lindsted, K. D. (1989). Determinants of long-term (24 year) diet recall ability using a 21-item food frequency questionnaire. *Nutr. Cancer*, **12:** 151–60.
40. Pickle, L. W. (1985). A comparison of frequency and quantitative dietary methods for epidemiologic studies of diet and disease. *Am. J. Epid.*, **121:** 776–8.
41. Block, G. (1982). A review of validation of dietary assessment methods, *Am. J. Epid.*, **115:** 492–505.
42. Borrud, L. G., McPherson, S., Nichaman, M. Z., Pillow, P. C., and Newell, G. R. (1989). Develoment of a food frequency instrument: ethnic differences in food source. *Nutr. Cancer*, **12:** 201–12.
43. Mullen, B. J., Krantzler, N. J., Grivetti, L. E., Schutz, H. G., and Meiselman, H. L. (1984). Validity of a food frequency questionnaire for the determination of individual food intake. *Am. J. Clin. Nutr.*, **39:** 136–43.
44. Hankin, J. H., Rawlings, V., and Nomura, A. (1978). Assessment of a short dietary method for a prospective study on cancer. *Am. J. Clin. Nutr.*, **31:** 355–9.
45. Tillotson, J. L., Kato, H., Nichaman, M. Z., Miller, D. C., Gay, M. L., Johnson, K. G., and Rhoads, G. G. (1973). Epidemiology of coronary heart disease and stroke in Japanese men living in Japan, Hawaii and California: methodology for comparison of diet. *Am. J. Clin. Nutr.*, **26:** 177–84.
46. Barker, D. J. P., Morris, J. A., and Nelson, M. (1986). Vegetable consumption and acute appendicitis in 59 areas in England and Wales. *Br. Med. J.*, **292:** 927–30.
47. Freudenheim, J. L. and Marshall, J. R. (1988). The problem of profound mismeasurement and the power of epidemiological studies of diet and cancer. *Nutr. Cancer*, **11:** 243–50.
48. Balogh, M., Medalie, J. N., Smith, H., and Groen, J. J. (1968). The development of a dietary questionnaire for an ischaemic heart disease survey. *Israel J. Med. Sci.*, **4:** 195–203.
49. Willett, W. C., Reynolds, R. D., Cottrell-Hoehner, S., Sampson, L., and Browne, M. L. (1987). Validation of a semi-quantitative food frequency questionnaire: comparison with a 1-year diet record. *J. Am. Diet. Assoc.*, **87:** 43–7.
50. Pietinen, P., Hartman, A. M. Haapa, E., Rasanen, L., Haapakoski, J.,

Palmgren, J., Albanes, D., Virtamo, J., and Huttunen, J. K. (1988). Reproducibility and validity of dietary assessment instruments. II. A quantitative food frequency questionnaire. *Am. J. Epid.*, **128**: 667–76.

51. Boutron, M. C., Faivre, J., Milan, C., Gorcerie, B., and Esteve, J. (1989). A comparison of two diet history questionnaires that measure usual food intake. *Nutr. Cancer*, **12**: 83–91.

52. O'Brien, C. and Nelson, M. (1991). Validity of a dietary questionnaire for assessing anti-oxidant vitamin intake, in preparation.

53. Lee, J. (1980). Alternative approaches for quantifying aggregate and individual agreements between two methods for assesing dietary intakes. *Am. J. Clin. Nutr.*, **33**: 956–8.

54. Bland, J. M. and Altman, D. G. (1986). Statistical methods for assessing agreement between two methods of clinical measurement. *Lancet*, **i**: 307–10.

55. Nelson, M., Black, A. E., Morris, J. A., and Cole, T. J. (1989). Between-and-within-subject variation in nutrient intake from infancy to old age: estimating the number of days required to rank dietary intakes with desired precision. *Am. J. Clin. Nutr.*, **50**: 155–67.

56. Borrelli, R. (1990). Collection of food intake data: a reappraisal of criteria for judging the methods. *Br. J. Nutr.*, **63**: 411–17.

57. Liu, K., Stamler, J., Dyer, A., McKeever, J., and McKeever, P. (1978). Statistical methods to assess and minimize the role of intra-individual variability in obscuring the relationship between dietary lipids and serum cholesterol. *J. Chron. Dis.*, **31**: 399–418.

58. Snedecor, G. W. and Cochran, W. G. (1967). *Statistical Methods*, sixth edn. Iowa State University Press, Iowa.

9. Measures of disease frequency and exposure effect

Carol A. C. Wickham

9.1 INTRODUCTION

Quantitative measures are used in epidemiology to describe the distribution of disease in populations. To investigate whether exposure to a potential risk factor is related to the frequency of a disease, these measures are compared among people with varying levels of exposure to the risk factor, for example, varying levels of intake of a nutrient.

Three measures of disease frequency will be discussed in this chapter; the incidence rate, the prevalence, and the cumulative incidence. Of these, the incidence rate is the measure most frequently used in epidemiological studies.

The method of standardization is often employed to compare disease frequencies in different populations separated geographically or by time. Standardization produces summary measures of disease for the populations; these allow for differences in the structures of the populations that could otherwise distort the comparisons.

Measures of exposure effect describe how a disease frequency changes according to the amount or level of exposure to a possible risk factor. These measures are either absolute effects, measuring differences in disease frequencies, or relative effects, which are ratios of disease frequencies. The proportion of a disease in the population caused by a specific risk factor, known as the population attributable proportion is another measure of exposure effect to be discussed.

9.2 MEASURES OF DISEASE FREQUENCY

The distribution of disease in a population can be summarized by absolute numbers of disease cases. This may be useful for planning the allocation of resources but to make comparisons of disease frequencies between populations, measures that incorporate the sizes of the populations at risk of disease are used. The measures are either rates or proportions, two terms that are frequently misunderstood. A full definition is given by Elandt-Johnson.[1] In summary, a rate measures how one quantity is changing with respect to another, usually time, at a specific instant. For example, the rate of bone loss in an elderly person measures how their bone mass changes with time at specific moments in time. Relative rates are usually more appropriate in biological situations because they incorporate the magnitude of the variable that is changing with time. A relative rate of bone loss would measure the rate of bone loss relative to the remaining amount of bone at a point in time. Strictly, a true rate applies to a precise moment, but rates are usually estimated by average rates that are calculated for short periods of time or periods during which the rates are assumed to be reasonably stable such as a year. Rates can take any value from minus to plus infinity.

A proportion is the quotient of two values in which the numerator is a subset of the denominator, for example, the proportion of vegetarians in a population is given by dividing the number of vegetarians by the total number of people in the population. A proportion can only take values between zero and one.

Ratios are used widely in epidemiological studies to express the effects of risk factors. A ratio generally denotes division of one term by another and is frequently used more specifically to denote a quotient in which the numerator and denominator are exclusive of each other, such as the P:S ratio in which the polyunsaturated fatty acid intake is divided by the saturated fatty acid intake.

9.2.1 Incidence rates

The incidence rate is the rate at which new cases of disease occur amongst individuals who are initially free from the disease in question. The incidence rate is a relative rate incorporating both new cases of disease and the size of the population at risk. It is usually calculated for a given period of time, such as a year, making it an average of the instantaneous rates throughout the year.

Incidence rates are non-negative because they only include new disease cases, not departures of old cases. They take the value zero if no new cases of disease are diagnosed in the time period, and can theoretically take any value up to infinity; rates would approach this value if an entire population contracted a disease almost instantaneously.

The calculation of an incidence rate involves selecting a suitable time interval and a population of interest that is free from the disease at the beginning of the time interval and at risk of the disease throughout the time interval. A count is made of the number of new disease cases that arise in that interval among members of the population. This number is divided not by the number of individuals in the population but by the sum of the time periods during which each individual was disease-free, alive and under observation. Thus

$$\text{incidence rate} = \frac{\text{number of new disease cases}}{\Sigma \ (\text{disease-free time periods})}$$

where Σ denotes the summation over all subjects in the population under consideration.

The denominator is referred to as the person-time, or subject-time, of observation or risk, and as person- or subject-years where incidence rates are expressed for yearly intervals. As an incidence rate has a denominator with units of time, it is not simply the proportion of individuals who develop the disease in a given time.

As an example, suppose that 1000 people are disease-free at the start of a year. They are observed throughout the year, during which time twelve new cases of disease occur, but some individuals die from other causes or are otherwise lost from the study. Suppose that the total length of time for which subjects were disease-free, alive, and under observation is 800 years. The incidence rate for this year is 12 per 800 person-years, that is 0.015 per person-year or 15 per 1000 person-years.

In practice, incidence rates are often approximated in geographically defined populations, such as countries, by counting all new disease cases that occur in the population in a given year and dividing by the estimated mid-year population, which approximates the person-years of observation for that population over the year. The approximation would be better if the mid-year population was replaced by the number of individuals free from the disease in question at the middle of the year. This number is usually less readily available and, with rare diseases, the difference is small. The approximation would also be improved if the mid-year population estimate contained only those individuals at risk of the disease. For example, rates of cervical cancer are most accurately estimated by including in the denominator only those women who have not had a hysterectomy, this being particularly important in countries such as the USA, where hysterectomy rates are relatively high.

The incidence rate given by dividing all new disease cases by the person-years at risk for all individuals in a population is called the crude incidence rate. It is usually more informative to present incidence rates subdivided by sex and age group. These are known as age–sex-specific incidence rates. The calculations remain as described above, except that the disease cases and person-years are counted separately for each age and sex stratum. However, individuals may contribute person-time to more than one stratum as they age during the period of observation.

Incidence rates may change over time. Investigations into whether these changes relate to changes in dietary habits, for example, may generate hypotheses as to potential causes of a disease. Calculation of incidence rates over time involves observation of a population over an extended period. Disease occurrences and person-years of observation are counted specifically to the year of diagnosis of disease and of observation. A complete summary of rates can be given by presenting rates specific to age at diagnosis, year of diagnosis, and sex. As individuals age they will contribute person-years of observation to several age and calendar year strata. The age group and calendar time divisions can be thought of as forming a grid. Rates can be calculated by counting the number of disease cases and person-years in each cell as the subjects move diagonally across the grid (Fig. 9.1).

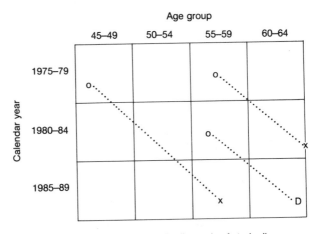

o, entry into study; D, diagnosis of study disease;
x, loss from study or end of study.

Fig. 9.1. Calculation of incidence rates over time.

Official statistics can be used to produce approximate age-, sex- and time-specific rates if both disease cases and mid-year populations are categorized by sex and the appropriate age groups and calendar years. The rates are then produced by dividing the number of new disease cases by the mid-year population for each stratum.

Throughout this section, incidence rates have been described in terms of disease onset. The same calculations can be used to produce mortality rates from specific diseases or all causes. The data required for the calculation of these rates may be more readily available than morbidity data. Mortality rates, however, are influenced by death certification practices, medical treatments, and other factors that affect survival once a disease has been diagnosed. Thus, mortality rates may not be associated with exposure to risk factors as closely as incidence rates. If incidence data are available, it is preferable that they should be used in studies investigating the causes of disease.

9.2.2 Prevalence

The point prevalence (prevalence) of a disease is the proportion of a population affected by the disease at a specific moment in time. It is calculated by dividing the number of diseased individuals in the population by the total number of people in the population. As prevalence is a proportion it can take values between zero (when no one has the disease) and one (when the entire population is affected by the disease). The prevalence is not a rate, although the term prevalence rate is frequently, but incorrectly, used.

The prevalence includes in its numerator both newly diagnosed cases and long term survivors. Prevalences are affected by changes in treatment of the disease and individuals' survival characteristics. Incidence rates are more closely linked to a disease's risk factors as they only include new cases of disease, identified before forces affecting the duration of the disease exert their influence. This is why, in studies of the cause of disease, incidence rates are used by epidemiologists in preference to prevalences, although they may be harder to obtain, especially for rare diseases of long duration (e.g. multiple sclerosis). Studies that aim to test aetiological hypotheses using prevalences can be misleading. A factor that appears to increase the prevalence of a disease may be prolonging survival or delaying recovery among people contracting the disease rather than causing the disease.

For a steady-state population, that is, one that individuals enter and leave over time, but for which the population size remains stable, the prevalence is approximately equal to the product of the incidence rate and the mean duration of the disease, until death or recovery, as long as it is reasonably small, say less than 10 per cent. That is:

Prevalence ≈ Incidence rate × mean duration of the disease

Thus, it can be seen that the prevalence is affected both by the disease incidence and by the disease's duration.

The period prevalence of a disease is the proportion of a population affected by a disease during a certain interval of time. It is a combination of point prevalence and incidence, in that it contains both prevalent cases at a certain point in time and incident cases arising during a given interval starting from that time point. All these cases are divided by the total number in the population at the start of the interval.

The point and period prevalence of a disease have limited use in aetiological studies as measures of disease frequency, although they are sometimes used when incidence data are not available, but the findings should always be interpreted with caution.

Prevalence is a useful measure of disease frequency in investigations into where best to target health resources, since existing cases of disease require these resources as well as new cases of disease arising in the population.

9.2.3 Cumulative incidence

A measure of disease that is frequently of interest is the risk, or probability, that an individual will develop a disease during a specified time period or age range. It is imperative that the time period is stated for the risk to be interpretable.

The cumulative incidence of a disease is the proportion of a population, initially free from the disease, that will get the disease in a given time period, and is therefore a measure of the average risk of the disease for members of that population over the time period. It is assumed that the disease is such, or that the time period is small enough, that the disease will be contracted no more than once during the period of interest. Cumulative incidence can be estimated in a fixed population (i.e. a population that is fully enumerated at the start of the period and to which no new subjects are added during the period) that is free from the disease in question by counting the number of disease cases that arise during the period of interest and dividing by the number in the population at the start of the period.

Age-specific incidence rates can be used to estimate the cumulative incidence by combining them over several age groups to give a summary measure of disease frequency, known as the cumulative incidence rate.[2] Cumulative incidence rates are calculated by summing the age-specific incidence rates over the age range of interest. For example, the cumulative incidence rate for subjects aged 45–64 would be given by summing the incidence rates for each year between and including 45 and 64. If rates are available only for five- or ten-year age groups, rather than for individual years, then these rates are multiplied by the length of the period before summing.

In mathematical notation, if i_t is the instantaneous incidence rate for individuals at some time, t, then the cumulative incidence rate between times 0 and T inclusive is:

$$\text{Cumulative incidence rate} = \int_{t=0}^{T} i_t \, dt$$

This is approximated by the cumulative incidence rate, based on annual incidence rates I_t:

$$\text{Cumulative incidence rate} = \sum_{t=0}^{T} I_t$$

and if the rates apply to intervals of length l_t then:

Cumulative incidence rate $= \sum_{t=0}^{T} I_t l_t$

The cumulative incidence rate between two points in time (or two ages) T_1 and T_2 is:

$$\sum_{t=0}^{T_2} I_t l_t - \sum_{t=0}^{T_1} I_t l_t = \sum_{t=T_1}^{T_2} I_t l_t$$

If P_t denotes the cumulative incidence of disease from time 0 to t, for some time t in the interval $[0,T]$, and if i_t is the incidence rate at time t, then it follows from the definitions that:

$$i_t = \frac{1}{1 - P_t} \frac{dP_t}{dt}$$

and integrating over the interval $[0,T]$ gives:

$$P_T = 1 - \exp\left(- \int_{t=0}^{T} i_t dt\right)$$

where P_T is the cumulative incidence of disease by time T.

The term $\int i_t dt$ is approximated by the cumulative incidence rate $\sum I_t l_t$. Thus, the cumulative incidence is equal to one minus the exponential of the cumulative incidence rate over a given time interval. In addition, for rare diseases with a cumulative incidence rate of less than, say, 0.1, the cumulative incidence is approximately equal to the cumulative incidence rate, because:

$$1 - \exp(-x) \approx x \text{ for small values of x}$$

So, for rare diseases, the cumulative incidence rate over some time period or age range can be interpreted as the average risk or probability that an individual will develop the disease during that period. For this reason, the terms rate and risk are often used interchangeably.

With more common diseases, the cumulative incidence can be calculated from the cumulative incidence rate using the formula:

$$P_T = 1 - \exp\left(- \sum_{t=0}^{T} I_t l_t\right)$$

As an example of the calculation of cumulative incidence and cumulative incidence rates from incidence rates, consider the following incidence rates for colon cancer in Finland 1977–81.[3]

Table 9.1. Average annual incidence rates per
100 000 by sex and age group for colon cancer in
Finland 1977–81.[3]

Age group	Males	Females
0	0.0	0.0
1– 4	0.0	0.0
5– 9	0.0	0.1
10–14	0.4	0.3
15–19	0.2	0.9
20–24	0.9	1.7
25–29	0.8	1.6
30–34	1.9	1.9
35–39	3.0	4.0
40–44	4.2	7.6
45–49	7.8	8.6
50–54	14.4	13.3
55–59	21.8	20.8
60–64	38.0	31.9
65–69	46.9	48.8
70–74	82.6	77.1
75–79	105.1	107.1
80–84	127.8	171.7
85+	178.5	175.1

The crude incidence rate for men is 11.6 per 100 000 and for women it is 18.3 per 100 000. The cumulative incidence rate for males aged 0 to 74 is

$$(1 \times 0.0 + 4 \times 0.0 + \ldots + 5 \times 46.9 + 5 \times 82.6)/100\,000 = 0.0111.$$

Thus the cumulative incidence for men up to the age of 74 is:

$$1 - \exp(-0.0111) = 0.0110 = 1.1 \text{ per cent}$$

Similarly, for females the cumulative incidence rate is 0.0109 for ages 0–74 and the cumulative incidence is:

$$1 - \exp(-0.0109) = 0.0108 = 1.1 \text{ per cent}$$

Thus, the proportion of men or women in Finland developing cancer of the colon by the age of 74 is about 1 per cent, which can be interpreted as the average risk of a Finnish man or woman developing cancer of the colon by the age of 74.

Implicit in the interpretation of cumulative incidence is the assumption that individuals at risk of the disease in question are free from competing risks, i.e. risk of death from other causes. This is only true for all-cause mortality, otherwise the cumulative incidence is a hypothetical quantity. It can be adjusted to allow for deaths from other causes which would be more realistic. However, unadjusted values are more useful for comparisons of disease frequencies in different populations because they reflect incidence rates for the disease in question only and not differences in mortality rates due to other diseases.

9.3 STANDARDIZATION

Associations between diseases and their potential risk factors are frequently explored by comparing disease experiences amongst populations with differing levels of exposure to the risk factors or by investigating how changes in disease incidence over time relate to changes in exposure to the risk factors. The populations to be compared are likely to differ in many ways other than their exposure to the risk factors of interest, and these differences may affect their disease incidence. Two factors that often affect disease frequencies are age and sex. These factors, possibly with others, should be considered before comparing the disease frequencies.

A comparison of crude disease incidence rates does not allow for differences in the age and sex structures of populations. One way of comparing disease frequencies allowing for age and sex differences is to compare the age–sex-specific rates. This can be a difficult task when there are many populations to compare with many age strata, but modelling techniques have recently been devised for this purpose.[4] A more traditional approach is to form summary values from the disease rates for either sex in each population under consideration—this allows for differences in the age structures of the populations—or one value may be calculated for each population, which allows for differences in both the age and sex distributions. The method of standardization is employed to produce these values. Two types of standardization are most frequently used—direct and indirect. Indirect standardization has been in use for at least two-hundred years.[5] It was used to compare mortality in various occupations by William H. Farr in the 1855 annual report of the Registrar General of Great Britain. As methods of standardization have been developed through investigations into mortality, the following descriptions will be in terms of mortality data. The calculations are identical for incidence data. The examples presented address standardization, allowing for differences in age distributions, but can be extended to allow for other factors that may otherwise distort comparisons.

9.3.1 Direct Standardization

The approach of direct standardization is to apply the age-specific incidence or mortality rates of a population under consideration to a 'standard' population, i.e. a population with an age distribution considered to be a suitable basis for the comparisons. The age-specific rates are 'weighted' by the age distribution of the standard population to produce a standardized rate that is the crude rate that would be observed in the study population if it had the same age structure as the standard population. This rate is called the directly standardized rate. Such a rate may be calculated separately for each sex, or may have been standardized to allow for differences in both age and sex distributions.

Consider a population under investigation with rates calculated for J strata, i.e. J divisions of age, and possibly other factors such as sex. The mortality rate in the jth stratum is denoted by r_j, where r_j is equal to the number of deaths, d_j, in stratum j divided by the person-years or mid-year population, n_j. Let the standard population comprise a total of N person-years, or individuals with N_j in the jth stratum. Then the directly standardized rate is:

$$\sum_{j=1}^{J} \left(\frac{r_j \times N_j}{N} \right)$$

which is the sum over all J strata of the number of deaths that would be expected in the standard population during a specified period if it had the same age-specific mortality rates as the population of interest, divided by the total number of subjects in the standard population to produce a rate. The rates, r_j, are said to be weighted by the terms N_j/N.

Table 9.2 presents incidence rates of stomach cancer in men for Norway and Cali in Colombia and a world standard population on which to base comparisons.[3] Although the age-specific rates in Norway are lower than in Cali, the crude rate is higher because Norway has an older population (18.0% of men in Norway are aged 60 and over compared with 4.6% in Cali).

The directly standardized rate for Norway

$$= (12\,000 \times 0.0 + \ldots + 500 \times 274.6)/100\,000$$

$$= 18.1 \text{ per } 100\,000$$

The directly standardized rate for Cali

$$= (12\,000 \times 0.0 + \ldots 500 \times 613.6)/100\,000$$

$$= 48.3 \text{ per } 100\,000$$

Now as expected the standardized rate for Cali is higher than for Norway.

9.3.2 Indirect standardization

Indirect standardization involves the selection of a suitable 'standard' set of age-specific disease rates. These are applied to the age structure of the

Table 9.2. Average annual incidence rates of stomach cancer by age group in men from Norway and Cali (Colombia) plus a world standard population[3]

| Age group | World standard population | Stomach cancer rates per 100 000 | |
		Norway (1978–82)	Cali (1977–81)
0– 4	12 000	0.0	0.0
5– 9	10 000	0.0	0.0
10–14	9000	0.0	0.0
15–19	9000	0.0	0.0
20–24	8000	0.1	0.4
25–29	8000	0.5	2.5
30–34	6000	1.0	4.8
35–39	6000	2.9	7.8
40–44	6000	8.9	23.0
45–49	6000	12.3	29.2
50–54	5000	23.6	72.2
55–59	4000	35.8	139.9
60–64	4000	67.5	197.1
65–69	3000	101.4	291.7
70–74	2000	168.1	277.9
75–79	1000	220.1	595.1
80–84	500	251.3	750.5
85+	500	274.6	613.6
All ages	100 000	29.7	23.2

population of interest, producing the number of deaths from the disease that would be expected in the study population if it had the same age-specific mortality rates as the standard. The number of deaths actually observed in the study population is then compared with the expected number of deaths. These calculations may be performed separately for each sex, or can be used to standardize for both age and sex.

Consider a population under investigation with a total of n person-years, with n_j in the jth stratum of age and possibly other factors such as sex, and with J strata in total. Let the total number of deaths observed in this population be d. Denote the age-specific rate in the jth stratum of the standard population by R_j. Applying the standard rates to the population of interest gives the expected number of deaths

$$e = \sum_{j=1}^{J} (R_j \times n_j)$$

where the summation is over the J strata.

The ratio of observed to expected deaths d/e, usually multiplied by 100, is known as the standardized mortality ratio (SMR) (or standardized incidence ratio (SIR) with incidence data). It compares the true mortality of a population with the experience that would be expected if it had standard mortality rates. An SMR in excess of 100 indicates that mortality rates are higher in the study population than in the standard population. For example, if the age-specific mortality rates are all 50 per cent higher in the study population than in the standard, then the SMR of the study population will be 150.

The SMR may be multiplied by the crude death rate in the standard population to give an indirectly standardized rate.

The following example investigates whether mortality rates from acute myocardial infarction amongst men and women over the age of 25 in the metropolitan county of Greater Manchester were higher than in England and Wales as a whole for 1979 (Table 9.3).[6]

Table 9.3. Mortality from acute myocardial infarction for Manchester and for England and Wales (1979)[6]

| | Manchester | | | | England and Wales | |
| | Males | | Females | | Males | Females |
Age group	Deaths	Mid-year population ('000s)	Deaths	Mid-year population ('000s)	Death rate per million	Death rate per million
25–34	19	189.7	1	184.7	48	10
35–44	116	155.5	18	151.3	420	66
45–54	446	148.4	99	149.2	2118	383
55–64	1021	140.0	340	154.9	5524	1524
65–74	1587	102.4	921	140.7	12 009	4924
75–84	810	36.1	1064	78.1	20 962	11 578
85+	166	5.1	371	18.6	30 185	20 091
All ages	4165	777.2	2814	877.5		

The expected number of deaths among men in Manchester (if Manchester had the same death rates from myocardial infarction as the whole of England and Wales) would be:

$$(48 \times 189.7 + 420 \times 155.5 + \ldots + 30\,185 \times 5.1)/1000$$
$$= 3302$$

So the SMR for men $= 100 \times 4165/3302$
                      $= 126$

and the SMR for women $= 100 \times 2814/2276$
                      $= 124$

9.3.3 Comparison of direct and indirect standardization

Until recently, direct and indirect standardization have been thought of as quite distinct techniques, although they are part of the same general procedure.[7,8] In direct standardization, rates in the population under study are standardized to or weighted by the age distribution of a standard population. In indirect standardization, the rates in the standard population are standardized to or weighted by the age distribution of the study population.

Both methods of standardization require a standard population. This should be carefully chosen, as it greatly affects the results. Tables of European, African or World standard populations are published and these can be used for direct standardization.[3,9] Within a country, comparisons can be made by standardizing to the age distribution of that country or study area using census data. The standard rates used for the calculation of SMRs may be overall rates for the country or district within which comparisons are to be made, or the rates for one particular country or district against which the others are to be compared. When comparisons are made of mortality rates over time, it is usual to take the population distribution or rates of a particular year within the period under investigation as standard for direct or indirect standardization respectively. Standardized rates or ratios are then calculated for the remaining years.

Standardization is a quick and easy way of comparing disease frequencies but it is not without its drawbacks. When the number of deaths in certain strata of a population is small, the directly standardized rate becomes very unstable, such that small changes in the data can lead to large changes in the directly standardized rate. This is not the case with indirect standardization, which uses the total number of deaths in the population, but direct standardization uses the individual stratum deaths to produce stratum-specific rates. Thus, when certain strata have small numbers of deaths indirect standardization is preferable.

The SMR, although less variable than the directly standardized rate, may be misleading. Suppose that mortality rates in several different populations are to be compared. Then the same set of standard rates is weighted by the age structures of these populations to form an SMR for each one. However, each SMR is based on a different age distribution for each study population, so these SMRs are not comparable with each other. As a hypothetical example of this consider the situation in Table 9.4.

Table 9.4. Comparison of mortality rates in two hypothetical populations

Age group	Population 1			Population 2		
	Deaths	Person-years	Rate	Deaths	Person-years	Rate
25–44	240	8	30	75	3	25
45–64	45	1	45	120	3	40
65–84	200	1	200	720	4	180

Rates are per 10 000 and person-years are in 10 000s. The standard rates are 20, 40, and 80 per 10 000 for increasing age group.

For population 1 the SMR

$$= 100 \times 485/(20 \times 8 + 40 \times 1 + 80 \times 1)$$

$$= 173$$

For population 2 the SMR

$$= 100 \times 915/(20 \times 3 + 40 \times 3 + 80 \times 4)$$

$$= 183$$

While both SMRs correctly indicate that mortality in the study populations is higher than in the standard population, the SMR for population 2 is higher than that for population 1, although all the age-specific rates are lower. This situation arises because population 1 is much younger than population 2 and standardization has not fully accounted for this. Such an inconsistency would not arise if the age-specific rates for each study population were in constant proportion with those in the standard population for all age groups. The interpretation of the SMR is only valid if this is the case, whether comparing one population with a standard or with several other populations. Before calculating any SMRs, the age-specific rates should be inspected to check that this assumption holds.

In practice, direct and indirect standardization usually produce similar results; but it has been proposed that only direct standardization should be used for comparisons of more than two groups, and then only when numbers of deaths are reasonably large in all strata.[7] However, as long as the age-specific rates are checked for proportionality, indirect standardization is valid for comparisons of more than two populations and is preferable when numbers of deaths are small in some strata.

Finally, both direct and indirect standardization may obscure important differences that should be preserved. This is the result of producing one summary value from a set of rates. The specific rates should be inspected before summarizing them to make sure that standardization is sensible. If, for example, one population has mortality rates that exceed those in another population at younger ages, but are lower at older ages, then both direct and indirect standardization will obscure these differences and, according to the standard chosen, one population could appear to have either higher or lower mortality than the other. In such a case, methods of standardization should not be used, but modelling techniques that preserve these differences should be employed.

In conclusion, standardization techniques are useful for summarizing sets of rates, but before comparisons are made the stratum-specific rates should be inspected to check for inconsistencies. If there are any, standardization is not a suitable procedure and modelling techniques should be used.

9.4 PROPORTIONAL MORTALITY RATIOS

In some investigations into a disease and exposure of interest, data are only available in the form of numbers of deaths by age group for the disease in question and for all causes combined. No person-time or population data are available for the calculation of mortality rates. The approach in this situation is to investigate how the proportion of total deaths attributable to the disease in question varies between populations, and whether exposure to some potential risk factor may explain the variation. Age is likely to be an important factor in determining proportions of deaths attributable to certain diseases and it is usually necessary to standardize for this, and possibly other factors, before comparing different populations.

Suppose that, in a population of interest, there are d deaths due to the disease in question out of a total of t deaths. In the jth of J strata, there are t_j deaths from all causes. In a standard population in the jth stratum let there be D_j deaths due to the disease in question and T_j from all causes.

If the disease caused the same proportion of deaths in the study population as in the standard population, then the expected number of deaths due to the disease (out of the t_j deaths observed) in the jth stratum of the study population would be:

$$t_j \times D_j/T_j$$

Summing over strata gives an expected number of deaths due to disease in the population of interest.

$$\sum_{j=1}^{J} (t_j \times D_j/T_j)$$

In a similar way to the SMR, the proportional mortality ratio (PMR) compares the observed deaths due to the disease with the expected number. Thus:

$$PMR = \sum_{j=1}^{J} (d_j) \Big/ \sum_{j=1}^{J} (t_j \times D_j/T_j)$$

$$= d \Big/ \sum_{j=1}^{J} (t_j \times D_j/T_j)$$

The PMR is usually multiplied by 100, thus a PMR in excess of 100 indicates that the disease accounts for a greater proportion of total deaths in the study population than in the standard population.

Proportional mortality ratios are difficult to interpret. An increased ratio could be due to high mortality from the disease in question, or low mortality from another cause. For this reason, PMRs tend to be used only in early exploratory studies, although the results given by using PMRs are usually similar to those produced using SMRs.[10]

9.5 MEASURES OF EXPOSURE EFFECT

Measures of exposure effect are used to express the magnitude of the association between a disease and a suggested risk factor by comparing disease rates over different levels of exposure to the risk factor. In epidemiological studies, such comparisons are usually presented in the form of ratios such as the relative risk or the odds ratio. Under certain circumstances the absolute difference between rates may be more appropriate, this is known as the excess risk. The contribution of a dichotomous risk factor to the overall disease incidence in a population is assessed by the evaluation of the population attributable proportion. For risk factors with more than two levels, the preventable proportion can be calculated.

Confidence intervals can be calculated for each measure of exposure effect. These indicate the precision with which an exposure effect has been estimated. The width of the confidence interval depends on three things:[11] (i) the size of the study; (ii) the distribution of the exposure variable; and (iii) the level of confidence required. To assess the effect of a risk factor upon disease, both the magnitude of the effect and the confidence interval should be considered. Formulae are available for calculating confidence intervals for the measures of exposure effect to be discussed below.[12,13]

9.5.1 Relative risk

The relative rate, or rate ratio, associated with exposure to a risk factor is defined as the incidence rate of disease amongst exposed individuals divided by the incidence rate amongst individuals who are not exposed. As risks and cumulative rates are very similar for rare diseases, the relative rate is usually called the relative risk or risk ratio. Relative risks may be calculated for each stratum, such as age group and sex and, if they are stable over these strata, they can be combined into one summary figure.

To ascertain a relative risk, the exposure status of a group of individuals is determined and the subsequent disease experience amongst those individuals is then observed. From this, incidence rates amongst exposed and non-exposed individuals can be calculated and the relative risk can be derived. For a continuous exposure, such as a nutrient intake, a common approach is to divide the distribution of the exposure into intervals and assess risks relative to that in one such interval (often the highest or lowest). An example from a cohort study investigating the relationship between serum cholesterol and cancer is given in Table 9.5.[14]

Table 9.5. Relative risks of cancer by fifths of serum cholesterol in women[14]

Cancer	Number	Serum cholesterol (mg/dl)				
		<185	185–207	208–228	229–255	>255
Breast	1088	1.03	1.00	0.92	1.01	1.00
Uterus	448	1.13	0.94	0.99	1.10	1.00
Cervix	455	1.66	1.35	1.23	1.45	1.00
Colon	339	1.16	0.80	0.68	0.82	1.00

9.5.2 The odds ratio

In general, if there is a probability, p, attached to the occurrence of a particular event within a certain time interval, then the odds of that event occurring in the time interval are:

$$p / (1 - p)$$

For a risk factor with two levels, if the risk of disease is p_1 for one level over a given period, and p_2 for the other level over the same period, then the odds of disease are $p_1/(1-p_1)$ for level 1 and $p_2/(1-p_2)$ for level 2. The odds ratio for level 1 compared with level 2 is thus:

$$\frac{p_1/(1-p_1)}{p_2/(1-p_2)} = \frac{p_1(1-p_2)}{p_2(1-p_1)}$$

The odds ratio is the measure of exposure effect used in case-control studies. In such studies, the risk of individuals developing disease cannot be estimated because different proportions of diseased and disease-free subjects are sampled from the population of interest for study as cases and controls. For example, with a rare disease, all new cases of disease arising in a certain population during some interval of time may be selected for study as cases, but only a small proportion of healthy individuals will be selected as controls. For a more common disease, only a proportion of diseased individuals may be selected and another proportion of healthy individuals sampled. The cases can be compared with controls as regards exposure, but the incidence of disease amongst exposed and unexposed persons cannot be calculated for the determination of relative risk because the same sampling fraction has not been applied for selection of cases and controls from the population.

The probability that a diseased person was exposed to a risk factor and that a disease-free person was exposed to the risk factor can be ascertained in a case-control study, and so the odds of exposure for cases and controls can be calculated. If cases are representative of the diseased population and controls of the non-diseased population in terms of exposure, then the odds of exposure in cases divided by the odds of exposure in controls is equal to the odds ratio for disease in exposed versus unexposed individuals. If cases and controls are sampled differentially according to their exposure then the above will not be true and bias is introduced.

For rare diseases and short time intervals, in which the cumulative incidence of disease is small, the odds of disease are approximately equal to the risks of disease because:

$$p_1 / (1 - p_1) \approx p_1$$
$$\text{and} \quad p_2 / (1 - p_2) \approx p_2 \text{ for small } p_1 \text{ and } p_2$$

In this situation, the odds ratio is approximately equal to the relative risk (which is easier to interpret). Thus, in case-control studies, the odds ratio is often called the relative risk, although neither disease incidence rates nor the true relative risk can be calculated, only the odds ratio which approximates the relative risk for rare diseases.

As an example of the calculation of an odds ratio in the simplest situation with a dichotomous exposure, consider Table 9.6:

Table 9.6. Calculation of an odds ratio with dichotomous exposure

	Exposed	Unexposed	
Diseased	150(a)	150(b)	300
Disease-free	200(c)	400(d)	600
	350	550	900

The probability that a diseased person is exposed

$$= 150/300 = 0.5$$

The odds that a diseased person is exposed

$$= 0.5/(1 - 0.5) = 1.0$$

The probability that a disease-free person is exposed

$$= 200/600 = 1/3$$

The odds that a disease-free person is exposed

$$= (1/3)/(2/3) = 2.0$$

Therefore, the odds ratio for exposure in diseased relative to disease-free subjects = 2.0, which is the same as the odds ratio for disease in exposed versus unexposed individuals.

It can be shown that the odds ratio in a table such as the one above is calculated using the formula:

$$\text{Odds ratio} = \frac{a \times d}{b \times c}$$

As with relative risks, odds ratios can be calculated for exposure variables with several categories by designating one of the categories to be a baseline with which the others are compared.[13]

9.5.3 Excess risk

The excess risk, also known as the attributable risk or the rate (or risk) difference, is the difference between the incidence rate of a disease in exposed persons and the incidence rate in unexposed persons. Excess risks may be calculated separately for each stratum and combined if they have similar values.

Both the relative risk and the excess risk are used by epidemiologists to summarize the changes in incidence rates over differing levels of exposure to potential risk factors. The relative risk is used more frequently in aetiological studies because the ratio of rates over several age groups, time-periods, or populations tends to be more stable than the difference.[15] Situations in which the relative risk is not stable over strata can often be explained by consideration of the biological mechanisms of the disease.

The relative risk is the better measure for assessing the strength of an association, as the larger the relative risk, the less likely it is that the association observed between exposure and disease is due to bias.[16] This is not necessarily true with the excess risk. The relative risk also has the advantage of being approximated by the odds ratio, which can be estimated in case-control studies, while the excess risk cannot. For these reasons, the relative risk is a more suitable summary measure of exposure effect than the excess risk in many epidemiological studies.

The excess risk is the more useful measure in policy making. A risk factor will cause more cases of disease for a common disease than a rare disease if the relative risks are the same for the two diseases. The excess risk would show this effect and indicate where preventive measures could produce the greater impact.

9.5.4 Attributable proportion

Once an association has been established between a risk factor and a disease, and is believed to be causal, then the impact of that risk factor on a population can be evaluated by calculating the attributable proportion. The attributable proportion measures the proportion of the disease in a population that is caused by a risk factor, and can be used to estimate the potential effect of eliminating exposure to the risk factor on the disease incidence.

If exposure to a risk factor is rare, then even if it has a large effect on disease risk, its impact on a population will be small. Disease incidence might be more effectively lowered by reducing exposure to a factor that carried smaller risks but was more widespread.

Let I_0 and I_1 denote the disease incidence rates for unexposed and exposed individuals respectively, and suppose that a proportion, p, of a population is exposed. The relative risk, r, due to exposure is:

$$I_1/I_0$$

The proportion of disease among exposed individuals caused by their exposure to the risk factor is:

$$\frac{I_1 - I_0}{I_0} = \frac{r-1}{r}$$

known as the attributable proportion in exposed persons.[17]

In an entire population of exposed and unexposed individuals the proportion of disease due to exposure is:

$$\frac{p(I_1 - I_0)}{(1-p)I_0 + pI_1} = \frac{p(r-1)}{1 + p(r-1)}$$

known as the population attributable proportion, the population attributable risk, or the aetiologic fraction.[18] This term may be multiplied by 100 and called the population attributable risk per cent. The numerator of the population attributable proportion is the reduction of disease incidence in the total population that would occur if the entire population was to become unexposed to the risk factor. This is divided by the total disease incidence of both exposed and unexposed individuals.

The above expression can be calculated from a case-control study if the disease is rare, so that the odds ratio approximates the relative risk and if the proportion of controls exposed is likely to be the same as in the general population. Alternatively, if p_c is the proportion of cases exposed, and the disease is rare, then the expression

$$\text{Population attributable proportion} = p_c \, (r - 1)/r$$

can be used.

It is unfortunate that there is no consensus on the nomenclature for either the excess risk or the population attributable proportion. In particular, the term attributable risk is used to refer to both the excess risk and the population attributable proportion. It seems best that the terms 'attributable proportion in exposed persons' and 'population attributable proportion' are used as defined here. Where excess risk is used it should be accompanied by a brief definition for clarity.

9.5.5 Preventable proportion

In studies of nutrition, the attributable proportion is not usually appropriate for assessing the effect of a nutrient on disease incidence in a population because it requires the use of a dichotomous risk factor. A more suitable measure is the preventable proportion, which considers risk factors with more than two levels of exposure and measures the proportion of disease that could be prevented by a shift in the distribution of the variable.[19]

Suppose there are $(K + 1)$ possible levels of exposure to a risk factor for some value K, or that the distribution of a continuous variable has been subdivided into $(K + 1)$ levels. Let the proportions exposed to each level be $p_0, p_1, \ldots, p_K$ and the corresponding relative risks be $r_0 = 1.0, r_1, \ldots, r_K$. If a shift in the distribution occurs such that the proportions exposed to each level are $p_0^*, p_1^*, \ldots, p_K^*$, then the proportion of disease prevented by such a shift, known as the preventable proportion (PP), is:

$$PP = \frac{\sum_{i=0}^{K} p_i r_i - \sum_{i=0}^{K} p_i^* r_i}{\sum_{i=0}^{K} p_i r_i}$$

Note that this expression is identical to the population attributable proportion when the risk factor has two levels (i.e. $K = 1$).

As an example, consider the relationship betweeen dietary calcium intake and hip fracture in Hong Kong (Table 9.7).[20]

Table 9.7. The relationship between dietary calcium intake and hip fracture in Hong Kong[20]

Sex	Calcium intake (mg/day)	Number of controls	Relative risk
Female	<75	137	1.9
	75–82	72	1.9
	83–128	105	1.1
	129–243	126	1.2
	≥244	120	1.0
Male	<75	67	2.1
	75–82	30	1.4
	83–128	44	1.7
	129–243	40	1.5
	≥244	59	1.0

Assuming that the distribution of calcium intakes in the controls is the same as in the Hong Kong population, then for women $p_0 = 0.21$, $p_1 = 0.23$, $p_2 = 0.19$, $p_3 = 0.13$ and $p_4 = 0.24$, with corresponding risks of 1.0, 1.2, 1.1, 1.9, and 1.9. If a general shift in dietary calcium intakes were to occur such that, for each category below the highest, all the individuals move up to the next category (100 per cent shift) so $p_0^* = 0.44$, $p_1^* = 0.19$, $p_2^* = 0.13$, $p_3^* = 0.24$ and $p_4^* = 0$, then PP $= (1.40 - 1.27)/1.40 = 9.3$ per cent. Similarly in men PP $= 17.7$ per cent.

For a shift such that 50 per cent of individuals move up to the next category of intake (50 per cent shift), in women PP $= 4.6$ per cent and in men PP $= 8.9$ per cent.

Thus, a 100 per cent shift in dietary calcium intakes in Hong Kong would prevent almost 10 per cent of hip fractures in women and 18 per cent in men and a 50 per cent shift would prevent 5 per cent of hip fractures in women and 9 per cent in men.

Preventable proportions can be calculated according to several possible shifts in order to ascertain a range of preventable proportions that could be produced by various changes in nutrient intake distributions.

REFERENCES

1. Elandt-Johnson, R. (1975). Definition of rates: some remarks on their use and misuse. *Am. J. Epid.* **102**: 267–71.

2. Day, N. (1976). A new measure of age standardized incidence, the cumulative rate. In Waterhouse, J. A. H., Muir, C. S., Correa, P., and Powell, J. (eds). *Cancer incidence in five continents*, Vol. III, pp. 443–52. International Agency for Research on Cancer (IARC Scientific Publications No. 15), Lyons.

3. Muir, C. S., Waterhouse, J. A. H., Mack, T., Powell, J., Whelan, S., Smans, M., and Casset, F. (eds). (1987). *Cancer incidence in five continents*, Vol. V. International Agency for Research on Cancer (IARC Scientific Publications No. 88), Lyons.

4. Breslow, N. E. and Day, N. E. (1987). Fitting models to grouped data. In Breslow, N. E. and Day, N. E. (eds.). *Statistical methods in cancer research*, Vol. II, The design and analysis of cohort studies, pp. 120–76. International Agency for Research on Cancer (IARC Scientific Publications No. 83), Lyons.

5. Keiding, N. (1987). The method of expected number of deaths, 1786–1886–1986. *Int. Stat. Rev.* **55**: 1–20.

6. Office of Population Censuses and Surveys. (1981). 1979 Mortality Statistics: England and Wales area. Series DH5, No. 6. Government Statistical Service, London.

7. Rothman, K. J. (1986). Standardization of rates. In Rothman, K. J. (ed.). *Modern Epidemiology*, pp. 41–9. Little, Brown and Company. Boston.

8. Chan, C. K., Feinstein, A. R., Jekel, J. F., and Wells, C. K. (1988). The value and hazards of standardization in clinical epidemiologic research. *J. Clin. Epid.*, **41**: 1125–34.

9. Waterhouse, J. A. H., Muir, C. S., Correa, P., and Powell, J. (eds). (1986). *Cancer Incidence in Five Continents*, Vol. III. International Agency for Research on Cancer, (IARC Scientific Publications No. 15), Lyons.

10. Roman, E., Beral, V., Inskip, H., McDowall, M., and Adelstein, A. (1984). A comparison of standardized and proportional mortality ratios. *Stat. Med.*, **3**: 7–14.

11. Gardner, M. J. and Altman, D. G. (1986). Confidence intervals rather than *P* values: estimation rather than hypothesis testing. *Br. Med. J.*, **292**: 746–50.

12. Morris, J. A. and Gardner, M. J. (1988). Calculating confidence intervals for relative risks (odds ratios) and standardised ratios and rates. *Br. Med. J.*, **296**: 1313–16.

13. Breslow, N. E. and Day, N. E. (1980). Classical methods of analysis of grouped data. In Breslow, N. E. and Day, N. E. (eds). *Statistical methods in cancer research*, Vol. I. The analysis of case-control studies, pp. 122–59. International Agency for Research on Cancer, (IARC Scientific Publications No. 32), Lyons.

14. Hiatt, R. A. and Fireman, B. H. (1986). Serum cholesterol and incidence of cancer in a large cohort. *J. Chron. Dis.*, **39**: 861–70.

15. Breslow, N. E. and Day, N. E. (1980). Fundamental measures of disease occurrence and association. In Breslow, N. E. and Day, N. E. (eds). *Statistical methods in cancer research*, Vol. I, The analysis of case-control studies. pp. 42–81. International Agency for Research on Cancer, (IARC Scientific Publications No. 32), Lyons.

16. Cornfield, J., Haenszel, W., Hammond, E. C., Lilienfield, A. M., Shimkin,

M. B., and Wynder, E. L. (1959). Smoking and lung cancer: recent evidence and a discussion of some questions. *JNCI.*, **22:** 173–203.

17. Cole, P. and MacMahon, B. (1971). Attributable risk percent in case-control studies. *Br. J. Prev. Soc. Med.*, **25:** 242–4.

18. Levin, M. L. (1953). The occurrence of lung cancer in man. *Acta Unio. Int. Cancer*, **9:** 105–15.

19. Wahrendorf, J. (1987). An estimate of the proportion of colorectal and stomach cancers which might be prevented by certain changes in dietary habits. *Int. J. Cancer*, **40:** 625–8.

20. Lau, E., Donnan, S., Barker, D. J. P., and Cooper, C. (1988). Physical activity and calcium intake in fracture of the proximal femur in Hong Kong. *Br. Med. J.*, **297:** 1441–3.

PART C

The design of nutritional epidemiological studies

10. Ecological studies

Janet E. Hiller and A. J. McMichael

10.1 INTRODUCTION

In ecological studies of the association between nutrition and disease, population or group indices of dietary intake or nutritional status are related to population or group indices of health status. The unit of analysis is not an individual but a group defined by time (calendar period, birth cohort), geography (country, province, or city), or by sociodemographic characteristics (e.g. ethnicity, religion, or socio-economic status).

Ecological studies are frequently the first stage in constructing an epidemiological picture of the differential distribution of diseases among people with different risk profiles. Variation in disease risk between different categories of persons can indicate differences in genetic composition, differences in environmental exposures (for example, diet), or differences in genes and environment. Ecological studies of migrant populations have been widely used to partition causation between genetic and environmental factors.

In nutritional epidemiology, ecological studies have predominantly examined geographic relationships of indices of nutritional status and health. An important example is the early series of ecological observations, suggesting the importance of blood cholesterol and dietary fats in the aetiology of coronary heart disease,[1] and showing the association between plasma cholesterol, dietary intake of saturated fats, and coronary heart disease rates. These comparisons usually take advantage of routinely collected data and are therefore considered relatively inexpensive.

Similar techniques can be used to investigate correlations over time. For instance, the age-standardized mortality rate from coronary heart disease which has decreased in the United States since the mid-1960s, has been linked to the increase in the per capita alcohol consumption over the same period (Fig. 10.1).[2]

Using what was essentially a cross-sectional analysis, Gregor also demonstrated that as per capita food intake increases over time, mortality rates for intestinal cancers also increase, while those for gastric cancers decrease.[3] Even more information may be obtained by simultaneously examining variations in both space and time, as shown by Dwyer and

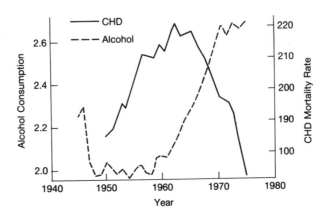

Fig. 10.1. Time trends in the age-standardized coronary heart disease (CHD) mortality rate (per 10^5 population) and per capita alcohol consumption (gal/yr), US, 1945–1975. Source: Kuller et al.[2]

Hetzel[4] in their examination of time trends in coronary heart disease mortality in three countries in relation to changes in major risk factors.

Ecological analyses are only of value when the groups or communities being compared are relatively heterogeneous in the exposure of interest, in this case, dietary variables. For this reason, they have been used most extensively for intercountry rather than intracountry comparisons. For example, although extensive maps, indicating regional differences in disease incidence,[5] are available for the United States, regional variations in most components of dietary intake in that country are limited. It has been estimated that 90 per cent of adults in the United States eat between 30 per cent and 44 per cent of their calories in fat, while, world-wide, 90 per cent of adults eat between 11 per cent and 42 per cent of their calories as fat.[6] Thus, ecological analyses are of relatively limited value in examining the association between dietary fat and disease in the USA.

The same limitation applies to most other Western countries. However, Joosens[7] has carried out population-based work in Belgium, examining the relationship of differences in saturated fat intake to the health status of the Flemish and Francophone populations. The French-speaking southern region of Belgium has had higher rates of coronary heart disease, in tandem with higher estimates of mean serum cholesterol and increased dietary fat consumption, relative to the northern Dutch-speaking population.

China offers a particular opportunity for the application of ecological techniques in the examination of the association between diet and disease because there are wide variations in disease rates from one region to another, accompanying substantial differences in culture, behaviour and life-style. For example, the geographic variation in incidence of nasopharyngeal cancer within China (which has the highest rates in the world in the southern provinces, while lower rates occur in the northern regions), has led to speculation about the role of differential patterns of dietary intake of salted fish or of an interaction between the Epstein–Barr virus, fatty acids, and croton oil—a plant-derived cancer promoter that is used in Chinese herbal drugs in southern China.[8]

The ecological approach is necessarily limited because of the inability to determine whether the index of dietary intake of interest is actually associated with health status at the level of the individual. The 'ecological fallacy' is a term applied to errors of inference that may result from making inferences about exposure–effect relationships at the level of individuals on the basis of relationships observed at the group level.[9] In addition, data about factors that are potential confounders are usually not available at the group level.

Nevertheless, ecological studies frequently provide a useful first look at relationships. When used in a frankly exploratory context, (for example, the study by Armstrong and Doll[10] on international variations in cancer incidence and mortality), they may suggest new hypotheses worthy of further study. Further, they are frequently the only research method of value in the investigation of the association between various aspects of diet and disease risk, either because exposure (i.e. dietary) data are not available at the individual level (for example, fluoride in drinking water), or because intrapopulation variations in exposure may be insufficient to be reflected in intrapopulation variations in disease risk.[11]

10.2 INDICES OF DIETARY INTAKE

10.2.1 Average consumption

Estimates of average individual intake can be made from pre-existing (usually commercially-oriented) data or from population survey data collected *de novo*.[12]

National food supply or food 'disappearance' statistics The Food and Agricultural Organization (FAO) publishes annual estimates of the food available per person on a daily basis. The FAO Production Year Book lists calories available per capita per day for a variety of foods, e.g. milk, meat, fats.[13] These 'food disappearance' statistics are calculated by estimating the quantity of food produced in a given country, added to the quantity of food imported, and subtracting the food exported, lost in storage, fed to animals or used for non-dietary purposes. The resulting figure is converted to an estimate of per capita consumption by dividing by the total population. These data tend to reflect food purchasing (that is, food 'availability')

Table 10.1. Estimates of per capita consumption

Parts of the food chain surveyed	Type of data published	Scope and limitations of survey data
National food supply	Food balance data collected by agriculture ministries, collated by FAO	Allows for home production, imports and exports, changing food stocks
Market distribution	Industrial data	Limited to specific sectors
Household budget	Economic statistics	Limited to financial outlay of whole households on food: costs do not relate to nutritional value of purchases
Household consumption	Household food survey	Often fails to allow for food eaten elsewhere; food waste assumed
Individual nutrition	Individual food and nutrition intake	Numerous methods available of varying reliability

From James *et al. Healthy Nutrition.*[12]

patterns rather than actual dietary intake and they are, therefore, a reflection of food wastage as well as of food consumption.

National governmental agencies tend to collate similar data, and make similar estimates of per capita 'food disappearance'. For example, in Australia,[14] national surveys of food consumption have been completed—again concentrating on purchases rather than intake *per se*—providing a national database estimating food 'disappearance'. Such surveys provide crude estimates of average national consumption; there is seldom sufficient information to estimate consumption for subgroups, such as people of a given age or gender.

Despite these shortcomings, national food 'consumption' statistics have proved useful in preliminary examinations of hypotheses. Dwyer and Hetzel[4] used these types of data in their examination of the time trends in ischaemic heart disease mortality and its major risk factors in Australia, the United Kingdom, and the USA. They inferred that the absence of a decline in mortality in the 1970s in the United Kingdom—in contrast with the marked declines in Australia and the USA—reflected the lack of change in national indicators of a number of risk factors, including per capita consumption of dietary fat based on national food disappearance data. Between-country comparisons that include both rich and poor nations may, however, be subject to biases in the quality of data collected at national levels.

Household or population survey data National population surveys have been used to collect more detailed dietary information on subgroups of the population. Presuming appropriate sampling techniques have been used, these data are then extrapolated to the general population. In Australia, detailed 24-hour dietary data have been collected on samples of the population as part of cross-sectional studies of changes in risk factors for coronary heart disease undertaken by the National Heart Foundation.[15] It has been argued that 24-hour recalls are only suitable for ecological studies, such as those being described in this chapter, and not for individual-based investigations of the association between disease and diet. The wide daily variation in an individual's diet (especially in micronutrients) renders a 24-hour recall more subject to error in estimating that individual's intake than is an instrument based on usual consumption of foods.[16] On the other hand, 24-hour dietary data may provide a reasonable estimate of the diet of a given population, enabling comparisons to be made with other populations.

The National Food Survey, in Great Britain, records food purchases over a 7-day period for a sample of 7500 households, although data are only available on a household basis and are not analysed by age or gender categories,[17] limiting their usefulness in examining associations with age- or gender-specific disease rates. Methods to overcome these limitations are discussed in Chapter 5.

On other occasions, small-area data collected on individuals (e.g. dietary histories from a sample of the population in a given town) are presumed to typify intake in the area or region as a whole. These data are often collected in the form of household food inventories in which food intake for a given time period is estimated by trained field-workers who visit the participating households. Average per capita intake is calculated by dividing the total household intake by the number of individual family members. Inferences are then drawn about the effect of regional differences in dietary intake on regional differences in indices of health status.

When analysing the health status of different subgroups in the population, indirect methods of estimating per capita consumption derived from aggregate data for the population as a whole must be interpreted with caution. In particular, associations between age- or gender-specific disease rates and per capita dietary consumption (for example, examining the correlation between national death rates from breast cancer in women and per capita consumption of dietary fat) presume that dietary patterns are relatively constant in all population subgroups. However, population-based dietary information is seldom published in disaggregated form that would enable the calculation of average dietary intake in these specific population subgroups. The United States Health and Nutrition Survey (HANES) is an exception, in that the surveys are designed so that intake can be estimated for various age-, gender- and ethnic-group-specific populations.

10.2.2 National indirect indicators of consumption

In the absence of the above mentioned types of more direct measures of dietary consumption, various indirect markers have been used. For example, sales or tax records have been used to estimate per capita consumption of alcohol. Such an indicator was used to examine the relationship of laryngeal cancer mortality time trends to those of alcohol consumption in the UK and Australia.[18]

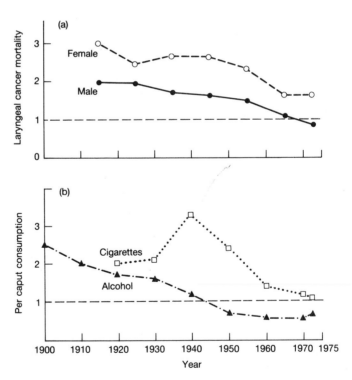

Fig. 10.2. Time trends in ratios of British versus Australian age-standardized laryngeal cancer mortality, by sex; and of British versus Australian consumption of alcohol and cigarettes. Source: McMichael.[18]

Estimates of alcohol consumption derived from 1960 tax receipts, for the various states within the USA, have been correlated with average age-adjusted cancer mortality rates for 1950–67.[19] However, this method may either under-estimate true intake because estimates of consumption do not include illegally purchased alcohol, exempt beverages, and home-brew, or it may overestimate intake by not accounting for wastage. However, if this type of unmeasured alcohol intake is a relatively constant proportion of all alcohol intake between the compared populations or time periods, then variations in the population marker of consumption may be a reliable indicator of changes in average individual consumption.

Another example of an indirect indicator of consumption is that of applying estimates from a source population to some derivative (presumably representative) subpopulation. For example, in comparing disease rates among migrant groups in Australia, the typical diet in the country of birth (derived from Food and Agricultural Organization data) was used as an indicator of the likely diet of those groups upon arrival in Australia.[20] Differences in mortality from cancer of the large bowel between migrants to Australia from the United Kingdom/Ireland and those from Southern Europe, within specified time intervals after arrival in Australia, were then correlated with the typical, per capita saturated fat and fibre consumption in the country of origin. Caution is needed in such an analysis because of the lack of information about post-migration secular trends in patterns of dietary behaviour.

10.2.3 'Macroscopic' generalization

Occasionally, statements are made about dietary patterns in populations, based on observations of subgroups that have not been specifically sampled for the purpose. Thus, generalizations about dietary intake in the population are global statements not founded in sampling procedures. A well known instance of this reasoning is the work of Burkitt and Trowell.[21] Stimulated by the large differences in disease profiles between eastern African and Western populations, they made casual observations about the traditional African diet replete with high fibre, unprocessed foods; they presumed that this diet typified that of all non-urbanized Africans. They then inferred that this dietary fibre was the crucial factor protecting African populations from the prevalent chronic diseases of Western countries, where fibre formed a much less significant component of the typical diet.

10.2.4 Average food/soil concentrations of micronutrients

The intake of various micronutrients may be inferred from known deficiencies or excesses in the food or soil of a particular region. This estimate of intake is particularly appropriate when most food sources for a region are local. In the event of importation of food from outside the local area, estimates of dietary intake derived from food or soil concentrations are likely to be misleading.

For example, the prevalence of goitre in Tasmania, an Australian island State with large areas of iodine deficiency, was demonstrated to have fallen in parallel with the introduction of dietary iodine supplementation, iodization of bread, and the growth in the importation of food from the Australian mainland.[22] Other health status indicators that varied in conjunction with the iodine supplementation programme were thyrotoxicosis, which temporarily increased, and stillbirths and infant deaths due to congenital anomalies, which decreased.

In China, ecological analyses have demonstrated that areas with low soil levels of molybdenum (and low nitrate uptake) have higher rates of oesophageal cancer.[23] In addition, molybdenum levels analysed in hair samples were low in the high risk regions. Soil supplementation programmes in areas of China at high risk have been noted to increase the molybdenum level of vegetables and to decrease their nitrate levels.[24] Thus, these analyses have correlated disease rates with the soil and food deficiencies and have also been able to demonstrate that changes in molybdenum content of locally grown foodstuffs occurred with supplementation programmes.

Concentrations of micronutrients can be influenced by changes in production processes. Changes in flour milling procedures during the Second World War, increased the amount of fibre in flour.[25] This change correlated with reduced mortality from colon cancer in affected countries some 15 years after this dietary change (although the confounding effect of other wartime dietary changes was not excluded in the analysis).

The concentration of chromium and other trace elements in drinking water has been linked with cardiovascular disease rates[26] in ecological studies that are inter- and intracountry. The analysis of the effect of drinking water quality on health is one that lends itself to ecological studies. In most communities, it is unlikely that drinking water to individual households would be supplied from a variety of sources (unlike London in the days of John Snow). Thus, any potential effect would need to be estimated by comparisons among communities with different water sources. The British Water Research Centre collected data on drinking water, in England, Wales, and Scotland by visiting divisions and contacting all relevant water authorities and companies to estimate the average concentrations of approximately 40 different constituents.[27] This study succeeded in estimating both water content and disease rates at the town level. Some socio-economic and environmental measures were also available for the same unit of analysis and therefore could be used in multivariable analyses to adjust for counfounding.

10.2.5 Average food/water concentrations of toxins

Variation in the amount of toxins in the local diet can be correlated with variations in disease occurrence in a group of communities. Again, such an analysis is only valuable in communities that do not consume foodstuffs that are grown elsewhere in any significant quantity. Investigations of dietary causes of liver cancer have correlated the aflatoxin contamination of peanuts with liver cancer rates in east Africa.[18] A similar effect has been noted in reports of N-nitroso compounds in maize beer consumed by African groups with high incidence of oesophageal cancer.[29] The motoneuron disease, lytico, that occurs commonly in Guam, has been associated with the consumption of the cycad, a palm-like plant that is the source of edible starch.[30] These plants contain a non-protein amino acid (BMAA) that, in monkeys, has been found to cause a motor neurone disease that resembles the Guam disorder.

10.2.6 Biological indices of dietary intake or nutritional status

Biological indices have not been widely used in ecological studies, in part because of the time and expense involved in collecting and analysing these data and, in part, because of our limited understanding of those specific aspects of the metabolism of dietary components that relate to disease aetiology. Further, because current disease rates presumably reflect environmental exposures in the past, the biological specimen will have maximum validity if it is an indicator of past consumption. Despite these limitations, the analysis of blood, urine, faeces, saliva, and even toe-nail clippings, has provided useful information about presumed dietary intake of a range of foods. In particular, these biological specimens appear to provide useful measures of micronutrient intake, estimates of which are probably less readily available from questionnaire data than are estimates of fat, protein, or carbohydrate intake.[31]

Since some disturbances of biological indices may reflect an aspect of the disease process itself, and not merely the causal pathway, ecological studies have one advantage over case-control studies in the interpretability of biological indices. In cases with disease, an abnormal profile of biological indices may reflect disease-induced metabolic derangements, or an abnormal exposure history. In ecological studies, using samples of predominantly healthy persons, no such ambiguity exists.

Blood   A study commencing in 1965 tracked changes in blood cholesterol in Japanese males residing in Japan, Honolulu, and California.[32] There was a gradient in serum cholesterol levels; the highest average level, in San Francisco, was 21 per cent higher than Japanese levels, while in Hawaii cholesterol was 12 per cent higher than in Japan. Coronary heart disease mortality rates followed a similar gradient, with San Francisco and Hawaiian rates being 2.8 and 2.7 times higher, respectively, than the Japanese rates. This combination of cross-sectional studies provided data that supported hypotheses concerning dietary differences among the communities being studied.

Urine   International differences in 24-hour urinary excretion of sodium have been related to average blood pressure levels as support for the dietary salt/hypertension hypothesis.[33,34]

It has been presumed that the international differences in breast cancer rates associated with differences in dietary fat intake, are mediated by hormone levels. Various investigators have measured urinary oestrogens in national groups at different risk of breast cancer, to refine the hypotheses regarding dietary fat and disease levels. However, these studies have yielded contradictory findings.[35]

Faeces   Examination of faeces has provided an indication of differences in dietary fibre intake between people experiencing different rates of a variety of diseases. In a series of studies sponsored by the International Agency for Research on Cancer (WHO), fibre consumption was compared in populations with differences in colorectal cancer incidence. In these Scandinavian-based studies, faecal chemistry, bacteria, and bulk were examined, as well as estimated average population intakes of dietary fibre.[36,37,38]

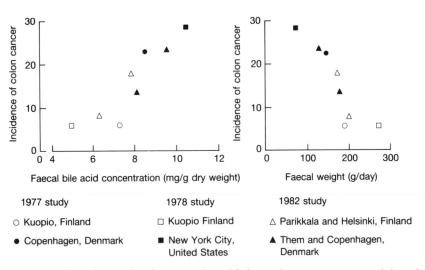

1977 study	1978 study	1982 study
○ Kuopio, Finland	□ Kuopio Finland	△ Parikkala and Helsinki, Finland
● Copenhagen, Denmark	■ New York City, United States	▲ Them and Copenhagen, Denmark

Fig. 10.3. The relationship between faecal bile acid concentration and faecal weight and the incidence of colon cancer in three studies, made in 1977, 1978, and 1982. Source: Muir.[38]

In examining causes of differences in colon cancer incidence between Northern and Southern India, Malhotra,[39] reported that the stools of Indians from the North, where colon cancer rates were low, contained more vegetable fibres than the stools of Indians from the south where colon cancer rates were higher. This finding was in agreement with what was already known about the typical diet of these two regions.

Toe-nails Analyses of the selenium content of toe-nail clippings have been used to assess selenium intake in different areas of the world. These specimens have the advantage of reflecting dietary intake over the previous year, are relatively protected and do not have the same storage and collection problems as sera or urine. Morris et al.[40] demonstrated that the analysis of toe-nail clippings collected from geographic areas with known differences in selenium intake reflected those dietary differences. However, given the vigorous physical and chemical cleaning procedures required prior to assay, only those trace elements tightly bound to the keratin molecular matrix (e.g. selenium) can be validly measured. Zinc, which is less tightly bound, appears to be a less valid assay via this method.

Saliva Geographic differences in stomach cancer in Great Britain have been hypothesized to be related to differences in nitrate levels. However, it has been reported[41] that preliminary attempts to clarify this association by examining nitrate levels in saliva in low and high stomach cancer incidence areas were not confirmatory.

10.2.7 Collection and analytical methods

The determination of mean values for indicators of dietary intake could theoretically involve the handling and analysis of many separate food samples or biological specimens from a particular geographic region. A less expensive approach is to use pooled samples to derive estimates of intake for each geographic region. This approach necessarily forfeits information about the underlying distribution among individual study subjects, and precludes calculation of standard deviations and standard errors. It also assumes that the pooled mean reflects the averages of the individual values of the specimens contributing to the pool.

For example, blood samples were collected from subjects residing in a variety of locations in the United States. These samples were pooled to determine mean zinc and copper concentrations for those sites. These values, in turn, were correlated with mortality rates from a range of cancers; the areas with high disease rates had high mean measures of zinc.[42]

A large ecological study of associations between diet, lifestyle, and disease[43] used pooled biological samples, instead of individual samples, to derive estimates of nutrient intake for given communes in China. This approach increased the size of the biological sample, enabling the investigation of a wider range of indices, and provided a substantial cost-saving (again permitting the investigation of more markers). Instead of analysing 50 individual samples to get an estimate for a given commune, far fewer analyses were necessary. Blood and urine specimens were combined into either gender-specific pools or age–gender-specific pools for each commune and then analysed. In the China study, the above-mentioned assumption about the pooled mean and mean of the component specimens were calculated and compared. Validation assays were conducted on a random subsample of 150 individual specimens, which were then placed into six pools of 25 specimens. The results of these assays indicated good agreement between the mean of the individual assays and the value derived from analysis of the pooled specimens.

An additional disadvantage is incurred if there is a non-linear association between the dietary component being estimated and disease risk. In such circumstances, pooled estimates of intake would not correlate with disease rates and the true association would be obscured. A further problem occurs if the intention is to use a standardized value (e.g. urine metabolite from casual specimens expressed per mg creatinine). Differences between groups may be obscured if there is large variation in the concentration of the standard between individual specimens (i.e. the denominator), which is not taken into account.

10.3 INDICES OF HEALTH STATUS

10.3.1 Routine measures of mortality and morbidity

Some of these measures have been alluded to in the section on indices of nutritional status. The measures of mortality or morbidity most frequently used in ecological studies include international, national, and small-area data[44] usually available through World Health Organization publications or from special reports from national governments. Age- and gender-specific disease rates or summary statistics (adjusted for age and, less frequently, gender) such as summary mortality rates or standardized mortality ratios can be used. These data have the advantage of routine availability, compatibility, and comprehensiveness, but are usually compiled only for the largest geographic unit, i.e. individual countries. Intra-country comparisons must rely on national and local data sources, which may not collect the required information on a routine basis. However, in addition to mortality data, various measures of morbidity typically exist within developed countries for a variety of disorders, such as cancer incidence and national estimates of decayed, missing, and filled teeth (DMFT).[45]

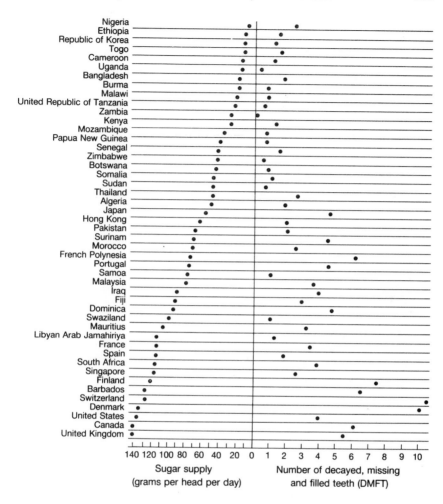

Fig. 10.4. Prevalence of dental decay, expressed as decayed, missing, and filled teeth (DMFT) in children aged 12 years, and per capita daily sugar supply in 47 countries. Source: Sreebny.[45]

10.3.2 Biological indices as (presumptive) disease-mediating processes

Biological specimens such as blood, urine, or faeces can be used as markers of stages in the disease process, or as direct measures of the presence of disease (for example, in diabetes). Such indices are not available routinely but must be collected as part of a special population survey. Data collected on representative subsamples of the population are presumed to be indicative of general associations.

Blood   Analysis of serum cholesterol was an essential component of the Japanese migrant study discussed in section 10.2.6.[32] A more direct measure of disease-mediating mechanisms has been provided in studies of the effect of marine oil ingestion on haemostasis in Eskimos, a group with a low death rate from coronary heart disease despite a high intake of animal fats.[46]

Faeces   IARC has completed two studies of regional variation in diet and faecal measures (concentration, absolute amounts, etc.) of primary and secondary bile acids as indicators of stages in the genesis of colon cancer.[36,37] It has been postulated that dietary fat and fibre induce changes in bile acid metabolism and concentration that influence the promotional stage of colon cancer. These studies indicate a limitation of the ecological approach. Although bile acid concentrations varied between areas with high and low incidence of colon cancer, the researchers were unable to identify definitively the dietary components that contributed to these variations in bile acids. The final unravelling of the causal pathway may rely on research techniques better able to control for the various non-dietary factors that affect colon cancer risk.

Other   Various other *ad hoc* methods of assessing the biomedical status of compared groups have been used. For example, the association of gall-stones with diet was investigated by an ultrasound survey of the prevalence of asymptomatic gallstones in vegetarians and non-vegetarians in Oxford;[47] a strong association was observed between meat-eating and asymptomatic disease. The work on aflatoxins and liver cancer in Africa[28] has been elaborated in a more recent study in which the presence of DNA-adducts in urine was correlated with liver cancer rates.[48] Although this analysis did not provide additional information concerning the relationship between aflatoxins and liver cancer, the tools of metabolic epidemiology can refine diet–disease associations being examined in ecological studies.

10.4 POPULATIONS OR GROUPS STUDIED

10.4.1 Migrants

Changes in disease patterns among migrant populations away from those of their country of origin and towards those in the host country, have provided opportunities for the exploration of the relative effect of genetic predisposition and environmental exposures on disease. National per capita dietary consumption data derived from FAO data can be used to infer usual diet in the host country and in the migrants' countries of origin. These dietary data can then be compared with disease rates experienced by the various migrant groups in the host country. In the analysis of gastrointestinal cancer mortality among recent European migrants to Australia,[20] migrants from countries with rates of stomach cancer that differed from the Australian rates initially had correspondingly different rates from those in the Australian-born population. However, with increased duration of residence in Australia and, presumably, concomitant acculturation in dietary pattern, the disease patterns increasingly reflected those experienced by the native Australian population.

More definitive studies of the effect of acculturation and passage of time on diet in migrant populations have provided direct evidence of the gradual cultural adaptation to dietary patterns of the host population. Such studies have occurred in Australia amongst Italian[49] and Greek migrants[50] and in the United States where first-, second-, and third-generation Japanese migrants have been compared with Japanese in Japan and the rest of the citizens of the United States. The number of generations of residence in the United States is used as a proxy for change in diet from a traditional low fat Japanese diet to an American pattern of food consumption. Comparisons between cancer sites of the generations taken for a migrant group to assume the disease profile of the host population may provide clues to carcinogenic processes. For example, colon cancer rates in migrant groups rapidly assume the pattern of the host population; stomach cancer rates take a little longer and breast cancer rates take one to two generations to assume a new pattern, thereby indicating different effects on the initiation and promotion stages of carcinogenesis.[51]

10.4.2 Religious groups

There have been many ecological studies of Seventh Day Adventists, who frequently follow a lacto-ovovegetarian diet. When their cancer mortality is compared with mortality data for the general population there are indications of reduced risk for colon cancer and equivocal results for breast cancer.[52,53] Similar analyses of Mormons, living in the state of Utah, who abstain from alcohol, tobacco, coffee, and tea and tend to eat moderate quantities of meat, indicate reduced incidence of colon and rectal cancers compared with non-Mormons in the same State.[54] This association persisted after removing smoking-related cancers from the analysis.

Ecological analyses of disease patterns among religious groups may even suggest covert patterns of social behaviour. For example, in analysing the high rates of oral cancer in Iran, which cannot be explained by reported alcohol and tobacco consumption (as they have been in studies of many other populations), undercover illicit alcohol consumption must be considered.

Vegetarian English nuns have similarly provided a unique social group for the investigation of the effect of dietary restrictions on disease risk.[55] This population has the added (investigative) advantage of being at high

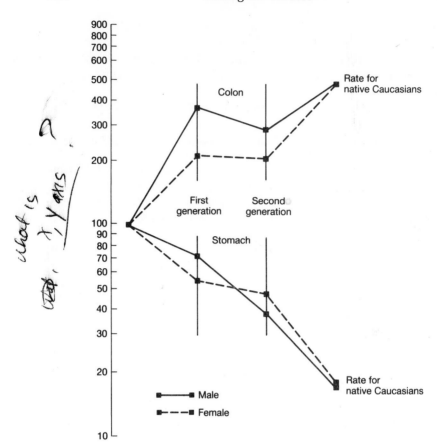

Fig. 10.5 Mortality from cancer of the stomach and colon in Japanese immigrants to the United States. Source: Wynder *et al.*[51]

risk of breast cancer by virtue of their distinctive, constant, reproductive behaviour.

10.4.3 Groups with distinct behaviour

Other subpopulations with distinctive dietary patterns have been investigated to determine whether these patterns are associated with similarly distinctive disease patterns. The work on vegetarians,[52,53] has been mentioned. Observations on Eskimo populations have revealed relatively low rates of coronary heart disease, despite the consumption of diets high in fat and cholesterol, which are presumed to increase the risk of this disease. The habitual consumption of large quantities of cold-water fish with long-chain polyunsaturated fatty acids of the omega-3 type, was presumed to be responsible, in part, for these low rates. The effect of this diet on thrombosis has been inferred by an examination of bleeding ti.nes in Eskimos and in Danish populations that have a different diet.[46] Eskimos were noted to have longer bleeding times.

10.4.4 Groups in cultural transition

Omran coined the term 'epidemiologic transition' to describe the changes, over time, in patterns of disease and health in different cultures.[56] In general, societies move from famine and pestilence, through an era during which infectious disease has the greatest impact on mortality, to a stage when degenerative or chronic diseases are the greatest health problems. Westernization has frequently been accompanied by dramatic increases in the rates of non-insulin dependent diabetes mellitus (NIDDM) and other chronic diseases.[57,58] In his early epidemiological observations on diabetes among the Pima Indians, West noted that diabetes, which had been uncommon before 1940 when most American Indians had been slender, became much more common as these populations became obese.[59] Zimmet and his colleagues have documented the effect of Westernization with its concomitant changes in diet, obesity levels, and physical exercise on various groups of Pacific Islanders, who now have some of the highest rates of NIDDM in the world.[60,61]

Although the effect on diseases of the cultural impact of Westernization has been most widely documented among aboriginal peoples and in developing countries, a similar pattern has been noted in Japan. The incidence of diseases associated (on an ecological basis) with high fat diets (cancers of the colon, pancreas, breast, prostate, ovaries, and endometrium, and coronary heart disease) is increasing in Japan as the traditional low fat diet undergoes increasing westernization.[62] Thus, these examples of ecological investigations of the association between diet and disease, associate changes in disease rates with knowledge of changes in cultural processes that are known to affect dietary patterns.

10.4.5 Subpopulations displaying sharp cultural differences

Hawaii has provided a natural setting for ecological studies of diet and disease because its multiethnic population, comprising five main ethnic groups, has a variety of diets.[63] For example, studies of generations of migrants amongst Japanese and, more recently, Filipino residents of Hawaii, have correlated changing disease patterns with changes in diet with increasing time in the United States. The first and second generation Japanese (Issei and Nisei) in Hawaii have increased their intake of dietary fat, meat, and animal protein while their intake of tofu, green tea, and vitamin A has decreased. In parallel, these first and second generations

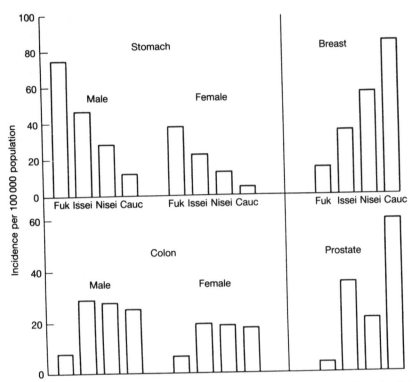

Fig. 10.6. Age-adjusted cancer incidence rates (World Population Standard) in Japanese migrants to Hawaii and indigenous populations, for the period 1973–77 (Hawaii) and 1974–75 (Japan). Fuk, Fukuoka Japanese; Cauc, Hawaii Caucasians; Issei first generation Japanese; Nisei, second generation Japanese. Source: Kolonel.[63]

Japanese increasingly experience stomach, breast, and colon cancer rates that are similar to those experienced by Caucasian Hawaiians.[63]

10.5 TECHNIQUES IN EXAMINING RELATIONSHIPS

10.5.1 Simple regression and correlations

The most direct method of examining ecological data is by the calculation of correlation coefficients between disease rates and regional indicators of dietary consumption.[10] Similarly, the relationship between meat/fat consumption and the incidence of colon or breast cancer can be plotted and depicted graphically with scattergrams. These types of data do not prove that the dietary component 'causes' the cancer, but they do indicate that there are systematic population-based patterns of association between diet and disease.

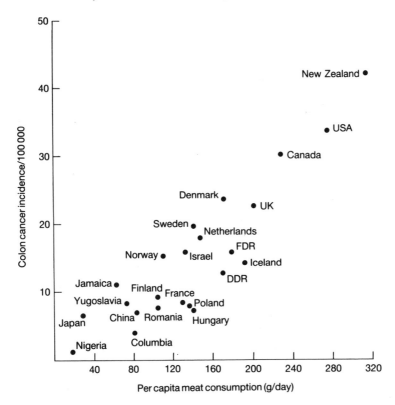

Fig. 10.7. Relationship between meat consumption in various countries and the risk, in those countries, of developing cancer of the colon. Source: Peto.[41]

Most ecological analyses rely on relatively simple statistical methods or correlation analysis. Analytical issues arise in deciding whether it is appropriate to weight each area by its relative size. In addition, contiguous areas are often similar in a variety of ways,[27,64] and therefore assumptions in a regression analysis of independent error terms are unlikely to be correct. However, since there are no recognized solutions to these problems, one can only bear in mind the limitations inherent in this type of analysis.

The simpler correlation analyses of ecological data can be refined by statistical methods designed to adjust for intercorrelations between indicators of dietary intake and other social indicators and amongst the range of dietary factors. Partial correlation coefficients[10] and stepwise regression techniques[65] have been used to examine the association between national age-adjusted cancer incidence and mortality rates and a variety of dietary and environmental variables (e.g. rainfall, population density, alcohol consumption, etc.) while adjusting for potential confounding variables.

The stepwise multiple regression procedure was also used by Pocock[27] because it gives adjusted regression coefficients and provides evidence for the relative importance of each of the items included in the model.

The use of correlation techniques in ecological studies has been criticized.[9,66] If the populations being compared are selected because they are heterogeneous with respect to an independent variable (for example, dietary fat), correlation coefficients tend to be inflated because these coefficients are dependent on the relative dispersion of the independent and dependent variables. The variance of the independent variable will be increased relative to the disease or outcome variable, thereby increasing the size of the correlation coefficient.

10.5.2 Time-lagging

Time-lagging techniques are valuable in the analysis of ecological data. In examining associations between diet and patterns of chronic disease morbidity and mortality where latency is known to be important, these time-lagging techniques may disclose the time of maximal aetiological influence of the dietary exposure. Rose used time-lagging techniques in an analysis of the association between blood cholesterol and coronary heart disease rates.[67] Data from seven countries on serum cholesterol levels recorded between 1958 and 1964, on men aged 40–59, were related to national mortality from coronary heart disease in the same age cohorts at 5-year intervals for a 15-year period. The correlations between serum cholesterol at baseline and coronary heart disease mortality rates increased with time, reaching a peak of 0.96 at 15 years.

Skog's analysis of the association between per capita alcohol consumption and liver cirrhosis mortality highlighted a major limitation to correlation analysis of the association between dietary intake and disease rates.[68] An individual's risk of dying from cirrhosis of the liver in a given year is a reflection of his/her drinking history, not merely their alcohol consumption in the last year of life. Similarly, inter- and intracountry ecological analyses relating alcohol consumption to cirrhosis mortality rates frequently display a time lag between the period of peak consumption and the time of peak mortality rates. When the regression equation is modified by the addition of a lag parameter, differential weightings are provided to exposures according to their proximity to the year of death or incidence of disease. This method is particularly appropriate when the median latency between exposure and diagnosis is known and can be used in the time-lagged analysis.

10.5.3 Cohort analysis

Government policy, or some other major social change (e.g. war) may affect the dietary intake for particular areas resulting in a sudden change in diet for the population. The effect of that change can be examined by investigating disease rates prior to the change and disease rates in population cohorts following the change. For instance, the introduction of bread iodization in Tasmania in 1966 resulted in a change in dietary intake of iodine for a cohort of the population. Disease rates for the cohort that was not exposed to the dietary supplement (or deficiency) can be compared with those for the subsequent cohorts that have experienced the effects of government intervention.[22] A birth cohort-based analysis of changes in age-specific oesophageal cancer rates in Australia highlighted a decline in risk from cohort to cohort commencing around the turn of the century with a recent increase in rates at younger ages.[69] Graphs of time trends in per capita consumption of alcohol in beer, wine, and spirits for 1900–1975 suggested that the drop in alcohol consumption (especially of spirits consumption) in the first third of this century was associated with the changing pattern of oesophageal cancer rates in successive cohorts. Plummer–Vinson syndrome, the rare disorder associated with prolonged iron and multivitamin deficiency in Scandinavian populations, declined following the fortification of the food supply.[70]

10.5.4 Adjusting for confounders

Ecological analyses are frequently criticized because they lead to spurious and often curious associations. Unlike study designs, in which data can be collected on the individual level and the effect of measured confounders estimated, analysis of the effect of confounding variables in ecological studies is not possible at the individual level, creating an additional source of error. This complication has been documented in studies of water hardness and cardiovascular disease, in which disease rates are not only associated with soft water, but with three other well documented risk factors for cardiovascular disease—smoking, high blood pressure, and serum cholesterol.[44] Certainly, it has been claimed that associations between dietary fat, or total calories, and chronic diseases associated with economic development, are confounded by other indicators of gross national product. Is the putative association between national diet and national disease rates merely a consequence of an association between some other factor affected by socio-economic development and the disease in question?

Adjustment for confounding variables is a problem in the analysis of ecological data because these data are often not available or easily measured on a geographic basis.[27] In the analysis of liver cirrhosis death rates by Qiao et al.,[71] partial correlation coefficients for a variety of dietary constituents and disease rates have been adjusted for alcohol consumption because data were available on a per capita basis for all dietary constituents examined. Unfortunately, data on confounding factors are not always available covering the same geographic units included in the ecological analysis.

Another approach to controlling the confounding effect of socio-economic differences has been followed by Barker and Morris,[72] who used data on the percentages of households without amenities as an indicator of both hygiene and of social class. The observed positive association between potato and sugar consumption and acute appendicitis rates was reduced after controlling for the percentage of households without a bath in each of the 90 areas of England, Wales, Scotland, and Eire. The inverse relationship between vegetable consumption (other than potatoes) and appendicitis was also weakened following the adjustment, via partial correlations, for social class. However, the partial correlation of −0.41 remained a strong indication of an inverse association between diet and appendicitis.

Occasionally, data are available that enable the calculation of appropriately adjusted rates from international correlation data. In investigating the association between dietary fat and lung cancer, Wynder et al. were able to adjust for the average number of cigarettes per day.[73]

Other creative adjustment methods may be available. Dobson[74] examined trends in cardiovascular risk factors in Australia, determined from serial risk factor prevalence surveys to determine their possible contribution to mortality declines. Proportional hazards models, derived from data from the Framingham study in the United States, were used as a source of coefficients to examine the contributions of average changes in risk factors among groups on group death rates. Beta coefficients were thus derived from longitudinal data collected on North American individuals and applied to changes in average cholesterol levels, systolic blood pressure, and cigarette smoking in Australia. Age- and gender-specific grouped data risk factor levels were available. This analytical method enabled the examination of the effect of each of these risk factors after adjusting for the other two in the equation.

10.6 LIMITATIONS

Beyond the logical problem of the ecological fallacy, there are a number of methodological difficulties in ecological studies. Confounding is an ever-present possibility in ecological studies, although numerous researchers have attempted to develop methods for adjustment. It is a particular problem in ecological studies of diet and diseases associated with industrialization. Unless the effect of confounding with level of development can be controlled, it will be impossible for ecological studies alone to disentangle the coexistent effects of diet and development. Studies conducted within a country can usually control for some of these other socio-economic factors, such as standard of medical care, quality of recording, and exposure to non-dietary risk factors.

Intercountry comparisons may be restricted by the absence of comparable data, usually on dietary intake, although cause of death may also be subject to international differences in data quality. On the other hand, intracountry comparisons (e.g. between Francophone and Flemish areas of Belgium, or between regions of the United Kingdom) that may not suffer from lack of compatibility of data, may yet be restricted by the limited size of the population in each region and the consequent instability in rates, as well as by homogeneity of exposures within the country as a whole.

Where there is marked individual variation in the dietary component of interest within each geographical region (i.e. heterogeneity of exposure), summary exposure measures (e.g. average consumption data) may have such large, but unknown, error terms associated with them that correlations with disease rates would be rendered useless. As a corollary to that limitation, there is a presumption that within a region of interest there are no systematic differences in dietary exposure between subregions. For instance, if only one county within a given region experiences unusual dietary intake patterns and disease rates, then this association may either be obscured, or else erroneous conclusions may be drawn about the region as a whole, i.e. a type of 'ecological fallacy' would occur.

As with other types of epidemiological studies, inferences are limited by the detail of the data. Studies indicating the association between water hardness (a composite chemical index) and cardiovascular disease cannot determine whether the beneficial effect is consequent upon the presence (or absence) of a particular trace element or mineral.

In addition, reports of ecological associations between chronic diseases and dietary indices have usually disregarded the long preclinical induction periods inherent in these diseases[64] and have examined correlations between contemporaneous indicators of dietary patterns and disease rates. Unless some time lag analysis is used there must be an assumption that current consumption patterns reflect past consumption, i.e. at the exposure time relevant to current disease rates. This assumption will be flawed when the exposure to the dietary factors being investigated has changed dramatically over time.

The population unit being used for analysis of morbidity or mortality is often inappropriate for the analysis of exposure to diet. In addition, one must ensure that the same geographical boundaries are used for all analyses. Mortality and incidence data may be available for different age, race, and gender groupings while dietary data may only be available for much larger aggregates.

Interactions between a variety of dietary exposures and a disease outcome or between diet and other exposure factors and disease cannot be assessed in ecological studies because data are not available about joint probabilities of exposure at the level of the individual.

10.7 CONCLUSION: WHEN ARE ECOLOGICAL STUDIES THE METHOD OF CHOICE?

Ecological studies are ideal for examining a new, but preconceived, hypothesis. However, the use of these studies for hypothesis generation can lead to the proliferation of nonsensical findings.

They have been particularly useful in situations where it is possible subsequently to study causal relationships at an individual level. An analysis of the relationship between dietary factors and liver cirrhosis death rates indicated a potential protective effect of calcium[71] that has not been documented previously and may warrant further investigation. Such investigation could be carried out at the individual level.

Ecological studies are invaluable when intake (or outcome) data are unavailable on an individual level. Despite the oft-stated proviso that ecological analyses can only generate hypotheses that should be tested subsequently using more rigorous observational or experimental methods,[66] it should be borne in mind that the ecological approach is frequently the only one available for the examination of hypotheses when exposure cannot be defined meaningfully on an individual level. For example, the association between the cumulative prevalence of dental decay in children aged 12 and sugar intake, can be readily documented by using FAO data on per capita daily sucrose utilization in 47 countries. It may not be possible (or at least practicable) to measure individual sugar intake because estimates should be based on total dietary intake including processed foods, although data may not be available for individual items.

Studies of the association between diet and coronary heart disease on an individual level are faced with difficulties. The collection and analysis of individual food records is difficult, may not reflect habitual intake, and cannot measure individual variability in the metabolic response to a given diet. Because of the innate (and/or acquired) variability in individual response to dietary 'exposure', the dietary risk factors for some diseases may be more evident for groups/populations than for individuals. The relationship between dietary salt and blood pressure is widely considered to provide an example of this important issue. The correlation between salt and blood pressure on an individual level may be further attenuated by the homogeneity of exposure among individuals within a given population. The ecological data are not easily dismissed given their strength and their concordance with experimental data.

These studies are also valuable in the investigation of the associations between dietary exposure and disease when, within a given population, there is insufficient heterogeneity in exposure experience. For instance, individual-based studies of the effect of water hardness (or even dietary fat) within a community may not be possible if all individuals within the community have similar exposures. Therefore, it may only be by inter-community comparisons that the effect of such exposures can be investigated.

Indeed, it has been claimed that the ecological investigation of the association between diet, especially dietary fat, and breast cancer may be more meaningful than analytic studies of individuals (case-control and cohort studies).[11] Studies of dietary fat undertaken on individuals identify those individuals within a given community who tend to be homogeneous in their dietary exposure. In a large prospective study of dietary fat and breast cancer risk,[75] the range of percentage intake of calories from fat among the nurse participants was only 32–44 per cent (a narrow 37.5 per cent range). In fact, it has been claimed that the cohort study mentioned above had statistical power of only 24 per cent to detect a true difference in disease risk.[76]

In addition, instruments assessing dietary intake on an individual level are subject to measurement error (as are instruments measuring population levels of dietary intake). Narrow gradients of exposure combined with the inherent limitations of measuring instruments reduce the power of cohort and case-control studies to detect an increase in risk. Fraser's illustration[77] of the limited variation in serum cholesterol levels within cultures demonstrates this phenomenon.

Ecological studies that are based on intracountry comparisons may be better placed to control for confounding factors. For example, Rosen et al.[78] looked at the association between diet and stomach, colorectal, and breast cancer mortality in the 24 counties of Sweden, a country in which there are few regional differences in socio-economic status (because, for

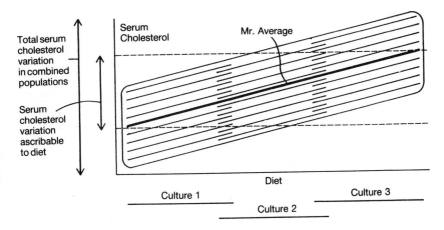

Fig. 10.8. A schematic representation of the variation of serum cholesterol ascribable to diet across three communities representing different cultures. Source: Fraser.[77]

example, of universal health care coverage) yet some regional differences in diet.

Thus, ecological studies may be invaluable not only for investigating diseases where there is no *a priori* method for measuring exposure on an individual level (and are therefore seen as the method of second choice) but, in certain circumstances, may even be the method of choice even when exposure can be measured at an individual level.

Criteria of 'proof' in ecological associations between diet and disease

The criteria for legitimizing the drawing of causal inferences are no different in ecological studies than in other epidemiological investigations, although emphases may differ. Particular attention should be paid to the biological plausibility of associations identified from ecological studies given the possibility of identifying associations that are nonsensical.

The consistency of an association can be a difficult criterion because it presumes that similar data will be available in different communities. For instance, small-area data on the composition of drinking water are unlikely to be available for many countries in the developing world.

The specificity of association is a criterion that can be readily tested. Is the association specific to the dietary component of interest and the disease of interest, or are there a variety of unconnected associations that may reflect the quality of data rather than true associations? An ecological analysis of the association between Alzheimer's disease and aluminium in drinking water determined that there was no association with another neurological disorder, epilepsy, although the risk for Alzheimer's disease in areas with higher aluminium concentration was 1.5 times the risk in low concentration areas.[79]

The calculation of correlation and regression coefficients, and the use of time series analysis to test covariation, incorporate the notion of the dose–response criterion.

Temporal relationships can be evaluated by investigating disease rates following changes in exposures. For example, the association between dental decay and fluoridation can be documented by examining indicators of dental health prior and subsequent to the introduction of a fluoridation programme.

Despite the numerous limitations to the interpretation of data derived from ecological studies, they have made and will continue to make an important contribution to our understanding of the relationship between diet and any number of diseases. Renewed interest in this type of study has resulted in the development of methodologies[11] that will enhance the contribution such analyses can make.

REFERENCES

1. McGill, H. C. Jr. (ed.). (1968). *Geographic pathology of atherosclerosis.* Williams & Williams, Baltimore.
2. Kuller, L. H., LaPorte, R. E., and Weinberg G. B. (1977). The decline in ischemic heart disease mortality: environmental and social variables. In Havlik, R. J. and Feinleib, M. (eds.). *Proceedings of the conference on the decline in coronary heart disease mortality*, pp. 312–39. DHEW Pub. No. (NIH) 79–1610 Government Printing Office, Washington DC.
3. Gregor, O., Toman, R., and Prusova, F. (1969). Gastrointestinal cancer and nutrition. *Gut*, **10:** 1031–4.
4. Dwyer, T. and Hetzel, B. S. (1980). A comparison of trends of coronary heart disease mortality in Australia, USA, and England and Wales with reference to three major risk factors—hypertension, cigarette smoking and diet. *Int. J. Epid.*, **9:** 67–71.
5. Blot, W. J. and Fraumeni, J. F. Jr. (1982). Geographic epidemiology in the United States. In Schottenfeld, D. and Fraumeni, J. F. Jr. (eds). *Cancer epidemiology and prevention.* W. B. Saunders, Philadelphia.
6. Wynder, E. L. and Hebert, J. R. (1987). Homogeneity in nutritional exposure: an impediment in cancer epidemiology. *J. Natl. Cancer Inst.*, **79:** 605–7.
7. Joosens, J. V., Brems-Heyns, E., Claes, J. H., Graffer, M., Kornitzer, M., Pannier, R., Van Houte, O., Vuylesteek, K., Carlier, J., de Backer, G., Kesteloot, H., Lequime, J., Raes, A., Vastesuger, M., and Verdonk, G. (1977). The pattern of food and mortality in Belgium. *Lancet*, **i:** 1069–72.
8. McMichael, A. J. (1983). Cancers of the head and neck. In Bourke G. J. (ed.). *Epidemiology of Cancer.* Croom Helm, Sydney.
9. Morgenstern, H. (1982). Uses of ecologic analysis in epidemiologic research. *Am. J. Public. Health*, **72:** 1336–44.
10. Armstrong, B. and Doll, R. (1975). Environmental factors and cancer incidence and mortality in different countries, with special reference to dietary practices. *Int. J. Cancer*, **15:** 617–31.
11. Prentice, R. L., Kakar, F., Hursting, S., Sheppard, L., Klein, R., and Kushi, L. H (1988). Aspect of the rationale for the Women's Health Trial. *J. Natl. Cancer Inst.*, 1988; **80:** 802–14.
12. James, W. P. T., Ferro-Luzzi, A., Isaksson, B., and Szostak W. B. (1988). Healthy nutrition: preventing nutrition-related diseases in Europe. WHO Regional Publications, European Series; No. 24, WHO Regional Office for Europe, Copenhagen.
13. United Nations Organization. (1976). Monthly Bull. Agri. Economics Statistics 25: No. 4 and No. 7, FAO, United Nations, Geneva.
14. Australian Bureau of Statistics. (1985). *Apparent consumption of foodstuffs and nutrients, Australia, 1983–84.* Catalogue No. 4306.0, Canberra.
15. Calver, G. D., English, R., and Wahlqvist, M. L. (1987). Changing eating patterns in Australia. In M. Wahlqvist, R. W. F. King, J. J. McNeil, and R. Sewell, (eds). *Food and Health Issues and Directions.* John Libbey & Company Ltd., London.
16. Beaton, G. H., Milner, J., Corey, P., McGuire, V., Cousins, M., Stewart, E.,

de Ramos, M., Hewitt, D., Grambsch, P. V., Kassim, N., and Little, J. A. (1979). Sources of variance in 24-hour dietary recall data: implications for nutrition study design and interpretation. *Am. J. Clin. Nutr.*, **179**: 2546–59.

17. Ministry of Agriculture, Fisheries, and Food. (1987). Household food consumption and expenditure survey 1985. HMSO, London.

18. McMichael, A. J. (1978). Increases in laryngeal cancer in Britain and Australia in relation to alcohol and tobacco consumption trends. *Lancet*, **i**: 1244–7.

19. Breslow, N. E. and Enstrom, J. E. (1974). Geographic correlations between cancer mortality rates and alcohol-tobacco consumption in the United States. *J. Natl. Cancer Inst.*, **53**: 631–9.

20. McMichael, A. J., McCall, M. G., Hartshorne, J. M., and Woodings, T. L. (1980). Patterns of gastrointestinal cancer in European migrants to Australia: the role of dietary change. *Int. J. Cancer*, **25**: 431–7.

21. Burkitt, D. P. and Trowell, H. C. (eds). (1975). *Refined carbohydrate foods and disease. Some implications of dietary fibre.* Academic Press, London.

22. Potter, J. D., McMichael, A. J., and Hetzel, B. S. (1979). Iodization and thyroid status in relation to stillbirths and congenital anomalies. *Int. J. Epid.*, **8**: 137–44.

23. Yang, C. S. (1980). Research on oesophageal cancer in China: a review. *Cancer Res.*, **40**: 2633–44.

24. Luo, X. M., Wei, H. J., Hu, G. G., Shang, A. L., Liu, Y. Y., Lu, S. M., and Yang, S. P. (1981). Molybdenum and oesophageal cancer in China. *Fed. Proc.*, **40**: 928, Abstract 3962.

25. Powles, J. W. and Williams, D. R. R. (1984). Trends in bowel cancer in selected countries in relation to wartime changes in flour miling. *Nutr. Cancer*, **6**: 40–8.

26. Masironi, R. (1970). Cardiovascular mortality in relation to radioactivity and hardness of local water supplies in the USA. *Bull. WHO*, **43**: 687–97.

27. Pocock, S. J., Cook, D. G., and Shaper, A. G. (1982). Analysing geographic variation in cardiovascular mortality: Methods and results. *J. Roy. Statist. Soc. Ser. A.*, **145**: 313–41.

28. Linsell, C. A. and Peers, F. U. (1977). Field studies on liver cell cancer. In Hiatt, H. H., Watson, J. D., and Winston, J. A. (eds.). *Origins of human cancer, book A.* Cold Spring Harbor Laboratory.

29. McGlashan, N. D., Walters, C. L., and McLean, A. E. M. (1968). Nitrosamines in African alcoholic spirits and oesophageal cancer. *Lancet*, **ii**: 1017.

30. Lancet (1987) (editorial). A Poison Tree. *Lancet*, **ii**: 947–8.

31. Hetzel, B. S. and Baghurst, K. I. (eds). (1981). The assessment of the nutritional status of the individual and the community. *Transactions of the Menzies Foundation*, **3**.

32. Marmot, M. G., Syme, S. L., Kagan, A., Kato, I. I., Cohen, J. B., and Belsky, J. (1975). Epidemiologic studies of coronary heart disease and stroke in Japanese men living in Japan, Hawaii, and California: prevalence of coronary and hypertensive heart disease and associated risk factors. *Am. J. Epid.*, **102**: 514–25.

33. Gleibermann, L. (1973). Blood pressure and dietary salt in human populations. *Ecol. Food and Nutr.*, **2**: 143–50.

34. Elliott, P. and Stamler, R. (1988). Manual of operations for "INTERSALT", an international co-operative study on the relation of sodium and potassium to blood pressure. *Controlled Clin. Trials*, **9**: 1S–118S.

35. MacMahon, B., Cole, P., Brown, J. B., Aoki, K., and Lin, T. (1974). Urine oestrogen profiles of Asian and North American women. *Int. J. Cancer*, **14**: 161–7.

36. Jensen, O. M., MacLennan, R., and Wahrendorf, J. (1982). Diet, bowel function, fecal characteristics, and large bowel cancer in Denmark and Finland. *Nutr. Cancer*, **4**: 5–19.

37. International Agency for Research on Cancer, Intestinal Microecology Group. (1977). Dietary fibre, transit time, faecal bacteria, steroids, and colon cancer in two Scandinavian populations. *Lancet*, **ii**: 2: 207–11.

38. Muir, C. S. and James, P. (1982). Diet and large bowel cancer in Denmark and Finland: report of the Second IARC International Collaborative Study. *Nutrition and cancer*, **4**: 1–79.

39. Malhotra, S. L. (1977). Dietary factors in a study of cancer colon from Cancer Registry, with special reference to the role of saliva, milk and fermented milk products and vegetable fibre. *Med. Hypotheses*, **3**: 122–6.

40. Morris, J. S., Stampfer, M. J., and Willett, W. (1983). Toenails as an indicator of dietary selenium. *Biol. Trace Elem. Res.*, **5**: 529–37.

41. Peto, R. (1986). Cancer around the World: evidence for avoidability. In B. Hallgren, O. Levin, and S. Rossner (eds). *Diet and prevention of Coronary Heart Disease and Cancer.* Fourth International Berzilius Symposium sponsored by the Swedish Society of Medicine. Raven Press, New York.

42. Schrauzer, G. N., White, D. A., and Schneider, C. J. (1977). Cancer mortality correlation studies—IV. Associations with dietary intakes and blood levels of certain trace elements, notably Se-antagonists. *Bioinorg. Chem.*, **7**: 35–56.

43. Junshi, C., Campbell, T. C., Junyao, L., and Peto, R. (1989). A preliminary study of dietary, lifestyle and mortality characteristics of 65 rural populations in The People's Republic of China. Oxford University Press, Oxford.

44. Pocock, S. J., Shaper, A. G., Powell, P. and Packham, R. F. (1985). The British Regional Heart Study: cardiovascular disease and water quality. In Thornton, I. (ed.). *Proceedings of the first international symposium on geochemistry and health*, pp. 141–57. Science Reviews, Middlesex.

45. Sreebny, L. M. (1982). Sugar availability, sugar consumption and dental caries. *Community Dent. Oral Epid.*, **10**: 1–7.

46. Dyerberg, J. and Jorgensen K. A. (1982). Marine oils and thrombogenesis. *Prog. in Lipid Res.*, **21**: 255–69.

47. Pixley F., Wilson D., McPherson K., and Mann J. (1985). Effect of vegetarianism on development of gallstones in women. *Br. Med. J.*, **291**: 11–12.

48. Autrup, H. and Wakhisi, J. (1988). Detection of exposure to aflatoxin in an African population. In Bartsch, H. Hemminki, K. and O'Neill, I. K. (eds). *Methods for detecting DNA damaging agents in humans: applications in cancer epidemiology and prevention*, pp. 63–6. International Agency for Research on Cancer, IARC Scientific Publications No. 89, Lyons.

49. Hopkins, S., Margetts, B. M., Cohen, J., and Armstrong, B. K. (1980). Dietary change among Italians and Australians in Perth. *Community health stud.*, **4**: 67–75.

50. Powles, J., Ktenas, D., and Sutherland, C. (1986). *Food habits in Southern European migrants: a case-study of migrants from the Greek Island of Levkada, Prahran, Victoria.* Department of Social and Preventive Medicine, Monash Medical School, Monash.

51. Wynder, E. L., McCoy, G. D., Reddy, B. S., Cohen, L., Hill, P., Spingarn, N. E., and Weisburger, J. H. (1981). Nutrition and metabolic epidemiology of cancers of the oral cavity, oesophagus, colon, breast, prostate and stomach. In G. R. Newell and N. M. Ellison (eds). *Nutrition and cancer: etiology and treatment*, pp. 11–48. Raven Press, New York.

52. Phillips. R. L. (1975). Role of life-style and dietary habits in risk of cancer among Seventh-Day Adventists. *Cancer Res.* **35**: 3513–22.

53. Phillips, R. L., Garfinkel, L., Kuzma, J. W., Beeson, W. L., Lodz, T., Brin, B. (1980). Mortality among California Seventh-Day Adventists for selected cancer sites. *J. Natl. Cancer Inst.*, **65**: 1097–107.

54. Lyon, J. L., Gardner, J. W., and West, D. W. (1980). Cancer risk and life-style: cancer among Mormons from 1967–1975. In J. Cairns, J. L. Lyon, and M. Skolnick (eds). *Cancer incidence in defined populations*, pp. 3–27. Banbury Report 4. Cold Spring Harbor Laboratory, Cold Spring Harbor, New York.

55. Kinlen, L. J. (1982). Meat and fat consumption and cancer mortality: A study of strict religious orders in Britain. *Lancet*, **1**: 946–9.

56. Omran, A. R. (1971). The epidemiologic transition: a theory of the epidemiology of population change. *Milbank Mem. Fund. O.*, **49**: 509–537.

57. Young, T. K. (1988). Are subarctic Indians undergoing the epidemiologic transition? *Soc. Sci. Med.*, **26**: 659–71.

58. Schooneveldt, M., Songer, T., Zimmet, P., and Thoma, K. (1988). Changing mortality patterns in Nauruans: an example of epidemiological transition. *J. Epid. Comm. Health.*, **42**: 89–95.

59. West, K. M. (1974). Diabetes in American Indians and other native populations in the New World. *Diabetes*, **23**: 841–55.

60. Zimmet, P. Z. (1979). Epidemiology diabetes and its macrovascular manifestations in Pacific populations: the medical effects of social progress. *Diabetes Care*, **2**: 144–53.

61. Zimmet, P. Z. (1987). Diabetes and other non-communicable disease in Paradise—the evolutionary and genetic connection. *Med. J. Aust.*, **146**: 457–8.

62. Hirayama, T. (1979). Diet and Cancer. *Nutr. Cancer*, **1**: 67–81.

63. Kolonel, L. N., Hankin, J. H., and Nomura, A. M. Y. (1986). Multiethnic studies of diet nutrition and cancer in Hawaii. In Y. Hayashi, M. Nagao, T. Sugimura *et al* (eds). *Diet, nutrition and cancer*, pp. 29–40. Japan Science Societies Press, Tokyo.

64. Stavraky, K. M. (1976). The role of ecologic analysis in studies of the etiology of disease: a discussion with reference to large bowel cancer. *J. Chron. Dis.*, **29**: 435–44.

65. Yanai, H., Inaba, Y., Takagi, H., and Yamamoto, S. (1979). Multivariate analysis of cancer mortalities for selected sites in 24 countries. *Environ. Health Perspect.*, **32**: 83–101.

66. Piantadosi, S., Byar, D. P., and Green, S. B. (1988). The ecological fallacy. *Am. J. Epid.*, **127**: 893–904.

67. Rose, G. (1982). Incubation period of coronary heart disease. *Br. Med. J.*, **284**: 1600–1.

68. Skog, O-J. (1980). Liver cirrhosis epidemiology: some methodological problems. *Br. J. Addict.*, **75**: 227–43.

69. McMichael, A. J. (1979). Alimentary tract cancer in Australia in relation to diet and alcohol. *Nutr. Cancer*, **1**: 82–9.

70. Wynder, E. L., Hultberg, S., Jacobssen, F., and Bross, I. J. (1957). Environmental factors in cancer of upper alimentary tract: Swedish study with special reference to Plummer-Vinson (Paterson-Kelly) syndrome. *Cancer*, **10**: 470–87.

71. Qiao, Z-K., Halliday, M. L., Coates, R. A., and Rankin, J. G. (1988). Relationship between liver cirrhosis death rate and nutritional factors in 38 countries. *Int. J. Epid.*, **17**: 414–18.

72. Barker, D. J. P. and Morris, J. (1988). Acute appendicitis, bathrooms, and diet in Britain and Ireland. *Br. Med. J.*, **296**: 953–5.

73. Wynder, E. L., Hebert, J. R., and Geoffrey, C. K. (1987). Association of dietary fat and lung cancer. *J. Natl. Cancer Inst.*, **79**: 631–7.

74. Dobson, A. J. (1987). Trends in cardiovascular risk factors in Australia, 1966–1983. Evidence from prevalence surveys. *Community Health Stud.*, **11**: 2–14.

75. Willett, W. C., Stampfer, M. J., Colditz, G. A., Rosner, B. A., Hennekens, C. H., and Speizer, F. E. (1987). Dietary fat and the risk of breast cancer. *N. Engl. J. Med.*, **316**: 22–8.

76. Greenwald, P. (1988). Issues raised by the Women's Health Trial. *J. Natl. Cancer Inst.*, **80**: 788–90.

77. Fraser, G. E. (1986). *Preventive cardiology*, p. 71. Oxford University Press, New York.

78. Rosen, M., Nystrom, L., and Wall, S. (1988). Diet and cancer mortality in the counties of Sweden. *Am. J. Epid.*, **127**: 42–9.

79. Martyn, C. N., Barker, D. J. P., Osmond, C., Harris, E. C., Edwardson, J. A., and Lacey, R. E. (1989). Geographical relation between Alzheimer's disease and aluminium in drinking water. *Lancet*, **i**: 59–62.

11. Case-control and cross-sectional studies

David Coggon

Case-control studies

11.1 INTRODUCTION

In a case-control or case-referent study, patients with a disease (cases) are compared with controls who do not have the disease. The prevalence of past exposure to known or suspected risk factors is measured in each group, and from this the relative risk associated with each factor can be estimated.

Case-control studies are usually quicker and cheaper than cohort studies, but difficulties arise in the choice of appropriate controls and in the unbiased ascertainment of exposure. By definition, exposure must be established retrospectively, and this poses problems in nutritional studies, especially when a disease has a long preclinical phase and the effects of diet are only manifest after a corresponding latent interval. Nevertheless, useful information has been obtained from nutritional case-control studies. For example, studies of stomach cancer have consistently shown a protective effect of fresh fruit and salad vegetables, thus pointing to possible preventive strategies.

The theory of the case-control technique has in the past been confused by its incomplete symmetry with the cohort method. Ideally in a cohort study, controls should be similar to exposed subjects in all ways other than their exposure to the risk factors under investigation. This has led to the erroneous recommendation that controls in a case-control study should be similar to cases in all respects other than their disease status. If carried to the extreme, the outcome of such a policy would be to ensure that the exposure pattern of cases and controls was identical, and no study would ever produce a positive result!

The case-control design is better understood if it is regarded as an efficient method of retrospective sampling within a (usually theoretical) cohort study. A weakness of the cohort method, particularly in the investigation of rare diseases, is that information about exposure must be collected for a large number of subjects who do not go on to develop the disease. The imbalance between the number of cases and non-cases in a cohort study is statistically inefficient. A case-control study attempts to overcome this weakness by measuring exposure in only a sample of non-cases.

There is no simple algorithm that can be followed when planning a case-control study. The important features of the method are discussed below under a series of headings, but the order in which these aspects are considered in the design of a particular investigation will depend upon individual circumstances.

11.2 STUDY POPULATION AND SELECTION OF CASES

Ideally, an investigator planning a case-control study should first formulate the questions that are to be asked in the study, and then select the best population in which to address those questions. The study population must be large enough and have a high enough incidence of disease to provide a sufficient number of cases over the course of the investigation. Furthermore, there should be adequate diversity of exposure to the risk factors under examination within the study population. If everyone in the study population eats a similar diet, then it will be difficult to identify and evaluate nutritional causes of disease. This is particularly so when (as is usual in retrospective studies) dietary habits can only be crudely assessed, because random errors in the measurement of exposure tend to obscure associations with disease (see Chapter 6).

In practice, the choice of a study population is often constrained by operational requirements. For example, the investigator may only have resources to conduct the study in the area where he normally works. In these circumstances it is still important to assess the suitability of the study population at the planning stage. If the population is too small or too uniformly exposed to the risk factors of interest, then it may be better not to waste time on the study.

Occasionally the study population is the starting point of an investigation, and the choice of risk factors for examination is decided secondarily. The trigger to such an investigation might be an unexplained focus of disease. For example, the observation of high rates of stomach cancer in South Louisiana prompted a case-control study to look for a possible dietary explanation.[1] This is a reasonable approach, but it will not be successful if the dietary factor underlying the local excess of disease affects all members of the population uniformly (e.g. the quality of a town's water supply).

Some case-control studies have exploited special circumstances leading to an unusually heterogeneous diet within a population. In Greece a gradual trend from a traditional Mediterranean diet to the consumption of western-style foods has produced a distinctive variation in eating habits. Manousos and colleagues took advantage of this situation to examine the role of diet in the causation of diverticular disease.[2] The associations that they found with high consumption of meat and low consumption of vegetables would have been much less easily demonstrated in a population with more uniform dietary habits.

In the simplest situation the study population is explicitly defined (e.g. all male residents of a town born between 1911 and 1930), and the cases comprise all members of the study population in whom the disease is newly diagnosed (according to specified criteria) during a defined study period. The cases might be identified from hospital or general practice records or perhaps from a cancer registry. Deaths or prevalent cases of disease are sometimes used as an alternative to incident cases because they are easier to ascertain, or are more numerous. However, if this is done, associations must be interpreted with care, because they may reflect an effect not on the rate of occurrence of the disease, but on survival after the disease has developed. For example, an association between mortality from lung cancer and low levels of serum β-carotene might occur not because the vitamin inhibits the development of the disease, but because it is associated with a higher cure rate or longer survival once a tumour is present.

Even when incident cases are used, interpretation may be complicated if the disease is not diagnosed uniformly throughout the study population. In a case-control study of acute appendicitis it would be reasonable to take as cases all members of the study population admitted to hospital as an emergency with histologically confirmed inflammation of the appendix. Acute appendicitis produces severe symptoms that almost always lead to hospital admission and operation. In contrast, diagnosis of uncomplicated duodenal ulcer does not automatically follow the development of disease. Some patients will be asymptomatic or insufficiently concerned about their symptoms to consult a doctor. Some doctors will treat dyspeptic symptoms without attempting to diagnose the specific underlying cause. If these influences that determine the recognition of duodenal ulcer were related in some way to diet (e.g. if stoical individuals tended to eat differently from those who readily complain to a doctor), then spurious associations might arise in a case-control study based on newly diagnosed patients. One way of overcoming this difficulty would be to set up an *ad hoc* surveillance programme within the study population to ensure that cases were ascertained by uniform criteria. Alternatively, it might be acceptable to use the cases that come to diagnosis through the normal channels, but to make allowance for the ensuing biases when interpreting the findings of the study.

Another consideration in the selection of cases is the specificity of the diagnosis. Any advantage from the larger number of cases that can be obtained with a broader definition of disease must be weighed against the loss of sensitivity that will result if an association applies to only a sub-category of the diagnosis under examination. If, for example, a vitamin protects against squamous carcinoma of the bronchus but not against other histological types, the effect will tend to be obscured in an analysis based on all lung cancers combined. If there is no clear *a priori* indication that an association is limited to a specific diagnostic subcategory, it may be better to use a broader definition but at the same time to collect more detailed diagnostic information. Insofar as numbers allow, analyses can then be carried out on subsets of cases to test whether the strength of associations varies for different diagnostic subcategories.

If the number of cases occurring within a study population is too large to be studied, it is quite acceptable to sample within the case group. Ideally, such sampling should be random, but it is often easier to use a non-random sampling method e.g. including only those patients who are admitted to hospital on specified days of the week. This type of systematic samp-ling does not usually create any problems, but the investigator should always consider the scope for bias if a non-random sampling method is employed.

So far it has been assumed that cases will come from a clearly delineated study population, but in practice this is often not so. A physician might wish to study newly diagnosed patients who present in his or her clinic, but the clinic may not receive all the cases that occur within the catchment population of the hospital. Some patients may be seen by colleagues working in the same or related specialities. Furthermore, the catchment population of the hospital may not be clearly defined. Patients living at the periphery of the catchment area may sometimes be referred to a different centre. In this situation one option might be to seek collaboration from the colleagues who are also seeing cases, and at the same time to restrict attention to cases resident in an area immediately around the hospital, from which referral to other centres would be unlikely. Such an approach may facilitate the choice of a control group (see section 11.4), but it is not essential that the study population be explicitly defined. If the cases do not come from an explicitly defined population, it is still helpful to think in terms of a theoretical study population in which individuals are each represented to the extent that they would be likely to be included as cases should they develop the disease under investigation. The arguments for using incident rather than prevalent or fatal cases, and the considerations regarding diagnostic specificity remain unaltered. Whether defined or theoretical, the study population can be thought of as a cohort that is followed for a finite period—the time over which the cases are diagnosed. The controls provide an estimate of exposure patterns in the members of this cohort who are at risk of becoming cases during the period of follow-up. Risk estimates then correspond to those that would be obtained if information about exposure were available for the complete cohort.

11.3 ASCERTAINMENT OF EXPOSURE

Exposure must be measured both to risk factors of interest and also to factors that might confound their association with the disease under study. If the disease has a long preclinical phase, the relevant exposures may have occurred many years before diagnosis, and in nutritional studies this can pose particular difficulties. Most studies rely on recalled dietary histories, but research has shown that people have difficulty in remembering past dietary practices and that answers to questions about previous diet are strongly influenced by current eating habits.[3] This will lead to error if the diet has changed, and particularly if cases and controls have altered their diet to a different extent. Changes in dietary practice are quite likely in diseases, such as cancer or renal failure, that affect the appetite and also where symptoms are aggravated or relieved by certain foods. Patients with gallstones may avoid fatty foods because they cause discomfort and patients with duodenal ulcer may increase their consumption of milk in order to relieve dyspepsia. In some diseases, dietary manipulation may form part of the treatment. For example, in a case-control study of renal stones it was difficult to obtain reliable measures of premorbid fluid intake because most patients with renal colic had been advised to increase their fluid consumption when they first presented to hospital.[4]

Sometimes it is helpful to ask subjects whether they are aware of having altered their diet, although information of this type can usually be only loosely quantified. Another approach has been to identify cases before their disease becomes symptomatic. For example, the relation of breast cancer to diet has been examined in patients diagnosed at screening clinics, and dietary risk factors for stomach cancer have been sought by comparing subjects with intestinal metaplasia of the stomach (a precursor of carcinoma) and controls. However, this strategy can only be employed when the disease has a preclinical phase that can be detected by cheap and ethically acceptable methods.

A common method of measuring diet in case-control studies is by a simple food frequency questionnaire or by a food frequency questionnaire with some estimate of portion size (see section 6.9.3). However, where the diet is constant and unaffected by the presence of the disease (e.g. in a study of early asymptomatic breast cancer detected by screening) it may be possible to use other techniques, such as 24-hour dietary recall or prospective food diary. If the study hypothesis concerns a specific nutrient, it may not be necessary to make a complete dietary assessment. In a study of fractured neck of femur in which calcium was the main nutrient of interest, intake of the mineral was estimated from the consumption of six key foods—milk, bread, cheese, puddings, cakes, and biscuits.[5] This was possible using a relatively simple questionnaire, the validity of which was assessed by comparison with duplicate portion analysis and a seven day weighed record.[6]

Occasionally, case-control studies have used biochemical measures of nutrition (see Chapter 7). For example, in a study to test the hypothesis that Perthes' disease of the hip is caused by deficiency of trace elements, levels of manganese were assayed in the blood (B. M. Margetts, personal communication). Again, there is an assumption that the variable measured has not changed as a consequence of the disease process. A particular advantage of biochemical measures is that they sometimes allow an assessment of long term nutritional status. For example, levels of selenium in toe-nail clippings reflect long term dietary intake.[7]

A confounding factor is associated with the risk factor under study and independently influences the risk of developing the disease. It may give rise to a spurious association when in fact the risk factor is not a cause of the disease, or it may mask a true causal association. Many non-dietary causes of disease, such as smoking habits, physical activity, personal hygiene, and exposure to infection are associated with diet and have the potential to confound its effects. A good example is the association between pancreatic cancer and coffee drinking, which has been demonstrated in several case-control studies, but which is thought to be due, at least in part, to a confounding effect of smoking.[8] In addition, one dietary variable may confound the effects of another. Interpretation of dietary associations in case-control studies requires that potential confounders be measured. However, the effects of a confounder will be large only if it is strongly associated both with the disease and with the dietary risk factor of interest.

11.4 SELECTION OF CONTROLS

The choice of a suitable control group is one of the most difficult aspects of case-control design. The aim is that controls should give a reliable estimate of exposure to risk factors and confounders among members of the defined or theoretical study population who are at risk of becoming cases during the period of study. This objective leads to two requirements:

1. The exposure of controls should be representative of that in members of the study population who are at risk of becoming cases.

2. The exposure of controls should be ascertainable with the same accuracy as for cases. (Ideally, exposure would be measured with complete accuracy in all subjects. In practice this ideal is rarely attainable but, if the

distribution of measurement errors is similar for cases and controls, the effect will tend to be conservative. It may mask a true association, but it will not give rise to spurious associations, see Chapter 3.)

It is in trying to reconcile these two requirements that problems are encountered. Two types of control are commonly used:

11.4.1 Patients with other diseases

Patients with other diseases are frequently a convenient source of controls, especially in hospital-based studies. They have the advantage that ascertainment of exposure can often be made comparable to that for cases. One of the dangers in studies based on anamnestic data is that, because of a natural interest in trying to find out why they have become ill, cases are more motivated to recall past exposures than controls. However, if the controls are also ill, they too will be seeking an explanation for their disease. It may be possible to blind subjects to the exact purpose of the study so that controls are not aware that their illness is not of prime interest. Furthermore, in studies that collect information at interview, it may be feasible to blind the interviewer as to whether he or she is dealing with a case or control, and so eliminate the possibility that, deliberately or subconsciously, questions are addressed differently to cases and controls. Another advantage of using other patients as controls in hospital-based studies is that control diagnoses can be chosen so that their catchment population is similar to that for cases. This is helpful where the boundaries of the catchment area of the hospital are ill-defined.

The main weakness of using patients with other diseases as controls is that their exposure may not be representative of that in members of the study population who are at risk of becoming cases. For example, controls with peptic ulcer or diabetes would be unlikely to have diets typical of those in the general population. It is, of course, open to the investigator to exclude from the control group diseases that have known dietary associations, but the possibility of unrecognized bias remains. The effect of such unsuspected biases is potentially greatest when all the controls have the same disease. For this reason, when using patients with other diseases as controls, it is better to include a range of control diagnoses.

11.4.2 Subjects selected from the general population

Various methods have been used to select controls from the general population. Some studies have used a predetermined algorithm to choose controls living in the same street or neighbourhood as cases; in Britain and Scandinavia population registers derived from censuses or health service records have been taken as a sampling frame and in countries such as the

United States and Hong Kong, where almost everyone has a telephone, controls have been obtained by random digit dialling.

In general, the exposures of controls selected in these ways are likely to be more representative of those in the population at risk of becoming cases, although biases may occur if there is a poor response rate from controls. (The exposure patterns of non-responders are often different from those of subjects who agree to take part in surveys.) The main problem with community controls lies in the ascertainment of exposure, since subjects selected from the general population will usually be less motivated than cases to put time and effort into helping with a study. Where such recall bias is a concern, its magnitude can sometimes be gauged by including dummy questions about variables that the investigator thinks are unlikely to be related to the disease under study. However, this technique does not eliminate the bias.

There is usually no perfect control group, and the choice of controls must be a compromise. Three general rules are worth bearing in mind:

1. Controls should always come from the study population, i.e. they should be people who would have become cases had they developed the disease during the period of study.

2. Where possible, the method used to ascertain exposure should be similar for cases and controls. For example, if controls are to be interviewed at home, it is better if cases are also interviewed at home.

3. If information is to be obtained at interview or by physical examination (e.g. measurement of height, weight, skinfold thickness), this should where possible, be carried out blind to the case/control status of the subject. Similarly, laboratory analyses should be performed without knowledge of whether specimens come from cases or controls. If it is not practical to keep an interviewer or examiner blind to a subject's status, then it is an advantage to keep him or her unaware of the exact purpose of the study. Subconscious biases in the method of questioning or examination are then less likely.

Having fixed on a control group, the investigator should try to assess the likely magnitude and direction of any resultant bias, and take that bias into account when interpreting the findings. Interpretation may sometimes be easier if two control groups are used such that any biases are likely to be in opposite directions (perhaps one comprising patients with other diseases and one from the general community). The true relative risk can then be expected to lie somewhere between the estimates obtained with each set of controls.

11.4.3 Matching

In many case-control studies, controls are chosen to match the cases in one or more ways. The matching may be on an individual basis (e.g. each case is paired with a control of the same age and sex) or in groups (e.g. controls are chosen to include similar proportions of current, ex-, and non-smokers to the case group). Matching is used in case-control studies for three reasons:

1. To permit allowance for complex confounders or for confounders that are difficult to define, e.g. by comparing within identical twin case/control pairs, it is possible to allow for ill-defined genetic confounders.

2. To make allowance for confounders statistically more efficient. Efficient analysis requires that there be a similar ratio of cases to controls at each level of exposure to the confounding variable.

3. To reduce biases in the ascertainment of exposure, e.g. if some cases are deceased, it may still be possible to elicit useful dietary histories from their spouses. However, such information is unlikely to be as accurate or complete as would be obtained from the subjects themselves. To make the collection of information for cases and controls comparable, deceased cases could be matched with deceased controls.

Unlike in a cohort study, matching in a case-control study does not in itself eliminate the effects of a confounder. On the contrary, if the factor matched is associated with the exposure under study, but is not itself a risk factor for the disease, then confounding may be introduced where none was previously present. Thus, when matching is employed in the design of a case-control study, it is essential to allow for the matching in the analysis. Matching for a variable that is associated with the exposure under study but not with the disease is statistically inefficient (in effect it removes some of the variation in exposure within the study population), and should be avoided if possible.

Once a variable has been matched it cannot be examined as an independent risk factor in the analysis (although it is still possible to explore whether it modifies the effect of other risk factors). Also, matching on more than two or three variables can become very time consuming and expensive, especially if effort is required to establish whether a potential control fulfils the matching criteria, and a high proportion end up being rejected because they do not meet the requirements. Matching is therefore usually limited to age and sex (which are almost always potential confounders) and perhaps one other variable.

A matched set in which exposure data are missing for all of the cases or all of the controls contributes nothing to the analysis. Any information about the exposure that has been collected for members of such a set is thus wasted. Insofar as such redundancy is more likely to occur with the smaller sets that are formed by individual matching, it is preferable to employ group matching if feasible. For example, it may be better to group match within 5-year age bands, rather than individually match to within 2 years of age.

When matching is employed, the exposures of controls should be representative of those at-risk members of the study population within each matching stratum.

11.4.4 Controls who are lost from the study

One common source of concern in the design of case-control studies is the control who is lost from the study because he/she cannot be contacted or refuses to participate. Is it permissible to replace lost controls? Clearly, if drop-outs have different exposure to risk factors from participants, their loss will introduce bias. However, replacing lost controls does not increase the bias, and may in some circumstances be advantageous. For example, when cases and controls are individually matched in pairs, failure to replace a lost control will lead to any information about the corresponding case being wasted.

11.4.5 Controls who go on to become cases

Another area of concern is the control who goes on to develop the disease. In a 3-year study of incident cases of myocardial infarction with controls selected from the general population, what should happen if a control chosen in the first year proceeds to become a case in year three? Understanding of this problem becomes clearer if the case-control study is viewed in the context of the cohort within which it samples. If the entire cohort was studied, subjects who developed the disease would contribute person-years at risk up to the time at which they became cases. Thus, in the case-control study it is quite legitimate that a control should contribute information about the exposure of persons at risk, even though he/she subsequently goes on to become a case. However, statistical calculations become more complicated if some subjects appear in the analysis as both cases and controls, and it may be simpler to discard controls who later become cases. In practice the event is usually so rare that it makes little difference whether they are included or excluded.

11.5 STUDY SIZE AND STATISTICAL POWER

The statistical power of a case-control study depends upon the number of cases and of controls, the distribution of the exposure of interest in the population at risk of becoming cases, and the relative risk of disease in those who are exposed. In the simple situation of an unmatched study with equal numbers of cases and controls, there is a formula whereby for a given prevalence of exposure in the population at risk one can calculate the number of subjects needed to detect a given relative risk (strictly odds ratio—see section 11.6) with specified Type 1 and Type 2 statistical errors.[9] Alternatively, if the number of subjects is given, the level of detectable relative risk can be derived.[10]

Where the aim of the study is to establish whether an association exists (i.e. whether the relative risk is different from one), and there is no constraint on the availability of cases and controls, the optimal ratio of controls to cases is 1:1. However, in some studies only a limited number of cases is available for study, or information can be obtained more cheaply and easily for controls than for cases. In these circumstances it may be better to have more than one control per case. However, there is a law of diminishing returns, and little is gained by having more than four controls per case (Fig. 11.1). Normally, a ratio of controls to cases greater than 4:1 would only be used if additional controls were very readily available. In a matched case-control study it is not necessary to have the same ratio of controls to cases in all matched sets or strata. Modern analytical techniques easily deal with a variable ratio.

There is no simple method for estimating statistical power when matching is to be used or allowance must be made for confounders. However, an

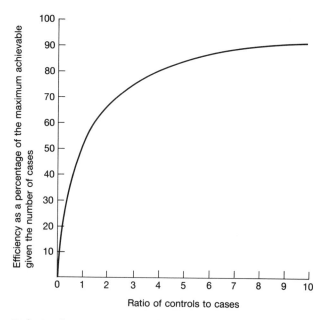

Fig. 11.1. Relation between statistical efficiency and ratio of controls to cases.

adequate approximation can usually be obtained by ignoring any confounders and assuming a simple unmatched design.

11.6 ANALYSIS AND INTERPRETATION

Two measures of association are commonly derived from case-control studies—the odds ratio and the attributable proportion. In most circumstances the odds ratio approximates closely to the relative risk. The attributable proportion, also known as the attributable risk per cent, is a measure of the proportion of cases in the study population that can be attributed to the risk factor (assuming that the effect of the risk factor is not confounded). Attributable risk and population attributable risk cannot be estimated directly from case-control studies.

In an unmatched study with dichotomous exposure distributed between cases and controls as in Table 11.1a, the odds ratio is estimated by the

Table 11.1. Distribution of exposure in case-control studies

(a) Unmatched study

	cases	controls
exposed	a	b
unexposed	c	d

(b) Matched study

	control exposed	control unexposed
case exposed	a	b
case unexposed	c	d

cross-product ad/bc. Approximate confidence limits for this estimate are given by the formula:

$$\exp\left\{\ln\left(\frac{ad}{bc}\right) \pm z_\alpha \sqrt{\left(\frac{1}{a} + \frac{1}{b} + \frac{1}{c} + \frac{1}{d}\right)}\right\}$$

where $100 - 2\alpha$ is the level of confidence. The statistical significance of the association is assessed by the chi-squared test.

In a similar study, but with pairwise matching, the distribution of exposures is displayed as in Table 11.1b, and the odds ratio is estimated by b/c. Approximate confidence limits for the estimate are given by:

$$\exp\left\{\ln\left(\frac{b}{c}\right) \pm z_\alpha \sqrt{\left(\frac{b+c}{bc}\right)}\right\}$$

where $100-2\alpha$ is the level of confidence. Statistical significance is assessed by McNemar's test.

More complex statistical techniques are needed when exposure variables have more than two levels or are continuous; when some matched sets have control:case ratios other than one; and to examine interactions between two or more exposure variables (including potential confounders). For further information readers should consult specialized texts, such as those by Rothman[11] and Breslow and Day.[12]

Computer software is now available to make even these complex statistical procedures relatively easy. Interpretation does not require complete understanding of the underlying mathematics, but the epidemiologist should at least be aware of any biological assumptions that are inherent in the analytical model. For example, in a logistic regression analysis there may be an assumption that, when risk factors are present in combination, their odds ratios multiply. The investigator must decide whether this supposition is justified. It is possible to test for interactions within the statistical model, but a final decision as to its acceptability will also rest on an understanding of the biological mechanisms that are thought to underlie the relevant associations. If two risk factors act at different stages in a carcinogenic sequence, then their effects might be expected to multiply. If they both act in the same way at the same stage, then an additive effect would perhaps be more likely.

It is also important that interpretation of the statistical analysis takes into account the possibility of biases in the study method and of unrecognized confounders. Measurement error is a special problem in dietary studies and can produce substantial bias (see Chapter 3). Assessment of whether an observed association is likely to be directly causal and not the result of unrecognized confounding depends upon several considerations:

1. The size of the relative risk. In general, higher relative risks are less likely to be explained by unknown confounders. The confounding exposure would have to carry an even higher risk and as such one might expect it to be recognizable.

2. The presence of a dose–response relation. The observation of a higher risk in subjects with greater exposure to the risk factor favours a direct causal relationship.

3. The existence of plausible biological mechanisms that might explain a causal relationship.

11.7 NESTED CASE-CONTROL STUDIES

The case-control approach has been presented as a method of efficient sampling within a theoretical cohort study. Occasionally, however, case-control investigations are 'nested' within real cohort studies. For example, in a study to examine the influence of vitamin status on subsequent cancer incidence, blood specimens might be obtained from a cohort of individuals who were then followed-up over a period of years. Rather than carrying out expensive assays for the whole cohort it might be preferable to store the specimens under appropriate conditions, and then at a later date analyse material from the cases of cancer and from a suitable sample of controls. The principles of the design are the same as in any case-control study. Controls chosen for a particular case should be members of the cohort who were themselves at risk of becoming cases at the time the case was diagnosed.

Cross-sectional studies

In a cross-sectional study, information is collected from a sample of a population at one point in time. The information may be about a disease state (e.g. obesity, iron deficiency anaemia) or about known or suspected risk factors for disease (e.g. dietary habits, smoking).

The main application of such data is in planning health promotion and health care. Rational design of health programmes requires information about the nature and scale of problems that are to be tackled. For example, if the aim were to prevent osteomalacia, it would help to know which sections of the population were prone to the disorder and what were the features of their diets. Appropriate advice could then be targeted most efficiently.

A second use is to characterize the diets of different populations in a way that can be related to their patterns of disease incidence. For example, Cade and colleagues surveyed eating habits among middle-aged residents of three English towns, and then looked to see how these correlated with death rates for coronary heart diease.[13] Such 'ecological' studies are discussed in Chapter 10.

Another application of cross-sectional surveys is to identify subjects with and without a disease for use in case-control comparisons. Sometimes, information about past exposures is obtained at the same time that disease is ascertained, i.e. for the complete study sample. Alternatively, cases and controls may be identified as a primary exercise, and exposure data sought secondarily for only this subset of subjects. The latter approach has merits if the disease is of low prevalence and exposures are costly to measure. Whichever method is adopted, the cases will be prevalent rather than incident, and care is therefore needed in the interpretation of associations (see earlier section on case-control studies).

Cross-sectional studies present fewer problems in design than case-control studies, but care may be needed with the sampling method if the findings from a sample are to be extrapolated to a larger population. Where possible, random sampling techniques should be used. Ascertainment of diet or nutritional status is often carried out prospectively (e.g. by a food diary or collection of duplicate portions), but the retrospective methods used in case-control studies may be more suitable in some circumstances.

REFERENCES

1. Correa, P., Fontham, E., Pickle, L. W., Chen, V., Lin, Y., and Haenszel, W. (1985). Dietary determinants of gastric cancer in South Louisiana inhabitants. *JNCI.*, **75**: 645–54.
2. Manousos, O., Day, N. E., Tzonou, A., Kapetanakis, A., Polychronopoulou, A., and Trichopoulos, D. (1985). Diet and other factors in the aetiology of diverticulosis: an epidemiological study in Greece. *Gut*, **26**: 544–9.
3. Wu, M. L., Whittemore, A. S., and Jung, D. L. (1988). Errors in reported dietary intakes: II long-term recall. *Am. J. Epid.*, **128**: 1137–45.
4. Power, C., Barker, D. J. P., Nelson, M., and Winter, P. D. (1984). Diet and renal stones: a case-control study. *Br. J. Urol.*, **56**: 456–9.
5. Cooper, C., Barker, D. J. P., and Wickham, C. (1988). Physical activity, muscle strength, and calcium intake in fracture of the proximal femur. *Br. Med. J.*, **297**: 1443–6.
6. Nelson, M., Hague, G. F., Cooper, C., and Bunker, V. W. (1988). Calcium intake in the elderly: validation of a dietary questionnaire. *J. Hum. Nutr. Dietet.*, **1**: 115–27.
7. Morris, J., Stampfer, M. J., and Willett, W. (1983). Dietary selenium in humans. Toenails as an indicator. *Biol. Trace Element Res.*, **5**: 529–37.
8. La Vecchia, C., Liati, P., Decarli, A., Negri, E. and Franceschi, S. (1987). Coffee consumption and risk of pancreatic cancer. *Int. J. Cancer*, **40**: 309–13.
9. Schlesselman, J. J. (1974). Sample size requirements in cohort and case control studies of disease. *Am. J. Epid.*, **99**: 381–4.
10. Walter, S. D. (1977). Determination of significant relative risks and optimal sampling procedures in prospective and retrospective comparative studies of various sizes. *Am. J. Epid.*, **105**: 387–97.
11. Rothman, K. J. (1986). *Modern epidemiology*. Little, Brown and Co., Boston.
12. Breslow, N. E. and Day, N. E. (1980). *Statistical methods in cancer research*. International Agency for Research on Cancer, Lyon.
13. Cade, J. E., Barker, D. J. P., Margetts, B. M., and Morris, J. A. (1988). Diet and inequalities in health in three English towns. *Br. Med. J.*, **296**: 1359–62.

12. Cohort studies

Michael L. Burr

12.1 GENERAL CONSIDERATIONS

Cohort studies have provided much valuable information about nutrition in relation to health. A cohort was a tenth part of a Roman legion and contained 300–600 men who marched together. The word has been adopted by epidemiologists to refer to a group of persons, identified at one point in time, who march off together into the future under the watchful eye of an investigator. The essence of a cohort study is that a group of persons is defined, certain characteristics about each individual are recorded, and they are then followed up in such a way that new events (such as disease and death) or other changes in their characteristics are detected. These new events and changes can then be related to the original observations in order to discover what aspects of the initial status of the subjects predict their subsequent experience.

The subjects in most cohort studies are followed up for the duration of the study, measurements and other observations are made on them when the study begins and information about new events is collected during the subsequent period or at some point in the future, when the original measurements may be repeated. Occasionally, however, a cohort is defined with reference to some time in the past (e.g. all the patients who attended a diabetic clinic 5 years ago) and followed up to see how they are now. These two approaches are sometimes called prospective and retrospective cohort studies, respectively. Unfortunately the terminology is somewhat confused in that some writers use the term 'prospective' of all cohort studies, in that the reasoning is always forwards in time, from causes to effects, even if not in execution of the study. In contrast, case-control studies usually look backwards from effects to causes.

The principal use of the cohort study is in the elucidation of aetiology. If we suspect that nutrition affects health in some way, we can assess the nutritional status of a group of people (by recording heights and weights, dietary intakes, or biochemical measurements), follow them up, and see whether their disease experience is related to their initial status. Investigations of this kind have been valuable in the study of ischaemic heart disease and other common conditions. Another use of cohort studies is in studying the natural history of a disease. Here the investigator defines a group of persons with a given disease, taking care to obtain a group that represents all patients with the disease, usually at the point of diagnosis. The patients are then followed up to investigate the course of the disease, e.g. in what proportion does the disease remit, and can its remission or advance be linked with anything in the patients' condition at the start?

There are important reasons for preferring the cohort type of study to the case-control approach. First, it enables the investigator to obtain accurate information about the individuals before the onset of the disease being investigated. This is particularly important in dietary enquiries, because a person's diet is liable to change over time and it is unrealistic to expect him/her to remember his/her dietary pattern of several years ago. The difficulty is even greater when the disease in question is likely to affect the subject's diet. For example, if we want to know whether diet affects the risk of ulcerative colitis, we are interested in the diet taken before the disease arose. A case-control design requires us to ask patients (and controls) about the diet they took some years ago. But the disease itself has probably affected their eating habits, and they may find it difficult to remember what they used to eat before their diet changed. A cohort design obviates this difficulty, in that the diet is recorded before the subjects acquire the condition.

Secondly, the information obtained prospectively is not only more accurate but is also less open to bias than that obtained retrospectively, when the outcome is known. And, thirdly, the cohort design allows us to detect unexpected effects of the initial factors, whereas a case-control analysis is restricted to the selected condition. A good cohort study provides a database that can be used afterwards to test hypotheses that were not thought of when it was set up. For example, the hypothesis that dietary fibre confers protection against various diseases has been tested on cohorts whose dietary intake was documented before dietary fibre was thought to be important.

The disadvantages of the cohort study are inherent in its design. It will inevitably take several years for aetiological factors to reveal their effects, so studies of this kind tend to be lengthy. Furthermore, the investigator usually assumes that the dietary information and other measurements at the start will continue to describe the subjects for the succeeding period of time. But it may happen that the subjects alter their eating habits, either spontaneously or as a result of changes in dietary fashion, to such an extent that the original observations are irrelevant. Other related disadvantages are the difficulties of tracing all the subjects, unforeseen changes in the personnel involved in the study, and the ultimate hazard that the hypothesis being tested becomes superseded, so that the investigator finds he/she has recorded the wrong baseline information. It must also be recognized that the cohort approach is unsuitable for the study of uncommon diseases, unless one is able to cope with very large numbers.

Occasionally, a 'hybrid' design is used, combining the cohort and case-control approaches. If a large cohort is being followed up, and a sample of every member's serum has been stored, a case-control analysis can be made within the cohort at a later date. Persons who acquire or die from a given disease are identified, and controls (usually two or three per case) are selected from the cohort, each control being matched with a case in respect of various characteristics such as age, sex, social class, etc. at entry. The sera of cases and controls are extracted and appropriate biochemical analyses are made. The sensitivity of the comparison is not much less than it would be if the specimens from all the subjects were used, and the time and expense of the analysis is greatly reduced. The advantages of the cohort method are thus retained, together with the greater efficiency of the case-control design.

12.2 PRACTICAL ISSUES

The design of a cohort study will, of course, depend on the hypothesis under investigation, but certain general principles apply in all cases. Since cohort studies are liable to involve large numbers of subjects and to require commitment of resources for several years, it is wise to obtain expert statistical advice at the planning stage so as to ensure that the study is likely to be large and long enough but not greatly in excess of the requirements.

The cohort itself is then defined, e.g. all babies born in a given hospital between certain dates; a random sample of 300 persons aged 65–74 years registered with general practitioners in a certain town; all the residents in homes for the elderly in a certain area. Permission is obtained from the consultants, general practitioners, and other appropriate authorities for their patients to be involved. Suitable forms are designed on which information can be collected and coded for easy computerization. Alternatively, portable computers can be obtained and programs designed to permit direct data entry. It is wise to conduct a short pilot study to test the procedures that will be used in the survey. At this point it may transpire (for example) that elderly people find difficulty with one type of dietary scales (because the digits are too small, or because it is calibrated in grams rather than ounces), and that a different type is more acceptable. The information is collected and checked at the time, and coded without delay (preferably by the person who interviewed the subject), so that ambiguities and obvious errors can be dealt with while memories are fresh. It is frustrating to find, months (or years) later, that data cannot be used because of some omission that could easily have been rectified at the time.

If the cohort is to be followed up for several years, it is inevitable that some of the subjects will change their diet, so that the initial information no longer applies. In so far as such changes occur as a consequence of alterations in the subjects' state of health, it is the previous diet that the investigators are usually interested in, and the cohort rather than the case-control design will have been chosen precisely to obtain information about it. But some of the changes in diet will occur for other reasons, and the investigator may wish to know to what extent the original data characterize the subjects during the whole period in question. It may not be feasible for the entire cohort to be re-examined periodically, but information can be obtained from a subsample and will provide some estimate of the stability of the original measurements in the group being studied.

Follow-up needs careful planning. It may be the intention to acquire information during the whole of the follow-up period (e.g. about illnesses experienced during the next two years). Contact will then have to be made with the subjects periodically, either by visiting or by telephone. If day to day information is required (e.g. on infant feeding methods) a diary may be used. In some studies the intention is to review the cohort at some time in the future rather than continuously. The problem then arises that some of the subjects will have moved or died, and information may not be easily obtained, particularly in a free-living population. Plans should be made at the start of the study about how the subjects will be traced. Persons who are 'lost to follow-up' are almost certainly different from the rest in several important respects, and if they are at all numerous some serious biases may arise. If the follow-up extends overs several years it may be very difficult to trace persons who moved soon after they entered the study.

Various techniques can be used, and the successful investigator has to acquire skills similar to those of private detective agencies. The cardinal rule is to anticipate the difficulties that will undoubtedly arise. It may be advisable to have periodic contact with all the subjects (say at annual intervals), by telephone or reply-paid card, simply in order to detect those who have left the area. Someone who moved recently is much easier to find than someone who moved several years ago: the neighbours may have forgotten or lost the information or moved themselves. Telephone directories and electoral registers are helpful in locating people whose where-abouts are approximately but not exactly known. If the study is hospital-based, the subjects' hospital numbers should be recorded. The next of kin is routinely recorded and may assist in finding people. Deaths can be traced via the National Health Service Central Registry, which can supply causes of death. It is a great help to have the subjects' National Health Service numbers, which should be obtained at the start. The NHS records of all the subjects can be flagged at the start of the study so that deaths (with causes) are notified automatically to the investigators.

Another way of minimizing the difficulties of finding subjects is to select them from certain occupations whose members are particularly easy to trace. Medical practitioners are all registered with the General Medical Council and listed in the Medical Registry; their names also appear in the

Medical Directory. Civil Servants can be traced through their pension arrangements. Several long term cohort studies have utilized these opportunities by enlisting subjects from these or similar occupational groups.

Other potential difficulties should be anticipated as far as possible. If the intention is to look for changes in biochemical variates (e.g. serum cholesterol), the study should be discussed with the biochemist at the start so as to avoid a change in laboratory methodology, which will invalidate comparisons. Changes in staff or collaborators may be more difficult to foresee and can have a disastrous effect if the newcomer does not have the same degree of interest or commitment as the person with whom the study was set up. If the final measurements (e.g. of blood pressure) are to be made by someone other than the person who made the initial measurements, attention should be paid to standardization and comparability. It may also be desirable for the person recording the final measurements or endpoints to be unaware of the initial data, so as to avoid bias.

A few examples will be given of cohort studies in different age groups to illustrate the use of this approach.

12.3 INFANCY AND CHILDHOOD

Infancy provides perhaps the best possible opportunity for cohort studies. A cohort of babies can easily be defined in terms of place and time of birth. Some information (e.g. regarding birthweight and initial mode of feeding) is collected routinely and can be supplemented with other details as required. The duration of such studies can in principle be extended indefinitely; even the longevity of the original investigators need not be a limitation!

Large national birth cohorts have been set up in which all the children born during a single week (or a random sample of them) were identified and followed up. The National Survey of Health and Development,[1] the National Child Development Study,[2], and the Child Health and Education Study[3] were based on children born in Britain during one week in 1946, 1958, and 1970, respectively, and have yielded much useful information. Nutritional aspects of these studies include longitudinal data on height and weight, and the relationship between mode of feeding in infancy with the subsequent development of various diseases.

Localized studies allow these issues to be looked at more frequently and in greater detail to see what nutritional and other factors affect development. For example, one cohort study monitored the growth of about a thousand babies in two South Wales towns up to the age of five years.[4] Length (or height), weight, head circumference, and skinfold thickness were measured six times up to 1 year and at 6-monthly intervals thereafter. It was found that those whose birth weight was less than 2500 g tended to be substantially smaller than the other children at the age of five, when growth in head circumference was a year behind that of the others, while height and weight were 25 and 40 weeks behind, respectively. The majority of the children 'tracked' along their growth centiles, more than 80 per cent remaining in the same or an adjacent quintile during the whole period of the study. Children in the different social classes tended to diverge after the age of 2 years, height and head circumference increasing more rapidly in those from the upper social classes than in the others. Maternal smoking had an important effect, particularly on birth weight.

Similar studies have been conducted in older children. A cohort of children in Harpenden[5] has been the basis for the construction of centile curves for height velocity and weight velocity, which (unlike simple height and weight centiles) require longitudinal rather than cross-sectional data. These curves have provided invaluable information about growth in children and form a frame of reference against which individuals can be compared so as to detect the unusual or pathological. In countries with a high childhood mortality, cohort studies are even more important in that they are likely to reveal the factors predisposing to death.

The investigation of the causation of specific conditions obviously calls for a special approach. As an example, we may consider the hypothesis that infant feeding affects the risk of acquiring allergic disease. The case-control approach is likely to be unsatisfactory; by the time the children have acquired allergic diseases, their mothers have probably forgotten the details of how they were fed in infancy. Furthermore, the mothers' recollections may be biased by what has happened since. The cohort design allows the relevant information to be collected prospectively, without risk of bias. The sensitivity of the study can be increased by selecting infants at high risk by virtue of a family history of atopic disease. Allergic conditions such as eczema and asthma are common, and it might be expected that a few cohort studies would easily establish whether or not these diseases are associated (positively or negatively) with breast feeding and early introduction of various foods.

Unfortunately, the results of numerous cohort studies show a remarkable lack of consistency:[6] several suggest that breast feeding protects against allergic disease, but some show no such effect, while at least one study shows a positive association between breast feeding and allergy. These inconsistencies illustrate the weakness of the observational approach in epidemiology; mothers who decide to breast feed their infants are different from those who decide to bottle feed, and these differences may be just as important as the mode of feeding in determining the risk of allergy. It may now be the case that, as breast feeding is believed to be protective, those babies who are most at risk of allergic disease (through having a strong family history) may be most likely to be breast fed, so creating a spurious positive association. Statistical methods such as multivariate analysis can allow for various confounding factors, but it is impossible to be sure that the right confounders have been identified or their effects completely eliminated. It may well be the case that different confounding variables operate in different populations, so that a study conducted in one area should not necessarily be an exact replica of one conducted somewhere else.

12.4 ADULTS

Cohort studies in adults have been very useful in elucidating the role of diet in the causation of disease. Nutrition is a major determinant of health, so it is obviously important to investigate its influence on morbidity and mortality. Everybody eats food, but not necessarily the same food, so there are ample opportunities for comparing the effects of different dietary habits within the same population.

Ischaemic heart disease (IHD) is a good example of a relationship between diet and health, and has been investigated in this way. Table 12.1 summarizes nine cohort studies that have reported associations between diet and heart disease. These studies showed considerable differences in methodology and analysis, and this summary of their findings is somewhat over-simplified. The various dietary methods have different degrees of reliability, which together with the wide range of numbers and the variety of countries, presumably explain the differences between the results. Thus, it is not entirely surprising that the same dietary factors do not emerge as important in every study. But some consistent features may be seen: no factor had a significant positive association in one study and a significant negative association in another; fat showed positive associations in several studies (although in the Puerto Rico study the association was with polyunsaturated rather than saturated fat); energy, fibre, and alcohol showed negative associations; while sugar was not associated with IHD in any study.

The interpretation of these findings illustrates the strengths and weaknesses of observational cohort studies. The investigators have had to assume that the information they obtained at the start would characterize the subjects throughout the follow-up period. This assumption will inevitably be partly false. First, most studies rely on dietary recall, which is particularly unreliable for people whose food is prepared for them: married men often have only a vague idea of what their wives give them to eat, or even what they ate yesterday. Secondly, if a precise account is obtained about intake over a short period of time (e.g. using weighed intake records), it may not represent habitual intake. And, thirdly, the subjects' eating habits may change during the period in which diet continues to influence the reported outcome. To this extent, therefore, the studies may fail to reveal associa-

Table 12.1 Some cohort studies of dietary factors associated with IHD incidence or mortality

Study	Dietary methods	No. subjects	Dietary factors		
			Positively associated	Negatively associated	Not associated
Framingham[9]	24 h recall	859		Energy, Alcohol	Fat, Sugar
Honolulu[9]	24 h recall	8006	Fat	Energy, Alcohol	Sugar
Ireland-Boston[10]	Food frequency	1001	Fat	?Fibre, Vegetables	Energy, Sugar
London[11]	Weighed intakes	337		Fibre	Fat
Puerto Rico[9]	24 h recall	9150	Fat	Energy	Sugar
Rancho Bernardo[12]	24 h recall	859		Energy, Alcohol, Fibre	Fat, Energy, Alcohol, Sugar
Seven Countries[13]	Weighed intakes (subsample)	12770	Fat		Sugar
Western Electric[14,15]	Detailed history	1900	Fat score	Fish	
Zutphen[16,17]	Detailed history	871		Energy, Fish	Fat

tions between diet and disease that would be found if more information were available.

A more profound issue concerns the interpretation of the associations that were reported. To what extent is an association likely to be causal, or could it be the result of confounding with some other dietary or non-dietary factor? In several of these studies, fibre has emerged as apparently protective. Is this because it is actually protective, or is the relationship attributable to a tendency for people to take a high fibre diet as part of a healthy life style, other aspects of which may be more important? The inverse relationship between IHD and energy intake presumably reflects a protective effect of exercise, although in some individuals inability to take exercise is a consequence (rather than a cause) of heart disease and related illnesses. The cohort design enables information about pre-existent illness to be recorded at the start, so that the analysis can be confined to persons who were then apparently healthy. This issue has been debated, especially in relation to alcohol: is the negative relationship between IHD and alcohol (which has been reported in several other studies) attributable to a protective effect of alcohol or to a tendency of people with early IHD to abstain from it? There is evidence to support both views, and the issue still remains open. Fat intake (as a percentage of total energy) is an adverse factor in several studies; to some extent it is confounded with other 'non-healthy' habits, such as smoking and lack of exercise. These difficulties of interpretation all arise because people who choose a diet high in fibre and low in fat are likely to differ from other people, and only a controlled trial can distinguish clearly between causal and non-causal associations.

Some cohort studies have examined one or two specific dietary factors rather than a wide range of foods. Intakes of coffee, tea, and alcohol are more easily described and likely to be fairly constant for any individual, so that drinking habits are sometimes available when other dietary information is absent. Coffee consumption has been positively related to IHD in several prospective studies.

If it is the intention to examine the causation of less common diseases, a larger cohort will be required to yield sufficient cases within a reasonable time. An example of a study involving several diseases is that undertaken amongst Californian Seventh-day Adventists, about half of whom are vegetarians.[7] More than 27 000 people over the age of 30 years completed a questionnaire that enquired about food and beverage consumption as well as other details of lifestyle. Deaths over the next 20 years were identified by means of record linkage with the local death certificate file. The vegetarians had a lower IHD mortality than the non-vegetarians among both men and women; in men, the vegetarians had a lower mortality from all causes (including diabetes) than the non-vegetarians. Frequency of meat consumption was significantly related to IHD mortality in both men and women. One advantage of this study was that all the subjects were non-smokers and non-drinkers and followed a generally similar life-style, so that many potential confounding factors were eliminated.

12.5 THE ELDERLY

There are several reasons for expecting cohort studies to be particularly easy and fruitful in the elderly. Old people tend to have fairly definite likes and dislikes so that the diet of any old person is likely to be more uniform (and therefore more easily characterized) than that of a younger person. Nutritional deficiency is more common in old age than at other periods of life, yet many elderly people eat very well. The dietary variation between individuals is therefore large in comparison with the variation within individuals. Furthermore, morbidity and mortality are very high in the elderly, so more endpoints will occur per person-year of follow-up than at younger ages.

Several nutritional cohort studies have been conducted in the elderly. The subjects' initial condition has been recorded in terms of body mass index, dietary intake, and various biochemical indices. For example, a sample of 830 persons over the age of 65 years was selected from general practitioners' lists in a certain area and stratified so as to provide relatively more over the age of 75 years.[8] Height, weight, plasma and leucocyte ascorbate concentration and certain other variates were measured, and the subjects were followed up and reweighed 8 years later. There was a tendency for initial ascorbic acid status to be inversely related to mortality, but it is not entirely clear how this should be interpreted. It may be that vitamin C deficiency is a common cause of ill-health in the elderly, so that a low vitamin C status results in a greater risk of death. Alternatively, the causal relationship may be in the opposite direction: old people who are in poor health for any reason are likely to have some impairment of appetite (and perhaps of their metabolism), such that their intakes and blood levels of various nutrients will be low.

The confounding effect of differential ageing is particularly important in old age, and is well illustrated by the paradoxical finding that obesity is a favourable prognostic index in the elderly.[8] Over the age of 65, people tend on average to lose weight as they grow older; this was noticed by Shakespeare in his description of the seven ages of man (*As You Like It*, Act II, scene 8): the fifth age is 'the justice, in fair and round belly', while the sixth age is 'the lean and slipper'd pantaloon, . . . his youthful hose well sav'd, a world too wide for his shrunk shank' (i.e. his old trousers are now too big for him). But not everybody ages at the same rate. Some enter Shakespeare's sixth age ahead of their contemporaries: they tend to be leaner and to die earlier, while those who are biologically young for their chronological age are on average fatter and less likely to die in the next few years. But it does not necessarily follow that thin old people would live longer if they managed to put on weight.

12.6 CONCLUSIONS

Cohort studies allow more rigourous testing of aetiological hypotheses than other observational studies. They also provide unique information about the natural history of disease. Their disadvantages firstly concern feasibility, because they tend to be large, long, and suitable only for the study of common diseases. Secondly, they share other weaknesses of the observational approach, in that the subjects determine their own nutritional status, which may therefore be confounded with various other relevant factors. This confounding is particularly important when the nutritional variables are likely to be associated with particular lifestyles or the initial state of health and senescence of the subjects. In so far as it is not possible to conduct long term randomized controlled trials of dietary changes in free-living populations, cohort studies provide the best available evidence of aetiology.

APPENDIX: CHECKLIST FOR PLANNING A COHORT STUDY

1 Purpose of the study

(1) What hypotheses will the study examine?

(2) What other specific questions will it address?

2 Value of the study

(1) If the hypotheses are confirmed, will we be any better off (e.g. in our ability to understand disease or treat patients)?

(2) If the hypotheses are not confirmed, will other scientists be interested?

3 Definition of the cohort

(1) Is the cohort to be identified retrospectively or prospectively?

(2) What are the inclusion criteria (age, sex, area of residence etc)?

(3) What exclusion criteria apply (e.g. presence of certain diseases, residence in institutions)?

(4) If the cohort is recruited over a period of time, at what point do the subjects have to meet the age and other criteria (e.g. at the start of the study, or when the subjects are seen)?

(5) Are there any ambiguities in the way the criteria are defined or recorded?

(6) Will the cohort comprise a total population defined as above, or will it be a sample of the population and if so how will the sample be selected (e.g. randomly or by volunteering)?

4 Numbers

(1) How large will the cohort be and how has its size been calculated (expected differences, statistical power, etc.)?

(2) What allowances have been made for non-response and migration of subjects?

5 Recruitment of the subjects

(1) How will the subjects be identified?

(2) How accurate and up to date is the sampling frame?

(3) Over what period will recruitment continue?

(4) Can we foresee any biases arising during recruitment (e.g. from selective identification or response of subjects)?

6 Baseline data

(1) What data are to be collected at baseline (including potential aetiological factors and possible confounders)?

(2) What checks should be conducted on reproducibility, validity, comprehensibility of questionnaires, etc. so that the findings will be accepted as true?

(3) How soon can the data be checked, coded, and computerized so as to allow early detection and correction of errors and omissions?

(4) If blood is to be taken, should specimens of serum/plasma be kept deep-frozen for future analysis in case further hypotheses are suggested?

7 Tracing of subjects

(1) How will the subjects be traced and when?

(2) What secondary methods of tracing are available for subjects who cannot be traced by the primary methods?

(3) What biases are likely to arise from incomplete tracing?

8 Collection of follow-up data

(1) After what interval(s) will follow-up data be collected?

(2) What information will be required (repeat baseline data, outcome events, new tests)?

(3) What checks should be made on the quality of the data to be collected (e.g. reproducibility, validity, comparability with the baseline data)?

(4) Can we ensure that the outcome events are recorded 'blind' with regard to the initial observations?

(5) If some subjects are not available (e.g. through migration or refusal), is there any useful information that we can obtain about them?

9 Analysis of data

(1) Is a statistician (preferably the person who will undertake the analysis) involved in the design of the study?

(2) What analyses of the data will be performed?

10 General considerations

(1) What ethical issues arise (e.g. concerning explanation and information given to subjects; signed consent forms for tests and follow-up procedures)?

(2) What issues of professional etiquette must be considered (e.g. whose permission needs to be obtained; who should be informed as a courtesy)?

(3) If the data collection could disclose abnormalities in the subjects (e.g. a high serum cholesterol), what is our criterion of abnormality and what do we do when we find it?

(4) What are the costs of the study and what personnel will be required?

(5) Is this the best time to start the study, or would it be better to wait (e.g. until the relevant technology has improved)?

(6) Should the methodology of the study be made comparable to that of any other study (e.g. by using similar questionnaires)?

(7) What experts should be consulted to increase the likelihood that the findings will be accepted as conclusive?

(8) Is somebody keeping a list of all the people we promise to inform about the conclusions of the study?

REFERENCES

1. Atkins, E., Cherry, N. M., Douglas, J. W. B., Kiernan, K. E., and Wadsworth, M. E. J. (1981). The 1946 British Birth Survey: an account of the origins, progress and results of the National Survey of Health and Development. In S. A. Mednick and A. E. Baert (eds). In *An empirical basis for primary prevention: prospective longitudinal research in Europe*, pp. 25–30. Oxford University Press, Oxford.

2. Fogelman, K. and Wedge, P. (1981). The National Child Development Study. In S. A. Mednick and A. E. Baert (eds). *An empirical basis for primary prevention: prospective longitudinal research in Europe*, pp. 30–43, Oxford University Press, Oxford.

3. Taylor, B., Wadsworth, J., and Butler, N. R. (1983). Teenage mothering, admission to hospital, and accidents during the first 5 years. *Arch. Dis. Child.* **58:** 6–11.

4. Elwood, P. C., Sweetnam, P. M., Gray, O. P., Davies, D. P., and Wood, P. D. P. (1987). Growth of children from 0–5 years: with special reference to mother's smoking in pregnancy. *Ann. Hum. Biol.*, **14:** 543–57.

5. Tanner, J. M., Whitehouse, R. H., and Takaishi, M. (1966). Standards from birth to maturity for height, weight, height velocity and weight velocity: British children 1965. *Arch. Dis. Child.*, **41:** 454–71, 613–35.

6. Burr, M. L. (1983). Does infant feeding affect the risk of allergy? *Arch. Dis. Child.*, **58:** 561–5.

7. Snowdon, D. A. (1988). Animal product consumption and mortality because of all causes combined, coronary heart disease, stroke, diabetes, and cancer in Seventh-Day Adventists. *Am. J. Clin. Nutr.*, **48:** 739–48.

8. Burr, M. L., Lennings, C. I., and Milbank, J. E. (1982). The prognostic significance of weight and of vitamin C status in the elderly. *Age Ageing*, **11:** 249–55.

9. Gordon, T., Kagan, A., Garcia-Palmieri, M., Kannel, W. B., Zukel, W. J., Tillotson, J., Sorlie, P., and Hortland, M. (1981). Diet and its relation to coronary heart disease and death in three populations. *Circulation*, **63:** 500–15.

10. Kushi, L. H., Lew, R. A., Stare, F. J., Ellison, C. R., El Lozy, M., Bourke, G., Daly, L., Graham, I., Hickey, N., Mulcahy, R., and Kevaney, J. (1985). Diet and 20-year mortality from coronary heart disease: the Ireland–Boston diet–heart study. *N. Engl. J. Med.*, **312:** 811–18.

11. Morris, J. N., Marr, J. W., and Clayton, D. G. (1977). Diet and heart: a postscript. *Br. Med. J.*, **2:** 1307–14.

12. Khaw, K-T. and Barrett-Connor, E. (1987). Dietary fiber and reduced ischemic heart disease mortality rates in men and women: a 12-year prospective study. *Am. J. Epid.*, **126:** 1093–102.

13. Keys, A. (1980. *Seven Countries: a multivariate analysis of death and coronary heart disease.* Harvard University Press, Cambridge, Massachusetts.

14. Shekelle, R. B., Shryock, A. M., Paul, O., Lepper, M., Stamler, J., Liu, S., and Raynor, W. J. (1981). Diet, serum cholesterol, and death from coronary heart disease. *N. Engl. J. Med.*, **304:** 65–70.

15. Shekelle, R. B., Missell, L. V., Oglesby, P., Shryock, A. M., and Stamler, J.

(1985). Fish consumption and mortality from coronary heart disease. *N. Engl. J. Med.*, **313:** 820.

16. Kromhout, D., Bosschieter, E. B., and Coulander, C. de L. (1982). Dietary fibre and 10-year mortality from coronary heart disease, cancer, and all causes: the Zutphen study. *Lancet*, **ii:** 518–22.
17. Kromhout, D., Bosschieter, E. B., and Coulander, C. de L. (1985). The inverse relation between fish consumption and 20-year mortality from coronary heart disease. *N. Engl. J. Med.*, **312:** 1205–9.

13. Experimental studies

Barrie M. Margetts and Ian L. Rouse

Experimentation is the optimal way of making causal inference. In an ideal experiment, treatments are compared concurrently in groups of adequate size, which are otherwise comparable and which are subsequently observed in the same way. In an experiment, one or more factors are altered under carefully controlled conditions and the effects of the changes on the outcome measure of interest are observed. Based on the observations it may then be possible to draw some inferences about the causes of the change in outcome.

Apart from the way subjects are randomly allocated by the investigator into treatment (or exposure) groups, the principles of experimental design are very similar to those that apply to cohort studies. As in all scientific investigations, it is essential to have a clear understanding of what research question the study can address. The development of the research protocol will then focus primarily on how to measure the effect of an exposure on an outcome with due consideration of the effects other factors have on the observed relationship. That is, we want to have precise measures of exposure and outcome free from bias (as discussed in Chapter 1).

In this chapter, we begin with a brief historical overview of the development of experimental studies, followed by a description of the types of experimental studies. The largest part of the chapter concerns general issues in designing experimental studies and the chapter concludes with a comparison of the commonly used types of study designs. As with other chapters in this book, the primary objective here is to provide an overview of issues relevant to the design of experiments in human nutrition. We will not attempt to consider all issues pertinent to the design, conduct and analysis of experimental studies and we will only refer to specific examples to clarify certain points.

13.1 HISTORICAL INTRODUCTION

Experimentation has been the method used to discover cause and effect for as long as humans have existed. Others have reviewed this literature in detail and it is beyond the scope of this chapter to repeat the detail of these historical accounts. Lind and Louis are two notable workers who used experimentation to attempt to objectively assess the effect of a treatment on a disease. In 1753, Lind (quoted in Carpenter[1]) described an experiment in which 12 sailors with scurvy were put on the same standardized diets, and then allocated to one of six treatment groups for 14 days. Those receiving oranges and lemons were much improved after 6 days. While Lind may have subsequently misinterpreted his findings, his study must be considered one of the first controlled clinical trials. It was some 80 years later, in 1834, that Louis (quoted in Pocock[2]) extended consideration of experimental design to consider the number of subjects required to show benefit of one treatment over another, the need to observe disease progress accurately in treated and controlled groups, the need for precise definition of the disease state prior to the experiment and the importance of observing deviations from intended treatments. While there were some advances in experimental designs during the nineteenth and early twentieth centuries, the first randomized controlled trials were not undertaken until the late 1940s, by the Medical Research Council. There were trials of streptomycin in the treatment of pulmonary tuberculosis (1948)[3] and antihistamines for the treatment of the common cold (1950).[4] This latter study was a double-blind placebo controlled trial.

In 1950 Cochran and Cox published an important textbook on experimental designs.[5] While drawing largely from agricultural experiments, this book clearly and simply described the major statistical considerations in experimental studies. Bradford Hill was also an important force in making the design of clinical trials more rigorous.[6] In his book, *Principles of Medical Statistics*, he has a lengthy chapter on clinical trials and this is still very relevant today. In 1959, Truelove summarized the current thinking on experimental design and he clearly described the essential elements of a therapeutic trial as follows:

1) The trial should be planned so that decisive answers can be given to one or more important questions.

2) Patients should be selected for inclusion in the trial before it is known into which group they will go. After admission to the trial, patients should be allocated at random to one or other treatment group.

3) Systematic and pertinent observations should be made on patients so that relevant data are available for analysis at the conclusion of the trial.

4) When possible, trials should be so arranged that neither the physician nor the patient knows which treatment is being used—the so-called DOUBLE-BLIND system. pp. 134–135.[7]

Since the early 1950s there has been a rapid expansion of the use of experimental studies in human nutrition. In section 13.3 we will expand on some of the points so clearly stated by Truelove in 1959, and still very relevant today. As it is not within the scope of this chapter to discuss in detail all aspects of experimental design the reader is referred to other texts.[8–10]

13.2 DEFINITIONS OF EXPERIMENTAL STUDIES

The terminology used to describe the different types of experimental studies is at times confusing. In terms of the principles we wish to consider in this chapter, there are only two major types of experimental study— the field or clinical trial and the community intervention trial. The clinical or field trial is an experiment in which individuals are assigned to different exposure or treatment groups, whereas in the community intervention trial the investigator assigns different communities (not individuals within the community) to different exposure groups. In addition to this major distinction there are a number of other ways in which experimental studies can be classified. For example, it is possible to classify types of experimental trials on the basis of the disease status of the person participating in the trial. Therapeutic trials assess the effect of a therapy or treatment on a group of subjects who have had the disease of interest. The aim here is to determine whether the new treatment modifies the further development of disease in those who already have the disease. Preventive trials assess the effects of treatment on individuals who are, at the commencement of the trial, apparently free from the disease of interest. The aim here is to determine what effect alteration in an exposure will have in a supposedly healthy group of individuals or in a group regarded as being at high risk, but who have not as yet developed the disease.

This classification in itself may be confusing, particularly if the outcome is based on an arbitrary classification of a variable that is continuously distributed, such as blood pressure or serum cholesterol. An investigator may be interested for example, to assess whether increasing the fat intake in the diet affects blood pressure. The choice of subjects for this trial could be those who are considered to be either normotensive or hypertensive. The former would be considered to be 'free of disease' and the latter could be considered either to actually have the disease 'hypertension' or if the investigator does not consider hypertension to be a disease, but only a risk factor for another endpoint called disease (such as stroke or ischaemic heart disease), then the subjects may be considered to be a high risk group. Someone with blood pressure of above the systolic blood pressure of 160 mmHg may be considered to be 'diseased', while somebody with systolic blood pressure of 159 mmHg may be considered to be 'normal'. The distinction between diseased/not diseased using harder endpoints, for example, acute myocardial infarction, may be just as arbitrary as for the example cited above for blood pressure.

Using the classification cited above, we would call the study of those with 'normal' blood pressure and at risk of disease as a result of higher blood pressure, a primary prevention trial; whereas if we considered hypertension to be a disease endpoint then we would call this a therapeutic or clinical trial. From the above it is obvious that the distinction is somewhat arbitrary when considering outcome variables like blood pressure or cholesterol. The level of the outcome measure considered high or 'disease' is arbitrary.

The distinction between types of experimental studies among individuals is less clear cut and important than the division cited above may indicate. The main points are that the disease state of all subjects should be carefully measured and that allocation to treatment (exposure) groups should not be influenced by the disease state of the subjects. All eligible subjects should be randomly allocated to treatments.

The other type of experimental study referred to is the Community Trial (quasi experimental study) where the unit of study is a population (community) and allocation to treatment is at the community level. For example, the Stanford Three Town study allocated two different treatments to two towns and had a third town as a control, where no treatment was given.[11]

In the community intervention trial, definition of the outcome may be either reduction in levels of risk factors (as, for example, in the North Karelia Project[12]) or in amount of disease (as in the Multiple Risk Factor Intervention Trial[13]) or both (as in the Lipids Research Clinics Coronary Prevention Trial[14]). Although the specific statistical methods used, and the interpretation of results from the community trial may differ from other types of experimental studies, the basic principle remains that change in outcome in the treatment group must be compared to any change in outcome measures that may have occurred in the control group. It is not appropriate to measure a 'statistically significant' reduction in an outcome measure in the treatment group and ignore any change that may have occurred independently of treatment in control groups.

Irrespective of the type of study, the main objective is to explore an exposure–outcome (cause–effect) relationship free from bias.

13.3 GENERAL CONSIDERATIONS IN DESIGNING EXPERIMENTS

There are a number of general principles that are relevant to all experimental studies. These include:

(1) selection of the study population;

(2) allocation of treatment regimes;

(3) length of observation;

(4) observer effects;

(5) participant effects;

(6) compliance;

(7) ascertainment of exposure and outcome;

(8) statistical power;

(9) analysis and interpretation.

13.3.1 Selection of study population

Chapter 1 devoted considerable time to the issues of internal and external validity. In all studies, the aim is to design a study so that it is free from bias and is therefore internally valid. Internal validity is the prime concern; the issue of external validity does not arise if the study is not internally valid. However, there is debate about the importance of external validity or generalizability. One view considers that external validity is important and that the selection of the study sample should be such that it is representative of a clearly defined population. The other point of view argues that the approach taken in experimental science is to demonstrate a phenomenon, not to make statements about the generalizability from the study sample to the population as a whole. This view argues that generalization is from the experience of the actual study to the abstract and is founded on judgement rather than statistical sampling and technical sample-to-population inference. In general, both points of view are similar in that they argue that one's view of whether the outcome is likely to be the same in another experiment in a different sample is based on a judgement about whether differences in study samples are likely to influence the result. For some situations, it is obvious that selection of a certain sample of people would, in the judgment of most people, have an effect on the result of an experiment. For example, feeding different diets to familial hypercholesterolaemics with metabolic defects in lipid metabolism could be expected to produce a different effect on lipids from the same diets fed to normal individuals. The postprandial effects of various carbohydrates in insulin dependent diabetics and normal subjects may also be reasonably expected to differ.

However, in many situations the extent to which the study population is likely to be representative of a larger population is more difficult to judge.

For example, if researchers are interested in the effectiveness of a vegetarian diet for reducing blood pressure, should one select normotensive,
hypertensive, or both types of subject for investigation? As already mentioned above, the definition of hypertension is arbitrary. Are the influences
of dietary factors on blood pressure control different at different levels of
blood pressure? Would someone with a blood pressure of 160 mmHg
(defined as hypertensive by most clinicians) be expected to respond differently from someone whose blood pressure is 159 mmHg and classified as
not hypertensive?

To conclude the above discussion, it is our view that it is critically
important to design and carry out a study that is internally valid. However,
in doing so one should always consider the influence that the selection of
subjects may have on one's judgement about the extent to which results
would be similar in other similar experiments.

The proportion of the eligible sample that participates in a study may
also influence one's confidence in the generalizability of the findings. It is,
usual for healthier, better educated, more motivated subjects to complete
studies. The trial of smoking and lung cancer by Doll and Hill[15] was
conducted in England because the researchers were able to define the
population of doctors and thereby assess participation rates within that
population. The results may not have been relevant to other populations,
but the study did demonstrate the effect of smoking on rates of lung
cancer.

For clinical trials where a therapeutic agent or procedure is to be tested,
consideration may need to be given to admission criteria. These criteria
may include certain demands for exclusion and inclusion, and may primarily
be intended for pragmatic and ethical purposes. In a clinical trial the
investigator may want to specify suitable clinical indications for treatment.
(It is not ethical to withhold a mandatory treatment or to give a potentially
harmful treatment.) It is not appropriate under any circumstances to allocate subjects within the study sample, however that sample is derived, into
treatments in a way that results in the treatment groups not being equivalent in clinical state and exposure to other variables.

Apart from the issues already raised, there may be other pragmatic
issues relating to sample selection. If the aim is to determine the effect of a
treatment on an outcome it may be important to consider whether the
selected subjects can complete the study and provide complete and reliable
information. If an intervention is to last several years it is important to
have a geographically stable sample, which is likely to have a lower loss to
follow-up. This pragmatic choice of study population limits the generalizability but is likely to give a more internally valid result.

In a community trial, the selection of towns may be influenced by the
treatment to be tested. If the treatment is a general media campaign it
will be necessary for the treatment and comparison communities to be

sufficiently discrete as to minimize exposure of the control community to the treatment. The selection of such towns may also be influenced by other pragmatic issues, such as ease of access to the town by the investigators or support from local community leaders in staging the research. Irrespective of these pragmatic issues, the towns should be randomly allocated to treatment group and monitored at baseline and followed-up in the same way.

13.3.2 Allocation of treatment regimes

Irrespective of how the study sample is selected, once selected, the optimal way of assigning subjects to treatment and comparison (control) groups is by randomization. Random assignment implies that individuals are allocated to each study group and that allocation of subjects to a group is independent of the allocation of other subjects. Randomization in a community trial occurs at the level of the community; subjects within a community are not randomly assigned to treatment or control group. The purpose of randomization is to ensure that differences between treatment and control groups in potential confounders and levels of other important variables arise by chance alone. Tables of random numbers (and computer programs) are available for the randomization of subjects.

The random allocation of subjects to groups also ensures that neither the observers nor the individual participating in the study can influence, by way of personal judgement or prejudice, who is allocated to receive which treatment. If the observer controls the allocation of subjects to treatment group there is the strong possibility of bias occurring. Whether consciously or subconsciously, it is possible that the observer may allocate into the treatment group all those people more likely to comply.

Where the study sample is small and a factor is known to be an important determinant of the outcome, it is common to block on that factor to ensure that differences between treatment groups for levels of that factor do not occur by chance. For example, subjects are often blocked on age and sex to ensure that groups are balanced for these factors. Within a block the allocation to a treatment or control group is still random. For large trials it is not usually necessary to block, because it is possible in the analysis to consider the treatment–outcome effect in subcategories of the factor of interest. While the effect of these blocking factors could be considered in the analysis, if the experiment is small and the chance variation large then it may be difficult to make a sensible adjustment for these effects in the analysis. For example, if all the old men were randomly allocated to one group and all the young women were allocated to another group.

Some studies make use of historical controls as a comparison group. For example, a new treatment may have been developed to the extent that it is considered unethical to withhold it from any subjects. How subjects responded to past treatments can be used in this situation. However, there are considerable limitations to this approach. We have repeatedly seen the effect that confounding can have on our interpretation of exposure–outcome relationships. It may be very difficult, using historical controls, to ensure that conditions other than the treatment of interest are comparable for the treatment and control periods.

It is also possible to use exclusion criteria and matching to take account of the effects of potential confounders. If, for example, smokers behave differently to non-smokers and this difference is believed to affect the way treatment affects outcome, it may be advisable to restrict the study to non-smokers.

While it may be ideal for subjects to be similar in their exposure variables prior to a study, unless a particular exposure level is a contraindication for the participation in the study, the subject should be included and randomly allocated to a treatment group. It is not acceptable to allocate the sickest children to a treatment and to allocate the less sick children to a control regime. While this may be the desired procedure to save lives, it is not appropriate for a study aiming to elucidate mechanisms. This bias in subject allocation may lead to either a falsely optimistic or falsely pessimistic outcome.

13.3.3 Length of observations

An experiment should be just long enough to allow the effect of exposure change to result in the hypothesized change in outcome. In deciding on the length of the study the investigator must have an idea as to the mechanism of action of the proposed treatment and thereby some idea as to how long it should take to affect the various steps in the pathway. The outcome of interest will affect the length of observation. If the aim is to assess the acute effects of food on, for example, catecholamines or glucose metabolism, the study may only last a few hours. For studies of diet and serum cholesterol or blood pressure the study may need to last weeks. For endpoints such as death the length of observation will need to be longer, perhaps many years.

It is clear that a careful consideration of the length of observation depends upon the hypothesis being investigated. We have recently carried out studies on the postprandial effects of a vegetarian diet on blood pressure and heart rate, where the period of investigation was several hours. On the other hand our trials on the longer term effects of diet on blood pressure have been able to demonstrate a change in blood pressure within six weeks.[16–18] However, for these studies it may be important to consider whether these short term changes are representative of what may occur when the diet is adopted over a longer period of time. The length of observation may also be influenced by statistical power considerations, which have already been discussed in Chapter 2 and which will be further discussed later in this chapter.

A worthwhile study must have sufficient events (outcomes), and the longer the observation in a large scale trial, the more events will occur and therefore the greater the statistical power of the study. From experience in recent trials, such as MRFIT,[13] the observed number of events (in both treatment and comparison groups) may be lower than expected because of a selection of healthier subjects into such a long study, or because of secular changes in disease rates, which may alter the expected number of endpoints in the control group. Under both of these circumstances, the original sample and length of observation may be insufficient to establish a cause–effect relationship. It may therefore be a sensible pragmatic precaution to underestimate the expected number of events. It may also be advisable to establish some rules whereby it would be permissible to extend the period of observation of a study in order to increase the number of endpoints and thereby its statistical validity. On the other hand, where a very substantial effect of a treatment emerges early in a clinical trial it may be unnecessary, or even unethical, to continue the trial. If the treatment (or lack of treatment in the control group) appears to be resulting in an increased rate of disease it may also be advisable to stop the trial. Where it may be considered likely that either of the above situations could occur, there should be clearly defined stopping rules incorporated into the study design. Readers are referred to other texts for more details about the implementation of stopping rules in clinical trials.[9,19,20]

13.3.4 Observer effects

If the observer knows to which group a subject has been allocated, it is possible that they may encourage or in some way alter the behaviour of the subject in the treatment group so that they react differently from a subject in a control group. If a subject knows they are in a treatment group their compliance may differ from their compliance if they were in the control group. It is therefore desirable that both the observer and the participants are blinded as to the participant's treatment group. Prior to the commencement of the study, all personnel involved must be carefully trained to ensure uniformity in the administration of the protocol. The instruments, be they for measuring height, weight, or blood pressure; biochemical assay methods; dietary questionnaires or any other source of ascertainment of information about the study subjects, must be carefully piloted to ensure that they measure what was intended, and also that they measure it in a way that gives reliable information.

It may not be possible for the same observer to make all the measurements in a multicentre trial. If different observers are involved, careful consideration needs to be given to the effect this may have on outcome. If one observer measures blood pressure in one centre and another measures it in another centre, and the centres produce different effects, it may not be possible to determine whether the effect was due to the different observers or to a real difference between the centres. If this type of problem can be thought of in the design stage it may be better to consider an observer-independent means of measuring the variable of interest. If this is not possible, it will be necessary to have a standardized comparison of the differences that should occur between observers in the training, pilot phase of the study. It is also important that a subset of subjects in each community be repeat-measured by an observer from another centre. By doing this it may be possible to establish the potential effect that observer differences may have on the outcome.

Where possible, analyses should be controlled by a central coordinating centre. For example, if blood, urine, or other tissue samples are being collected, they should be analysed in one centre, or at least in centres with identical analytical and standardization procedures.

When any measurement is being made, the observer should be blind as to the treatment group. This will ensure that any effect of the observer on the measurement will be random. As mentioned in Chapter 1, it is also important to have a measure of the size of the likely intraobserver variation (measurement error). This should also be established prior to the commencement of the study. An assessment of within-observer variation should also, where appropriate, be undertaken during the study.

13.3.5 Participant effects

The aim of an experiment is to establish whether an exposure causes an effect. For example, does the treatment reduce blood pressure in an individual. The aim, therefore, is to standardize the conditions under which the experiment is conducted so that the response of the participant to the treatment can be attributed to the treatment.

To be a participant in the trial a person must be recruited and give free and informed consent to participate. They should be aware of the general nature of the research and aware of what they will be expected to do, and have done to them. The provision of adequate information about the study for the participants is important to improve subject compliance. The exact detail given to the participants needs to be balanced with the requirement that, as far as possible, the subjects be blinded as to the treatment allocation. For some trials this is relatively simple where, for example, one drug is given compared to another or to a placebo. However, this is much more difficult for dietary interventions and it is likely that the subject will know the treatment group. This may affect their response to the treatment.

The way a subject passes through the research protocol should be carefully standardized. Any violation of the protocol should be noted. For example, if a subject is scheduled to have their blood pressure measured in the morning, they should always have their blood pressure measured at the same time. In practice this is not always possible and when violations occur they should be noted. Subjects should be given clear and consistent instructions for the completion of dietary records and questionnaires. If they are to provide urine or blood samples they should be given clear written instructions about what they need to do, for example, whether to fast the night before or, for a urine sample, how long the urine collection is for and when it is to start and stop.

We have already said that allocation to treatment groups should be random. This should ensure that other variables likely to influence outcome are randomly distributed. However, it is still important to measure these potentially important variables. While it is not appropriate to analyse for statistically significant differences between these variables at the baseline measurement (because of randomization, any differences that occur will, in any case, be by chance) it is appropriate to assess how changes in these variables may have affected the treatment–effect relationship. These variables need to be measured with sufficient reliability for their effect to be properly considered. Measurement error in potential confounders is just as important as in the exposure and outcome measures.

The way information is collected needs to take account of the within-subject variability. Just as repeat measures give an idea of observer effects, they also give an indication of subject variability. The aim in an experiment is to characterize the individual, and measurements need to be precise enough to achieve this. The prime concern must be the internal validity—that all aspects about subject participation in the study are comparable and that deviation from this ideal can be documented.

13.3.6 Compliance

Much of what we have already said with respect to participant effects relates to compliance. Deviation from the protocol needs to be documented in all subjects, not just those on the treatment. It may be that a comparison or control group alters their behaviour so as to make them more like the treatment group in their exposure status. Perhaps more commonly, participants will forget or deliberately fail to take drugs, or, if they have been placed on a dietary regime, they may occasionally 'break-out' and deviate from the protocol.

Measurement of compliance is essential in any clinical (dietary) trial. The study must be designed so that all important variables can be measured during the trial with sufficient precision to give a sensitive and specific (valid) indication of the level of each variable. The observer in many situations is reliant upon the participant honestly reporting whether they have deviated from the protocol. However, where possible, an independent measure of compliance should be used. For example, measuring changes in the levels of fatty acids in serum, red blood cells, or a fat biopsy enables the researcher to assess the compliance with dietary advice to alter fat intake. If a dietary intervention is increasing fibre intake, it may be possible to include a marker that in the fibre diet can subsequently be measured in faecal samples. The level in the faecal sample gives an indication of the amount of fibre supplement eaten. From our experience it is helpful to tell participants that we are checking their compliance by taking blood or urine samples.

It may be more difficult to measure individual compliance in a community trial but by random sampling of subjects within each study community it should be possible to at least measure whether subjects are aware of the community intervention and whether it has had any effect on their knowledge, attitudes, behaviours or levels of some outcome variables. It may not be reasonable to assume in a community trial that compliance will be similar in all centres and that it is therefore not necessary to go to the trouble of random sampling of subjects within the community. The efficiency of the treatment as measured by changes in community rates of disease may be adequate. However, not measuring the effect of the exposure on behaviour may give a misleading impression of the cause–effect relationship.

We have always had a run-in or familiarization period in our controlled clinical trials; this improves compliance. It gives the subjects time to adjust to the rigours of the study protocol. However, the diet during this period should not have any effect on the outcome measure. In theory, it should be similar to the subject's usual diet. If the trial is for a therapeutic agent, the run-in period should only use a placebo or usual care treatment. The run-in period should be before randomization, so that any dropouts that occur during this process do not affect the internal validity of the study.

There are situations where it may not be possible or appropriate to have a run-in period. For example, where the experiment is to see whether surgical procedure X or Y has a better effect on survival, or where the experiment is assessing the effect of treatment following an acute event such as angina or myocardial infarction, or the effect of oral rehydration therapy on survival in an acutely malnourished child.

13.3.7 Ascertainment of exposure and outcome

All subjects in an experimental study should complete the study protocol in the same way. This is particularly important for the ascertainment of levels of exposure and outcomes, which should be identical in all subjects irrespective of their treatment allocation. For example, it is not acceptable to use a 7-day weighed record to assess fat intake in the treatment group and to only use a restricted food frequency method in the control groups. It is not acceptable to use different outcome measures in treatment and control groups. Exposure in clinical and field trials must be measured in a valid way that correctly characterizes the individual participants. The measurement of exposure and outcome in a community intervention trial should correctly characterize the population distribution. The protocol must ensure that outcome can be objectively measured with minimal misclassification.

Measurement of exposure   A primary aim of a dietary intervention study should be to accurately characterize the diet of the individual at baseline and during the study. The change in diet can then be related to the change in outcome. The number of days of recording dietary information required to characterize an individual's intake varies according to the nutrient of interest. If the aim is to be able to assess intake for vitamin A or fatty acids, more days for recording will be required than if total fat intake is the exposure of interest. This is discussed in more detail in Chapter 6. It may be argued that the variability in the dietary factor of prime interest determines the number of days of dietary records required. However, if there is any concern that other dietary factors may influence outcome, and there almost always will be, then it is essential to measure these other factors with the same precision as is required for the primary exposure measure. Failure to do so may prevent an appropriate assessment of the confounding effect these other dietary variables may have on the cause–effect relationship being studied.

To characterize the overall diet of an individual it is also important to consider any differences that days of the week (or weekend) may have on intake. If dietary practices vary throughout the week then due consideration of this variation is essential. It may be that, for example, fish is only ever eaten at the weekend and, if dietary intake is only ever assessed during the week, the assessment of fatty acid intake will not reflect usual consumption. Missing days or periods of consumption of nutrient-rich foods (such as liver for vitamin A or carrots for β-carotene) will give misleading exposure levels.

While optimally it may be desirable to record intake for, say, 14–21 days, the effect that this arduous task may have on compliance needs to be considered. If subjects drop-out of the study, or only partially complete dietary records, the study protocol may be more compromised than by the use of a shorter, somewhat less precise method of assessing diet that can be more readily completed by the subjects. On the other hand it is possible that the task of recording diet may actually improve compliance by making the subject aware of what they are eating and whether or not they are deviating from the required regime. It is also possible that the act of recording diet alters a subject's usual intake, so while the subject accurately records what has been eaten, they have made significant changes on record days to that normally eaten. Estimation of food intake, irrespective of the number of days of recording, relies on the use of food tables to convert grams of food eaten into grams of nutrients. As has been shown in Chapter 4, this may impose considerable limitations on the precision of the estimate of intake. It may be considered more desirable to obtain duplicate portions of meals eaten and directly measure the levels of nutrients in these samples. However, this procedure itself may introduce different errors, which could affect the validity of the data (for example, by causing the subject to change their usual dietary patterns).

The way diet is measured depends on the type of study. If the subjects are in a well controlled metabolic ward study where the observer measures and prepares all the food, then all that is required for accurate measures of intake is to measure what food is not eaten.

Most clinical or field trials of dietary regimes assess diet during the experiment by the same method used for baseline assessment of diet, although this may not always be necessary. If the diet is controlled by the investigator (but not in a metabolic ward) a food frequency questionnaire may be adequate to monitor any deviation from prescribed meal patterns. Dietary modification in most field trials is usually by prescription, i.e. subjects are told to follow a particular dietary regime. This may be with or without food supplements provided by the investigator. Under these conditions it is desirable to monitor diet as accurately as possible.

Because of the limitations of assessing dietary intakes by subject-based recording methods, alternative methods of assessing intake have been sought. Biochemical markers of intake have been discussed in more detail in Chapter 7. While the actual variability of the marker may be much smaller than for a dietary intake measure, the relevance of these markers must be considered. For example, there is little point in precisely measuring a blood or urinary constituent that is not involved in or affected by the exposure of interest.

Measurement of outcome Outcomes in experimental studies are measured in the same way as in a cohort study. The outcome measures may be routinely collected data sources (death certificates or hospital activity/medical records), may be collected by the participant themselves (by completion of a questionnaire) or may be collected by the investigator (by personal interviewer or medical examination). The outcome of the study depends upon the completeness and validity of the information obtained. Where routinely collected data are to be used to measure outcome it must be possible to ascertain, for all subjects, whether they have died or been admitted to hospital. It may be relatively simple to determine vital status and obtain a death certificate where there is a central registry of deaths. It may be much more difficult to obtain complete hospital admission data in the absence of a suitable computerized system.

If the investigator finds that a subject has died or had an event of interest (in a hospital or elsewhere) they are then reliant upon the accurate ascertainment (usually by some other person) of the cause of death or clinical details on the hospital admission. For an outcome measure like, for example, fractured neck of the femur, which is not likely to be recorded on a death certificate as an underlying cause of death, under-ascertainment of outcome will occur if the death certificate is the only source of information about outcome. Even for common causes of death, the detail written on a death certificate may not accurately reflect the major underlying disease process that resulted in the death. If hospital records are to be used the investigator must be sure that all relevant hospitals to which the study subjects may be admitted are checked for any admissions. Where general practitioner's records are to be used the investigator must also be assured that subjects only attend that practice and that if an illness occurs they go to the same practitioner. The more subjects and information lost to follow-up the more likely it is that a biased result will occur.

Where outcome measures are obtained either by self report or observer measurement, it is essential that information is obtained in the same way for all subjects. Any under-ascertainment of outcome will effect the validity of the study. Observer blindness will reduce the risk of ascertainment bias and will also ensure that follow-up procedures to obtain outcome will not be influenced differentially in treatment groups. It is also essential that the measure of outcome is precise enough to categorize subjects correctly.

For example, the way blood pressure is measured needs to be carefully standardized. The method used should be very reliable and free from observer bias. In most of our studies we have used an automatic oscillometric device (the DINAMAP), which is free of observer influences and very reliable. For more subject self reported outcomes like, for example, feeling better, having fewer severe headaches, or number of diarrhoea-free days, there is considerable risk of outcome misclassification.

In designing an experiment with accurate ascertainment of outcome, there is no substitute for a clear understanding of the biological process under investigation and the potential errors associated with the outcome measure.

13.3.8 Statistical power/sample size

The aim is always to have a study with sufficient participants to ensure that the result obtained is likely, to the best of your knowledge, to be a statistically viable one; this has been discussed in detail in Chapter 2. An estimate of the study's statistical power is required before it commences. To estimate the statistical power the investigator needs to be able to estimate the likely random errors in the measurements being used and the number of events or the change in an outcome measure to be expected. The investigator also needs to specify the acceptable level of statistical significance and confidence.

It may be that, on the basis of the power calculations, the study cannot be undertaken with the population and finance available. It is wasteful, and in some cases unethical, to commence a study that is never going to produce a statistically and biologically meaningful result.

13.3.9 Analysis and interpretation

The analyses to be undertaken need to be specified before the study commences. This will ensure both that there are sufficient subjects available in subsets of the sample and that the data are collected in a way that is appropriate for the required analysis.

A sufficiently large sample, accurate and reliable assessment of exposure and outcome, and randomization are likely to ensure that the estimation of rates of disease in exposed and non-exposed group gives an unbiased estimate or risk.

In practical terms it is important to document the baseline characteristics of the treatment groups and show how the variables of interest have changed during the study. It is also desirable to present absolute and relative changes in variables and, where appropriate, outcome measures.

There are two major approaches to the consideration of the subjects in the analysis of the data. One view is that once subjects have been randomly allocated to treatment groups they should be included in the analysis irrespective of whether their compliance was good or bad or whether they dropped out or not. This is sometimes referred to as analysing on an 'intention to treat' basis. Excluding subjects who have a 'measured' compliance below a certain level is arbitrary and may give optimistically positive results. As it is not possible to measure compliance perfectly accurately, the decision to exclude those whose compliance measure is below a certain level may give misleading results.

A second view would argue that, if the aim of the study was simply to demonstrate that a treatment can effect an outcome, then it may be acceptable to use a restricted subset (on the basis of compliance) of the data. If this approach is taken, consideration must be given to the effect that breaking the balanced group allocation may have on any comparisons. It may be that those who comply sufficiently well to be included are either different in other important characteristics from those not adequately complying and/or the distribution of those characteristics may be different in treatment and control groups.

If the objective of the research is to see whether the offering of the treatment affects outcome, then all subjects must be included in the analysis, irrespective of compliance scores. This latter question is more relevant to public health issues, where the investigator wants to know whether the treatment works in the community. For more detailed consideration on statistical analysis, readers are referred to other more detailed texts. [5,8,21-24]

13.4 DESIGNS USED IN EXPERIMENTAL STUDIES

A basic premise for all experimental studies is that the effect of any treatment on an outcome must be compared with the effect of a control treatment on outcome. Uncontrolled studies of any design are very difficult to interpret. Without a control group being studied in the same way, and over the same period, it is difficult to estimate the effects that regression to the mean, familiarization, seasonality in response, and the effects other unknown factors may have on outcome. For example, in trials measuring blood pressure as the outcome, it is very common to see blood pressures falling in all groups throughout the study; without a control group it would be impossible to separate out the effect of the treatment from the general 'familiarization' effect.

Parallel and crossover designs are commonly used for clinical research. A parallel design is where subjects receive only one treatment and the change in outcome response in one group of subjects (receiving treatment of interest) is compared with that in another group of subjects receiving a different (or control) treatment. Every subject in a crossover design receives both (all) treatments and outcomes/response is compared within subjects. A factorial experiment may use either a parallel or a crossover design. Irrespective of whether the design is parallel or crossover, the general considerations already mentioned in this chapter must apply. Subjects should be randomly allocated to treatment groups, followed-up in the same way and observers and participants should be blinded as to group allocation. If appropriate, a run-in or familiarization period should also be included. In a crossover design (with one treatment) subjects should be allocated to treatment group so that half receive the treatment first and half receive the control diet first.

The effects of a number of different factors can be investigated at the same time in a factorial experiment. The basic design may be parallel or crossover, the treatments are formed by all possible combinations that can be formed from the different factors. For example, Burr and colleagues assessed the effects of a high fibre diet and a high fish oil diet on recurrence of infarction. Subjects were first randomly assigned to receive either the high fibre diet or control diet and then, within these groupings, they were randomly assigned to receive either the fish oil or the control diet. The advantage of this approach is that the investigator can assess the effect of the interaction between treatments as well as whether one treatment may be more effective than another. If treatments are considered to be acting independently, a factorial design is effectively a number of independent experiments that are being conducted at the same time, it is therefore a cost effective approach. However, it may be considerably more difficult for the researcher to keep control of the study and, generally, factorial designs are limited to only two factors.

An advantage of the crossover design over the parallel design is that subject characteristics are approximately constant for both treatment (exposure categories) groups and it is therefore possible to separate out the effect of the treatment from those that may be due to the individual. This is not the case in parallel studies where subjects do not receive all treatments. Another advantage of a crossover design is that, as all subjects receive the treatment under investigation, the statistical power of the study is greater than in a parallel study of equivalent size, where only a proportion of the subjects receive the treatment under investigation. These advantages of the crossover design need to be weighed against problems that may arise in using this approach. Louis *et al.*[25] consider that five factors should be considered in choosing either a parallel or crossover design:

(1) carry-over and period effects on treatment outcomes;

(2) treatment sequencing and patient assignment;

(3) crossover rules and timing of measurements;

(4) drop outs, faulty data, and other data problems;

(5) statistical analysis and sample size.

13.4.1 Carry-over and period effects

In a crossover design the effect of the first or earlier treatment may 'carry-over' into the second or subsequent period and hence influence treatment during that period. For a two-period design, this means that the response in period two may be affected by the treatment given in period one. The response of the treatment in period two will be affected by the second treatment as well as an additional residual effect of treatment in the first period. Some investigators use a wash-out period between treatments to minimize this carry-over effect. However, it may be difficult to interpret the effect of this wash-out period and it may not be clear what is an appropriate wash-out diet.

Having groups that receive the same treatment throughout, as well as alternate treatments, may allow for the assessment of potential carry-over effects, as well as familiarization effects. For example, it is possible to estimate the carry-over effect by taking the difference in response (e.g.

serum cholesterol or blood pressure) for the group with the sequence, treatment-control (d1) and adding that to the difference in response in the control-treatment (d2) group and then subtracting that from two times the response in the control–control (d3) group (d1 + d2 − 2d3) (P. Armitage, personal communication). If there is not likely to be any interaction between treatment and control diets (on the basis of previous experience), it is statistically inefficient to use a control–control group. Putting more subjects into the treatment groups improves the treatment estimate but makes the interaction estimate less precise. Having more subjects in the control–control group improves the interaction estimate, but reduces the treatment estimate.

The disease state may alter during long term trials. Disease status may progress, regress or have a cyclical pattern of response. If the subjects have been randomly allocated to groups (or blocked on disease state if disease state is considered important) these period effects are not likely to lead to a systematically biased outcome. It may be that overall response is different in latter periods where disease may have progressed.

Where it is not known what carry-over effects exist, and where it is not feasible to use the more complex designs required to assess its likely effect, it may be advisable to use a parallel design.

13.4.2 Treatment sequencing and patient assignment

All subjects in a simple one-treatment parallel design are allocated to their treatment group at randomization. In a two- or more treatment design, consideration needs to be given to the order in which treatments are given. The effect of treatment X followed by treatment Y may be quite different from the other way around. Some patients should receive treatments in the order YX and others should receive XY. If the subject response is different for treatment X after Y, rather then before it than this can at least be measured using the above procedure. Allocating all subjects to YX does not allow an assessment of the treatment order effect.

Subjects in many trials are not recruited all at once, but rather over time as they become available. For example, in our trial of the effects of a vegetarian diet in mild hypertensive subjects, subjects were recruited as they attended for screening at a National Heart Foundation risk factor prevalence survey. Each week about five subjects were eligible for inclusion in the study on the basis of their blood pressure level. They were then reassessed several times and, if their blood pressure had remained above a certain level, they were included in the trial. There were several ways that we could have then allocated subjects into treatment groups:

(1) by the same fixed sequence of assignment for all subjects;

(2) by random assignment;

(3) by deterministically balanced assignment;

(4) by uncontrolled haphazard assignment.

Method (1) does not allow assessment of any treatment ordering effects and, for this method to be used, the investigator needs to be assured that there is no treatment order effect. Random assignment (2) insures against bias. Methods (3) and (4) are not recommended because they are prone to introducing bias. We used a randomized block method to allocate subjects —blocking on age (5-year groups) and sex.

13.4.3 Crossover rules and timing of measurements

Decisions about treatment crossover can be either time or disease-state dependent. For the time dependent crossover design, subjects switch treatments after a predetermined time. As stated elsewhere the length of treatment should be sufficient to allow the treatment to affect outcome. In the disease-dependent approach, subjects change treatments when indicated by clinical characteristics. In this latter approach the length of treatment will vary for each subject, and may make it difficult to determine treatment-order effects and the effect of the other variables on outcome.

Whenever possible, observers and subjects should be blinded as to the timing of the crossover. In practice this is difficult and, if it is likely that the crossover will affect subject compliance it may be better to use a parallel design.

13.4.4 Drop outs

The validity of any study is affected by subjects dropping out or not providing complete data (such as missing appointments and so on). Crossover designs are longer than parallel studies and may therefore be more likely to lead to dropouts. It is acceptable to use whatever data has been collected on subjects who drop out, but consideration should be given to the possibility that the treatment has caused the subject to drop out. Ideally, the trial should be as short as possible and the treatments being tested should have no obvious side effects that will affect subject compliance.

11.4.5 Statistical analysis and sample size

The statistical power of a crossover design (of a given size) is greater than for a parallel study. This may not be a major consideration in choosing a parallel design if it is not difficult to recruit subjects. In a crossover design it is possible to eliminate within-subject effects as a subject acts as its own control. However, it is still important to analyse the change in effect in one group in relation to change in a control group. It may be that the outcome of interest falls in the treatment group, but if the outcome also changes in the control group the correct analysis is to look at the difference in the change between the treatment and control groups. Using this approach the analysis of the last period of a crossover trial will be the same as in a parallel trial. An advantage of a crossover study is that it is possible to see the effect of being on and off the treatment in the same individual. If, for example, treatment with a particular diet or drug effects serum cholesterol and, after withdrawal, levels of cholesterol return to baseline, this gives a strong indication of a treatment effect on response.

In summary, there are advantages and disadvantages in using either a parallel or a crossover design. Where it is possible to recruit sufficient subjects, a parallel study is easier to interpret, likely to have fewer dropouts and compliance problems and is quicker. For the same number of subjects, a crossover design has greater statistical power and control over within-subject factors that may affect the outcome. Crossover designs may need to be more complex to enable proper consideration of the effect that carry-over effects (and interaction) may have on treatment. Because they are usually longer they are more costly and dropout rates and subject compliance may be affected. In both study types, adequate baseline assessment and subsequent measurement of potential confounders should be incorporated in the study design.

13.5 DESIGNS USED IN EXPERIMENTAL STUDIES IN COMMUNITIES

The same basic principles apply in community trials as for field or clinical trials based on individuals (described in section 13.4). Communities should be randomly allocated to either treatment or control regime as far as is possible (and if not this should be clearly stated, with a justification) and they should be followed in the same manner throughout. Ideally, communities should be blind to the treatment regime. Communities should be followed up at the same time to minimize potential cohort effects in outcome measures that may either decrease or increase the prevalence of the outcome measures and artificially increase or decrease the apparent effect of the treatment.

Compliance with the experimental regime should also be checked in all communities throughout the study. This may be achieved by sampling a representative subset of individuals. However, it is less common to collect outcome measures on individuals. If communities are to be actually given a treatment or placebo like, for example, a vitamin A supplement, it is important to determine whether the capsules have been consumed. If a treatment is to be given by mass communication (television, radio, newspaper) it is important to ensure that communities are sufficiently separated so that the control community does not receive the treatment. If compliance with the treatment is only checked by looking at differences in the outcome measures between treatment and control groups, without checking for compliance with the treatment, potentially misleading results may be produced.

Generally, the design used in community trials is the parallel group, rather than the crossover design. It may be important to consider how outcome is to be assessed in the communities, and for how long the study needs to continue so that sufficient endpoints acrue from which a reliable assessment of the difference in effects between treatment and control regimes can be made. As in individual-based studies, the correct analysis is the comparison between change in outcome measures in the treatment community compared with change in the control community.

13.6 SUMMARY

A properly controlled, randomized experiment offers the best test of causality. If it is properly conducted it is less likely to give a biased estimate of the effect of an exposure on an outcome. However, experiments are not free from the problems of non-experimental studies. Measurement error and the effects of confounding variables may still affect the outcome.

A clearly defined aim for the research is essential and establishes the structure for the research protocol. The question being asked in the experiment needs to be clear, and exposure and outcome need to be measured with precision and freedom from the effects of other variables. The design used needs to be appropriate to the research question and population under study. All subjects, once included in the study, should be observed and followed-up in exactly the same way. Poor compliance, subjects dropping out, and incomplete ascertainment of outcome seriously affect the validity of the study. There should be sufficient subjects, observed for an adequate period of time, included in the study to allow appropriate analyses to be conducted.

REFERENCES

1. Carpenter, K. (1986). *The history of scurvy and vitamin C*. Cambridge University Press, Cambridge.
2. Pocock, S. J. (1983). *Clinical trials: a practical approach*. Wiley, New York.
3. Medical Research Council. (1948). Streptomycin treatment of pulmonary tuberculosis. *Br. Med. J.*, **2**: 769–82.
4. Medical Research Council. (1950). Clinical trials of antihistamine drugs in the prevention and treatment of the common cold. *Br. Med. J.*, **2**: 425–9.

5. Cochran, W. G. and Cox, G. M. (1957). *Experimental Designs*, second edition. Wiley, New York.
6. Bradford Hill, A. (1971). *Principles of medical statistics*, ninth edn. The Lancet Ltd., London.
7. Truelove, J. C. (ed). (1959). Follow-up studies. In L. J. Witts (ed.). *Medical surveys and clinical trials*, pp. 91–104. Oxford University Press, London.
8. Meinert, C. L. (1986). *Clinical trials. Design, conduct, and analysis*. Oxford University Press, New York.
9. Buyse, M. E., Staquet, M. J., Sylvester, R. J. (eds). (1984). *Cancer clinical trials: methods and practice*. Oxford University Press, Oxford.
10. Henneckins, C. H. and Buring, J. E. (1987). *Epidemiology in medicine*. Little, Brown and Co., Boston.
11. Macoby, N., Farquhar, J. W., Wood, P. D., and Alexander, J. (1977). Reducing the risk of cardiovascular disease: effects of a community based campaign on knowledge and behaviour. *J. Community Health*, 3: 100–14.
12. Hjermann, I., Holme, I., Velve-Byre, K., and Loren, I. (1981). Effects of diet and smoking intervention on the incidence of coronary heart disease. *Lancet*, ii: 1303–10.
13. Multiple Risk Factor Intervention Trial Research Group. (1982). Multiple risk factor intervention trial: risk factor changes and mortality results. *JAMA.*, 248: 1465–77.
14. Lipid Research Clinics Programme. (1984). The Lipids Research Clinics coronary prevention trial results. *JAMA.*, 251: 351–74.
15. Doll, R. and Hill, A. B. (1950). Smoking and carcinoma of the lung: preliminary report. *Br. Med. J.*, 3: 739–48.
16. Margetts, B. M., Beilin, L. J., Armstrong, B. K., Rouse, I. L., Vandongen, R., Croft K. D., and McMurchie, E. J. (1985). Blood pressure and dietary polyunsaturated and saturated fats: a controlled trial. *Clin. Sci.*, 69: 165–75.
17. Margetts, B. M., Beilin, L. J., Vandongen, R., and Armstrong, B. K. (1986). Vegetarian diet in mild hypertension: a randomised controlled trial. *Br. Med. J.*, 293: 1468–71.
18. Margetts, B. M., Beilin, L. J., Vandongen, R., and Armstrong B. K. (1987). A randomised controlled trial of the effect of dietary fibre on blood pressure. *Clin. Sci.*, 72: 343–50.
19. Armitage, P. (1975). *Sequential medical trials*, second edn. Blackwells Scientific Publications, Oxford.
20. Whitehead, J. (1983). *The design and analysis of sequential clinical trials*. Horwood, Chichester.
21. Hills, M. and Armitage, P. (1979). The two-period cross-over clinical trial. *Br. J. Clin. Pharmac.*, 8: 7–20.
22. Norman, G. R. (1989). Issues in the use of change scores in randomised trials. *J. Clin. Epid.*, 42: 1097–105.
23. Peto, R., Pike, M. G., Armitage, P., Breslow, N. E., Cox, D. R., Howard, S. V., Mantel, N., McPherson, K., Peto, J., and Smith, P. G. (1976). Design and analysis of randomised clinical trials requiring prolonged observations of each patient. i: Introduction and design. *Br. J. Cancer*, 34: 585–612.
24. Peto, R., Pike, M. G., Armitage, P., Breslow, N. E., Cox, D. R., Howard, S. V., Mantel, N., McPherson, K., Peto, J., and Smith, P. G. (1977). Design

and analysis of randomised clinical trials requiring prolonged observations of each patient. ii: Analysis and examples. *Br. J. Cancer*, **35:** 1–39.

25. Louis, T. A., Lavori, P. W., Bailar J. C., and Polansky, M. (1984). Crossover and self-controlled designs in clinical research. *N. Engl. J. Med.*, **310:** 24–31.

Index

abetalipoproteinemia 212
absolute intake 270–1
accuracy
    weighed and estimated records 156–8
    see also validity
acrodermatitis enteropathica 211, 212
acute appendicitis 356
acute myocardial infarction 212, 308
acute phase reaction 211, 212
adipose tissue 197
aetiologic fraction 316–17, 318
aflatoxins 331, 336
African diet studies 329, 331
age
    biochemical markers and 208
    as confounder 39–40, 41
    questionnaire completion and 278
age-specific incidence rates 299, 300
    standardization 305–7
alanine aminotransferase (ALT) 233
alcohol
    consumption from sales/tax records
        328–9
    heart disease and 323, 324, 377
    liver cirrhosis 342
    NFS results and 125–6
    nutrient status and 208
    observation period and intake 160
    oesophageal cancer 343
    under-reporting 170
allergic disease, breast feeding and 374
alpha errors 32, 62, 63
α-tocopherol 224–6
    see also vitamin E
alternative hypotheses 31–2, 64–5
aluminium 348
Alzheimer's disease 348
animal research 5–6
anthropometry 3–4, 98
anti-histamines 386
apolipoproteins 246
appendicitis 344, 356
ascorbate 229, 236–9
    see also vitamin C
aspartate aminotransferase (AST) 233
assay protocols 194–5
association, strength of 43–4
atom bomb survivors 88
attributable proportion 316–17, 365
attributable risk 315, 317
    see also excess risk; population
        attributable proportion

Australia 326, 327, 329, 343, 344
autopsy diagnosis 30
autocorrelation 275–6, 279–80
availability, biological 27, 106, 109, 207–8,
    209–10

balance studies 272
basal metabolic rate (BMR) 165–6, 252
Bayes theorem 87
Belgium 324
Berksonian errors 88–9
beta errors 32, 64
between-subject variance 59, 60, 62
    see also variance
bias 13, 34–7, 58–9, 83–5
    case-control studies 361
    confounding 84–5
    differential misclassification 84
    information 36–7, 84
    interviewer, *see* interviewer bias
    questionnaires with constant 281
    recall 36–7, 84
    selection 35–6
    weighed records and 154
    see also confounders; misclassification;
        variability
bile acid 336
bile salts 196
bioavailability 27, 106, 109, 207–8, 209–10
biochemical markers 29–30, 98, 192–254
    case-control studies 359
    dietary fibre 251
    energy 252
    experimental studies 398
    feasibility of intake prediction 192–213
        complicating factors 206–13
        reference materials 195
        temporal variations and factors
            affecting choice 195–206
        validity and reproducibility 193–5
    inorganic nutrients 213–18
    lipids 239–47
    protein 247–51
    vitamins 218–39
    see also under individual names:
        biological markers
biochemical standards 195, 272
bioequivalence 28
biological markers 29–30, 105
    dietary intake validity 154, 160–6, 248,
        249